NEUROLOGICAL PATHOPHYSIOLOGY

Neurological Pathophysiology

THIRD EDITION

Edited by

ALAN L. PEARLMAN

ROBERT C. COLLINS

New York   Oxford

OXFORD UNIVERSITY PRESS

1984

Library of Congress Cataloging in Publication Data
Main entry under title:

Neurological pathophysiology.

Includes index.
1. Nervous system—Diseases. 2. Physiology, Patho-
logical. 3. Neurology. I. Pearlman, Alan L. II. Collins,
Robert C. [DNLM: 1. Nervous system diseases—Physio-
pathology. WL 100 N49465]
RC347.N477 1984   616.8'047   83-23657
ISBN 0-19-503431-7
ISBN 0-19-503432-5 (pbk.)

The cover illustration is a cross section from the brain of a monkey having a focal seizure in the right temporal-limbic cortex.
During the period of epileptic discharges the monkey was given
an intravenous injection of radioactive deoxyglucose. The amount
of isotope taken up into different regions of brain is proportional
to the intensity of activity in that area. At the conclusion of the
experiment, autoradiograms were prepared from the brain slices
which serve to localize the areas of greatest activity. The autoradiograms were scanned and digitized by computer. In the illustration the most active areas are red. Less active areas are blue
or grey. There is a high degree of normal activity bilaterally in
the superior temporal sulcus in the cortex and in the inferior colliculi in the brainstem. This type of experiment can be used to
localize an epileptic focus, seen here as the red area in the posterior hippocampus (lower right). See Chapter 12. (From R. C.
Collins and A. W. Toga, Laboratory of Neuroimaging, Washington University.)

Printing (last digit): 9 8 7 6 5 4 3 2 1

Printed in the United States of America

Preface

The desire to understand and treat the neurological diseases is a major motivating force in the quest for information about how the nervous system works. At the same time, a great many clues about the system's normal function have come from studies of these disorders. This interaction between progress in understanding the normal function of the nervous system and understanding its abnormalities has been an important guiding principle in the preparation of this book. The book is meant to provide an introduction to the scientific foundations of clinical neurology. Like the two previous editions, it is directed toward medical students who are making the transition between their courses in neuroscience and their neurology clerkships. We hope that it will also be useful to graduate students and postdoctoral fellows in the neurosciences, who have become increasingly aware that the study of disease processes can provide valuable insights.

This book has come about largely through the efforts of our contributing authors, and we are very grateful to them for their enthusiasm and cooperation. We are also grateful for the support and guidance provided by Dr. William Landau, who played a major role in developing the stimulating scientific and clinical environment where we are privileged to work. Dr. Ed Kravitz, who has involved us both in the organization and teaching of the Neurobiology of Disease course for the Society for Neuroscience, has heightened our awareness of the interest in neurological diseases among neuroscientists. We would like to acknowledge the skillful efforts of Joe Hayes, who prepared many of the illustrations, Patti Nacci, Sue Eads, and Janice Weulling who typed and retyped the manuscript, and Susan Sunderman who helped with the editing. Our editor at Oxford University Press, Jeffrey House, deserves special thanks for his encouragement and patience.

St. Louis, Missouri   A.L.P.
October, 1983   R.C.C.

Contents

CONTRIBUTORS

LEONARD BERG, M.D.
Professor of Clinical Neurology
Washington University School of Medicine
St. Louis, MO 63110

MICHAEL H. BROOKE, M.B., B.Ch.
Professor of Neurology and of Preventive
    Medicine (Rehabilitation)
Director, Irene Walter Johnson Institute of
    Rehabilitation
Washington University School of Medicine
St. Louis, MO 63110

RONALD M. BURDE, M.D.
Professor of Ophthalmology, Neurology and
    Neurological Surgery
Washington University School of Medicine
St. Louis, MO 63110

JAMES E. CARROLL, M.D.
Associate Professor of Pediatrics and
    Neurology
Assistant Director, Irene Walter Johnson
    Institute of Rehabilitation
Washington University School of Medicine
St. Louis, MO 63110

DAVID B. CLIFFORD, M.D.
Assistant Professor of Neurology
Washington University School of Medicine
St. Louis, MO 63110

ROBERT C. COLLINS, M.D.
Professor of Neurology
Washington University School of Medicine
St. Louis, MO 63110

LESLIE J. DORFMAN, M.D.
Associate Professor of Neurology
Stanford University School of Medicine
Stanford, CA 94305

JAMES A. FERRENDELLI, M.D.
Seay Professor of Clinical Neuropharmacology
Departments of Neurology, Pharmacology and
    Ophthalmology
Washington University School of Medicine
St. Louis, MO 63110

LAWRENCE D. GELB, M.D.
Associate Professor of Medicine and of
    Microbiology and Immunology
Washington University Medical Service
Veterans Administration Medical Center
St. Louis, MO 63125

JUDITH L. LAUTER, Ph.D.
Research Associate
Central Institute for the Deaf
St. Louis, MO 63110

ERIC W. LOTHMAN, M.D.
Associate Professor of Neurology
University of Virginia Medical Center
Charlottesville, VA 22908

ERWIN B. MONTGOMERY, JR., M.D.
Assistant Professor of Neurology
Washington University School of Medicine
St. Louis, MO 63110

JOHN C. MORRIS, M.D.
Research Instructor in Neurology
Washington University School of Medicine
St. Louis, MO 63110

ALAN L. PEARLMAN, M.D.
Professor of Neurology and of Physiology and
    Biophysics
Washington University School of Medicine
St. Louis, MO 63110

WILLIAM J. POWERS, M.D.
Assistant Professor of Neurology and
    Radiology (Radiation Sciences)
Washington University School of Medicine
St. Louis, MO 63110

MARCUS E. RAICHLE, M.D.
Professor of Neurology and Radiology
    (Radiation Sciences)
Washington University School of Medicine
St. Louis, MO 63110

CLIFFORD B. SAPER, M.D., Ph.D.
Assistant Professor of Neurology and of
    Anatomy and Neurobiology
Washington University School of Medicine
St. Louis, MO 63110

JAMES W. SCHMIDLEY, M.D.
Assistant Professor of Neurology
University of California Medical Center
San Francisco, CA 94143

W. THOMAS THACH, JR., M.D.
Professor of Neurology and of Anatomy and
   Neurobiology
Washington University School of Medicine
St. Louis, MO 63110

STEPHEN G. WAXMAN, M.D., Ph.D.
Professor and Associate Chairman
Department of Neurology
Stanford University School of Medicine

Chief, Neurology Unit
Veterans Administration Medical Center
Palo Alto, CA 94304

JOHN N. WHITAKER, M.D.
Professor of Neurology and Anatomy
University of Tennessee
Center for the Health Sciences
Veterans Medical Center
Memphis, TN 38104

G. FREDERICK WOOTEN, M.D.
Professor of Neurology
University of Virginia Medical Center
Charlottesville, VA 22908

NEUROLOGICAL PATHOPHYSIOLOGY

Introduction

Anatomy, physiology, and pathology have changed dramatically since Hughlings Jackson defined them over 100 years ago as essential disciplines for understanding neurological illness. Similarly, neurological pathophysiology, a subject that is derived from all three, is currently enjoying a spurt of rapid growth as new techniques for studying the nervous system appear at an amazing rate. The definitions of Jackson's three "lines of investigation" must of course be expanded considerably to take account of remarkable advances in fields as diverse as molecular genetics and neuroradiological imaging. Nevertheless, the analysis of structure and function and the ways that they are altered by disease processes remain the cornerstones for both clinical neurology and the neurological sciences, and for the extensive interactions between them.

LOCALIZATION

When beginning the process of localization, clinicians use the symptoms and signs obtained in the history and physical examination in an attempt to answer the question that is fundamental to neurology and neurosurgery: where is the lesion? Although this process is important in all clinical fields, it takes on particular importance in neurology, since a lesion the size of a small coin can cause symptoms as diverse as hemianopia, paraplegia, or coma, depending on its location. To aid in the process of localization, it is often useful to think of the nervous system as many separate but interconnected systems: visual, motor, somatosensory, etc. The chapters in the first section of this book focus primarily on these functional systems, and consider how their normal function is disrupted by disease to produce the symptoms and signs that are used in localization.

Many disease processes affect the nervous system at a single locus, and the patient's symptoms and signs reflect dysfunction in the system or systems involved at that site (Table I–1). For example, the occlusion of small penetrating vessels on one side of the pons can cause a decrease in facial sensation on one side (nucleus and tract of the fifth cranial nerve) and ataxia (pontocerebellar fibers), along with weakness (corticospinal tract) or loss of proprioception (medial lemniscus) on the contralateral side of the body. Such a constellation of abnormal findings, together with the presence of normal function in neighboring structures, provides a precise localization of the lesion in three dimensions. In contrast, a patient whose only neurological abnormalities are unilateral

weakness and spasticity could have a single lesion within the corticospinal tract anywhere from the cortex to the upper spinal cord. If an involved system has a long traverse through the brain, precise localization usually requires evidence for involvement of contiguous structures at a specific level.

Determining the anatomic site of the lesion can provide clues to the nature of the disease process as well, since many neurological diseases have characteristic distributions. Dysfunction that is restricted to a single system often indicates that the disease is degenerative. Involvement of only the upper and lower motor neurons of the motor system, for example, would suggest the degenerative disease that affects these structures selectively—amyotrophic lateral sclerosis. Other diseases characteristically affect the nervous system at several discrete locations. Cerebral infarction from cardiac emboli and multiple metastasis from cancer are two examples. Signs and symptoms also can reflect disease processes spreading through the coverings or extracellular spaces of the brain, as occurs in subarachnoid hemorrhage and meningitis. Finally, widespread neurological dysfunction occurs whenever the blood supply fails to deliver essential nutrients or to remove toxic wastes, as occurs in the conditions catagorized as metabolic encephalopathies. The basic pathophysiologic features of these and other major categories of neurological disease are covered in the second section of this book.

Several new techniques have become available in recent years which are extremely helpful to the clinician in the localization process. Computerized tomography (CT) and nuclear magnetic resonance (NMR) imaging, in many instances, can provide very clear outlines of lesions within or adjacent to the brain and spinal cord. The introduction of the computer has also made it possible to record and analyze the electrical activity evoked by visual, auditory, and somatosensory stimuli. Evoked

Table I–1. Localization of Signs and Symptoms

Systems localization
1. Focal (infarct, tumor, abscess, etc.)
2. Multifocal (emboli, metastasis, multiple sclerosis, etc.)
3. Systems degeneration (motor, spinocerebellar, etc.)
4. Diffuse
   a. parenchymal (encephalitis, Alzheimer's disease, etc.)
   b. extracellular (hydrocephalus, meningitis, etc.)

Cellular and molecular localization
1. Metabolic encephalopathies
   a. substrate deficiency (O_2, glucose)
   b. toxins (ammonia, uremia, etc.)
   c. cofactor deficiency (B_1, B_{12}, etc.)
   d. enzyme deficiencies (inborn errors of metabolism)
2. Local neuronal circuits (focal epilepsy, migraine)
3. Neuronal (amyotrophic lateral sclerosis, polio, herpes zoster)
4. Synapse
   a. presynaptic (dopamine—parkinsonism)
   b. postsynaptic (acetylcholine receptor—myasthenia gravis)
5. Myelin (demyelination)

potentials recorded by these methods are useful in demonstrating the presence of lesions and their location.

Localization as an investigative method

Anatomical localization of the symptoms and signs of disease processes within the nervous system is also one of the oldest methods for studying normal functions of the brain. It came into full use as an investigative method at the turn of the century with the observations of Charcot, Gowers, Jackson, Broca, Wernicke, Déjerine, and many others. The method's underlying assumption is that the dysfunction resulting from damage to a particular structure indicates the function of that structure when it is intact. At a simple level of analysis this assumption is usually correct. For example, acute damage to a region of the precentral gyrus can cause loss of dexterity and weakness of the contralateral upper extremity. From such cases it can be safely inferred that this region is involved in the movement of the upper extremity. The problem comes in trying to determine *exactly* what this area does. Early observers invoked such concepts as "engrams," suggesting that specific anatomical areas contain memories or programs for individual functions. These notions were extended to explain such complex functions as perception, speech, and cognition. Although early clinical observations on the phenomenology of signs and symptoms that result from particular lesions have proven to be very useful, the explanations regarding the normal function of specific regions and systems have changed considerably as a result of the recent advances in neuroscience.

Until about thirty years ago, lesioning experiments in animals were the principal method for studying functional systems. Data from such experiments ran closely parallel to the observations of the effects of disease processes in man. Today, many new methods are providing considerable insight into functional systems. Neuroanatomical tract-tracing methods that make use of the intraneuronal transport of tracer molecules have increased our knowledge of the extent and specificity of pathways and connections. Refinements of physiological recording techniques in awake animals have made it possible to localize populations of neurons within those pathways that become active with highly specific sensory stimuli or during particular behaviors. Radioactive metabolic substrates and blood flow markers are being used to localize areas throughout the brain that are active during both simple and complex functions.

One result of these new methodologies has been to make us even more aware of the complexity of the nervous system. To return to our original example, we now know that a simple arm movement depends upon normal structure and function in many systems—corticospinal, muscle stretch, somatosensory, cerebellar, and the basal ganglia. Function is not localized to any one part. There is apparently no kinesthetic engram in one locus. Rather, normal function is the characteristic of integrated activity within the whole system, with individual parts adding specific modifications that are distributed in space and time. Symptoms and signs like hemiparesis or hemianopsia can indicate what part of a functional system has been damaged, while others, such as spasticity and tremor, are abnormal manifestations of the remaining parts of the system functioning without the contribution of the lesioned structure.

Although these considerations may offer new insights into how the signs and symptoms of disease express abnormal activity within a distributed functional system, it still remains unclear how this type of analysis can be applied to more complex neurological dysfunctions. As yet we have no easy way to infer from studies of patients with brain lesions who have cognitive, perceptual, or emotional deficits how systems subserving these functions are organized anatomically or physiologically in the brain.

Cellular and molecular localization

Advances in neuroscience have also greatly increased our ability to localize disease processes at the cellular and molecular level (Table I–1). In most instances our knowledge has been advanced by the rich interplay between basic and clinical neuroscience. This partnership was established long before such academic divisions were judged necessary. Historically, the first molecular localization of neurological disease was the discovery by Eijkman, working in Utrecht in 1925, that an amine purified from rice polishings could cure pigeon polyneuritis. Working with this first vital amine, or "vitamine" (B_1, thiamine) in the early 1930s, Rudolph Peters at Oxford discovered that brains from pigeons fed deficient diets were unable to oxidize pyruvate and suggested that this defect constituted a "biochemical lesion." At about the same time C.O. Prichett, a veterinarian in Alabama, produced brainstem lesions in rats and pigeons kept on a thiamine-deficient diet, but he was unaware of Carl Wernicke's description in 1881 of the same lesions (acute hemorrhagic polioencephalitis superior) in man. In 1938 Leo Alexander in Boston drew attention to the similarity between the brainstem lesions of pigeon polyneuritis and Wernicke's encephalopathy. Within three years, Joliffee, Wortis, and Fein, at the Bellevue Psychiatric Clinic, demonstrated that giving thiamine alone to malnourished alcoholics reversed the ocular palsies and improved the ataxia of Wernicke's encephalopathy.

Advances in neurological pathophysiology continue to come from such diverse roots as these. The progress that has been made in understanding myasthenia gravis, a profoundly debilitating disorder of the neuromuscular junction, is perhaps one of the best recent examples of the interplay between basic and clinical neuroscience (Chapter 4). Many years of study of the neuromuscular junction provided the framework for determining that the disease causes a decrease in the number of postsynaptic receptors for acetylcholine. One of the major breakthroughs came when investigators who were trying to produce antibodies to these receptors in rabbits in order to study receptor structure realized that some of the rabbits were developing a syndrome like myasthenia gravis. The discovery that patients with the disease have circulating antibodies to the receptor has led to new forms of treatment, while the serum antibodies from patients are being used in further studies of the receptor molecule. Other prominent examples include the studies of the dopamine receptor that are leading to new treatment strategies for movement disorders, including parkinsonism (Chapter 19), and the new concepts of dementing illnesses that have arisen from the analysis of the infectious agent causing scrapie in sheep (Chapter 13).

PHYSIOLOGY

The second principle of neurological pathophysiology is to determine what Jackson called "the functional effection of nerve tissue." How has neuronal function been altered by the disease? At the most basic level, we want to know whether the patient's symptoms represent an increase or a decrease in neuronal activity. At first glance, this might seem like an easy task, but in practice it can be very difficult.

In order to understand neurological symptoms and signs, clinicians originally divided them into negative and positive phenomena (Table I–2). They further suggested that negative phenomena, or loss of normal function (e.g. paralysis), always implied a decrease in neuronal activity and a destructive process. Positive phenomena, such as a seizure, were thought to result from excessive neuronal activity and

Table I–2. Physiological Basis of Signs and Symptoms

Negative Signs and Symptoms: Loss of Function	Examples
1. Decreased neuronal activity	Loss of sensation or movement from local destructive lesions such as infarct, tumor, or trauma
2. Increased neuronal activity	Symptoms associated with epilepsy, such as the interruption of behavior and consciousness that occurs with partial complex seizures
Positive Signs and Symptoms: Abnormal Function	
1. Increased neuronal activity	Clonic and tonic manifestations of epilepsy; fasciculations of motor neuron disease
2. Increased axonal activity	Parasthesias in demyelinating diseases
3. Decreased neuronal activity	Movement disorders such as tremor, rigidity, and chorea, which may result when a lesion in one structure "releases" or "destabilizes" other parts of the system

an "irritative" process. Today, advances in the study of pathophysiological mechanisms have shown that the interpretation of individual symptoms can be quite complex. For example, the negative symptom of transient bilateral leg weakness in an adult suggests ischemia of the pyramidal tracts in the spinal cord or brainstem, a destructive process causing a decrease in neuronal activity. Yet a transient loss of muscle tone in children can be a sign of an akinetic seizure, i.e., an "irritative" lesion, or excessive neuronal firing.

Positive signs can be particularly difficult to dissect. Tremor, spasticity, and rigidity are signs that reflect an imbalance within the motor system in which different neuronal centers may exhibit decreases or increases in neuronal activity (Chapter 9). In other situations positive clinical phenomena may arise from axons within fiber tracts rather than from a primary increase in activity in neuronal cell bodies. Partially demyelinated axons can initiate spontaneous action potentials or conduct action potentials abnormally (Chapter 1), producing such positive symptoms as sensory paresthesias or paroxysmal pain.

Focal destructive lesions can affect functional systems in several different ways. Acute lesions commonly depress activity within distant synaptic pathways. Trauma to the cervical spine, for example, can cause the negative symptoms of flaccid paraplegia and loss of sphincter control, which is called spinal shock. It might last a few hours or several weeks, eventually changing into a picture of spasticity with a variable degree of recovery of motor power. By contrast, infarction of the subthalamic nucleus causes a very striking positive symptom complex, a movement disorder called hemiballismus, characterized by wild flailing movements of the contralateral upper extremity. It has been suggested that the subthalamic nucleus normally inhibits distant synaptic pathways in basal ganglia, so that when it is injured these downstream pathways are released into excessive activity.

From these considerations one might conclude that there are no *a priori* rules for determining whether a particular positive or negative symptom complex represents an increase or decrease in neuronal activity at a lesion site or within its synaptic pathways. In a broad sense that is true. It reflects the present state of the art in which we have a rich knowledge of the phenomenology of disease but a relatively deficient understanding of disease mechanisms. In other words, we know from clinical experience which signs and symptoms commonly occur with different diseases at different sites, but we know considerably less about how abnormal physiological processes cause these signs

TIME-INTENSITY PROFILE OF NEUROLOGICAL ILLNESS

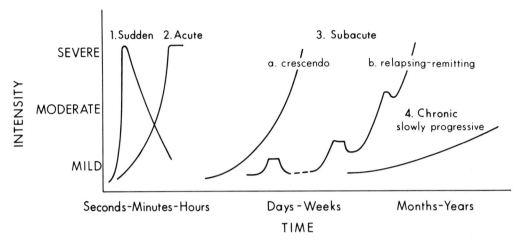

Fig. I–1. A diagrammatic representation of the time courses that characterize several types of neurological disease. 1. *Sudden:* Onset in seconds or minutes with rapid improvement. Implies the paroxysmal dysfunction of epilepsy, or the vascular phenomena of transient ischemic attacks or migrane. 2. *Acute:* Onset in minutes or hours. Implies metabolic dysfunction, as occurs with ischemia-infarction, toxins, and some infections. 3. *Subacute:* (a) Onset over days to weeks with crescendo worsening. Implies an expanding mass lesion such as tumor, abscess, and obstructive hydrocephalus. (b) Onset over days or weeks, with step-like progression or relapses and remissions. Implies recurrent processes like transient ischemic attacks leading to stroke, or multiple sclerosis. 4. *Chronic:* Slowly progressive over months or years. Implies gradual deterioration as occurs with degenerative illnesses like parkinsonism and Alzheimer's disease.

and symptoms. This situation is changing rapidly, however, with the development of new clinical and basic research methodologies.

A consideration of the onset of signs and symptoms and of how they change with time is a second type of physiological analysis. Constructing a time-intensity profile of a patient's individual symptoms is often an important method for discovering the cause of symptoms (Fig. I–1). The sudden onset of symptoms that subside over minutes suggests either epilepsy or vascular phenomena such as the prodrome of migraine or transient ischemia. Acute deficits reaching a maximum over several minutes or hours suggest metabolic failure, as occurs with vascular occlusion or with the local toxins of infec-

tions. Symptoms that progress over days or weeks and present with a crescendo of worsening are typical of an expanding mass lesion. A steplike quality to the progression, or clear evidence of relapses and remissions, suggests recurrent episodes of ischemia or multiple sclerosis. Slowly progressive neurological deficits, especially when confined to particular systems, imply a degenerative process.

PATHOLOGY

As Jackson's phrase "to find the alteration in nutrition" suggests, the central task of pathology is to determine the etiology of the neurological disorder. Until recently, pathology encompassed two basic approaches: post mortem localization of the disease process by gross examination and dissection of the brain, and attempts to determine the etiology by gross and microscopic analysis. In the last several years the methods used in determining location and etiology have been expanded considerably. Computerized tomography and NMR imaging have contributed greatly to the science of localization, and they also provide important clues to the histological pathology. Sophisticated techniques for the biochemical, immunological, and microbial analysis of cerebrospinal fluid and serum have made it increasingly possible to make accurate pathological inferences while the patient is alive.

Despite these advances several problems remain. First, the anatomical resolution of the new imaging techniques will never approach postmortem gross and microscopic analysis of the brain. Ultimately, our knowledge of where and how many disease processes affect the nervous system depends on these traditional methods. Second, many neurological disease processes do not cause anatomical lesions (Table I–3). At present we think that migraine prodromata and the generalized epilepsies reflect "electrophysiological lesions," or perhaps submicroscopic abnormalities in nerve membranes (Chapter 12). Metabolic encephalopathies can result from "biochemical lesions" such as those that occur in renal or hepatic failure (Chapter 16). Long-term treatment with certain drugs can cause "neuropharmacological lesions," as in the development of movement disorders like tardive diskinesias in patients treated with major tranquilizers. In these situations new techniques will be necessary to localize the "pathological" process. Experiments with positron emitting isotopes of substrates and neurotransmitters offer promise in this regard. It is becoming possible to give these isotopes to humans and scan the brain to localize sites of abnormal metabolism and synaptic function.

Thus, determining the etiology of a

Table I–3. Pathological Basis of Signs and Symptoms

Anatomical lesions
  1. Vascular
  2. Neoplastic
  3. Traumatic
  4. Infectious
  5. Immunologic
  6. Demyelinative
  7. Developmental and genetic
  8. Degenerative (usually advanced)

Neurophysiological (excitable membrane) lesions
  1. Generalized epilepsies
  2. Migraine
  3. ? Narcolepsy

Metabolic lesions
  1. Metabolic encephalopathies
      a. nutritional deficiencies
      b. toxins
  2. Developmental and genetic
  3. Degenerative

Pharmacological (synaptic) lesions
  1. Prolonged use of synaptic drugs
  2. ? essential tremor
  3. ? dystonia
  4. ? narcolepsy
  5. ? depression, schizophrenia

neurological disease now encompasses a very broad range of investigative activity, including biochemical and pharmacological studies of living patients as well as biopsy and post mortem material. In addition, new techniques for studying genetic and immunologic diseases, and for isolating infectious agents are under intensive investigation.

As the chapters of this book will indicate, there is still a great deal to be learned about the etiology of most neurological diseases. But the rapidly expanding set of investigative approaches and techniques that now constitute anatomy, physiology, and pathology offer great promise in providing new insight into the pathophysiology of neurological disorders. As our understanding of the effects of these diseases and their causes increase, so will our ability to diagnose and treat patients who are afflicted by them.

Robert C. Collins

Alan L. Pearlman

PART ONE

Functional and Anatomical Systems

1.

Conduction in Normal and Demyelinated Axons

STEPHEN G. WAXMAN

Myelinated axons carry information rapidly from one point to another in both the central and peripheral parts of the nervous system, often over very long distances. Loss of the myelin sheath, called demyelination, can disrupt the movement of neuronal signals along axons, and thereby produce profound neurological deficits. Demyelination of axons in the peripheral nervous system occurs in several of the neuropathies; it occurs most commonly in the central nervous system as a consequence of multiple sclerosis. Although the cells that produce the myelin sheath in the central and peripheral nervous systems are quite different, the role that myelin plays in the conduction of neuronal impulses is similar, as are the consequences of myelin loss. This chapter will review the basic principles of structure and function that underlie impulse conduction in axons, with emphasis on the role of myelin, before proceeding to a consideration of the abnormalities that occur with partial or total loss of myelin from segments of axons, and how this loss produces neurological systems and signs.

THE MYELIN SHEATH AND ITS CELLS OF ORIGIN

Nerve fibers (axons) in both the peripheral and central nervous system are either myelinated or nonmyelinated. Myelinated fibers are surrounded by a sheath of myelin, which consists of a compact spiral of closely apposed cell membranes. The cell of origin of myelin in the peripheral nervous system is the Schwann cell (named after its discoverer, Theodor Schwann, who together with Schleiden enunciated the cell theory). In the PNS, one Schwann cell produces myelin around a single axon. In the central nervous system, the cell of origin of the myelin is the oligodendroglial cell, a specialized glial element. One oligodendroglial cell produces myelin sheaths around an entire family of axons in its vicinity. The oligodendroglial cell body is connected to its family of myelin sheaths by thin cytoplasmic bridges. Estimates of the number of axons myelinated by a single oligodendrocyte vary between 3 and 200. The fact that one oligodendroglial cell body supports (via tenuous cytoplasmic strands) multiple myelin sheaths in the central nervous system has been cited as one possible explanation for the paucity of remyelination following demyelination in the central nervous system.

It is now established that the axon provides the signals as to whether myelination will take place. For example, if a nerve containing myelinated axons is transected and experimentally anastomosed with distal stump containing nonmyelinated fibers, the regenerating axons, which under normal conditions are myelinated, will regenerate into the distal stump containing Schwann cells that previously did not produce myelin. In such a situation, the distal Schwann cells will produce myelin, as is appropriate for the regenerating axons. The nature of the intercellular signal from axon to Schwann cell, while of great interest, remains unclear.

The myelin sheath consists of a spiral of compacted Schwann cell (PNS) or oligodendroglial (CNS) membranes surrounding the axon. Figures 1–1–1–4 illustrate the sequence of myelin formation in the PNS. As shown in these micrographs, the structure of the myelin is essentially that of a "jelly roll" of membranes. This structure imparts to the myelin a high electrical resistance and a low capacitance. These characteristics permit the myelin sheath to function essentially as an electrical insulator surrounding the axon. The myelin sheath is periodically interrupted at distances of 100 μm (small-diameter fibers) to slightly over 1 mm (larger fibers), at specialized structures which are called the *nodes of Ranvier*. The region between the nodes is called the *internode*.

Myelinated fibers conduct action potentials in an uneven or *saltatory* manner, with the impulse "jumping" from node to node. This mode of conduction in myelinated fibers is distinctly different from the continuous mode of conduction assumed to occur in most nonmyelinated fibers. In nonmyelinated fibers, conduction velocity is proportional to the square root

of the diameter. In contrast, conduction velocity is approximately proportional to the diameter in myelinated fibers. For any specified diameter (above a critical diameter where the conduction velocity-diameter relationships for myelinated and nonmyelinated axons cross), impulse conduction occurs at a greater velocity in a myelinated fiber than in a nonmyelinated fiber of the same size (Fig. 1–5). Thus, myelination is associated with an increase in conduction speed that does not require the large increase in diameter that would be necessary to support high conduction velocities in fibers without myelin. Myelinated fibers can also conduct impulses at higher frequencies, and consume less energy per impulse, than nonmyelinated fibers.

The presence of voltage-dependent sodium channels accounts for the excitability, or capability to produce a regenerative, propagated action potential, of mammalian myelinated fibers. At the normal resting potential (approximately −70 mV), the sodium channels tend to be closed. As an action potential approaches a given axonal region, the axon membrane in this region is depolarized by the oncoming impulse and voltage-sensitive sodium channels open. The concentration of sodium ions outside the axon is much higher than inside, and this concentration gradient provides an electrochemical driving force that tends to depolarize the axon by allowing sodium ions to enter. This causes further depolarization, resulting in the opening of still more sodium channels. If a threshold of depolarization is reached, the response becomes regenerative or explosive. This response propagates along the axon as an all-or-none action potential.

According to the classic Hodgkin-Huxley formulation of action potential electrogenesis, derived from studies of the giant axon of the squid, a second type of voltage-sensitive ionic channel, the potassium channel, is responsible for repolarization, that is, the falling phase of the ac-

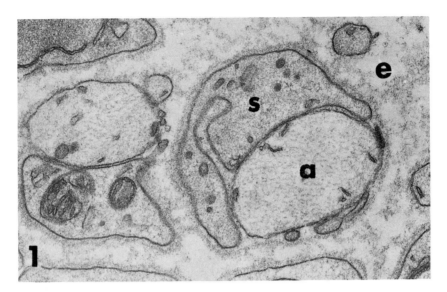

Fig. 1–1. Electron micrographs in Figures 1–1 to 1–4 show cross sections from developing sciatic nerve in the newborn mouse. This figure shows the earliest stage in myelin formation. An axon (a) is approached by a Schwann cell; S, Schwann cell; e, extracellular space. × 36,000

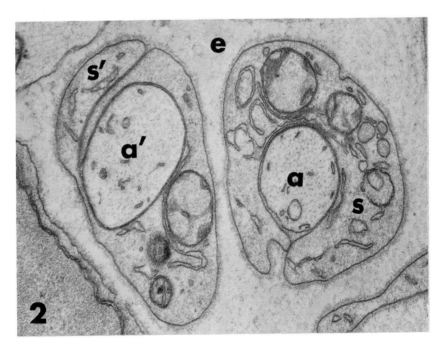

Fig. 1–2. Two axons at slightly more advanced stages of myelination. Axon (a) is surrounded by a Schwann cell (s), but spiral wrapping has not begun. Axon (a′) is surrounded by a Schwann cell (s′) that has begun to form the myelin spiral. × 36,000

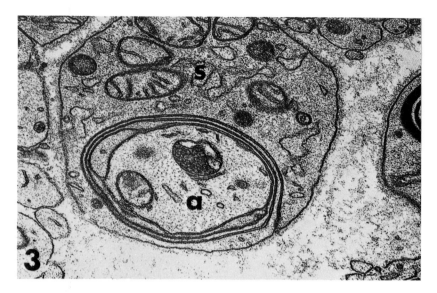

Fig. 1–3. At this stage, the Schwann cell has formed two spiral layers around the axon. × 36,000

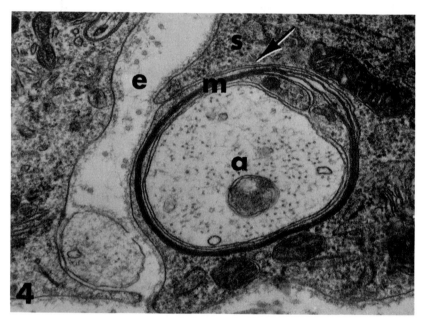

Fig. 1–4. With maturation of the sheath, the myelin (m) becomes compact. × 53,700

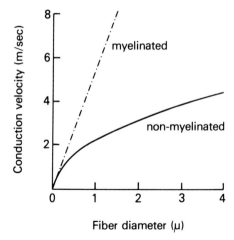

Fig. 1–5. Conduction velocity plotted as a function of diameter for myelinated (dashed line) and nonmyelinated (solid line) fibers. Above a critical diameter, conduction occurs more rapidly in a myelinated axon than in a nonmyelinated axon of the same size. (From S. G. Waxman and M. V. L. Bennett. Relative conduction velocities of small myelinated and non-myelinated fibers in the central nervous system. *Nature New Biol.* 238:217–19, 1972.)

tion potential. The concentration of potassium ions inside neurons is much higher than outside, resulting in an equilibrium potential for potassium that is close to the resting potential. According to this formulation, after the opening of sodium channels and depolarization during the onset of the action potential, potassium channels open *(potassium activation)*, allowing efflux of potassium from the axon, with a subsequent repolarization back to approximately the resting potential. Recent voltage clamp studies on mammalian myelinated fibers have shown, however, that there are very few, if any, potassium channels that function in this way at normal nodes of Ranvier. It has been postulated that repolarization in mammalian myelinated fibers is due to a rapid closing of the sodium channels, together with a "leakage" (nonspecific) conductance. Interestingly, it appears that there *are* potassium channels in the axon membrane in the internode, under the myelin sheath. While the function of these potassium channels has not been precisely determined, it has been suggested that they may play a role in stabilizing the axon and preventing repetitive discharge following the conduction of a single action potential. As will be discussed, this complex organization of the myelinated fiber has important implications for axonal pathophysiology.

In normal fibers (Fig. 1–6), the high-

Fig. 1–6. Conduction in normal (upper panel) and demyelinated (lower panel) regions of myelinated axon. The myelin sheath normally functions as a high-resistance, low-capacitance insulator, shunting current from one node to the next. In demyelinated regions, current is lost through the damaged myelin sheaths and underlying internodal axon membrane.

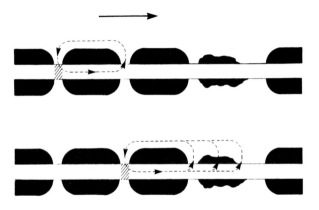

resistance, low-capacitance myelin acts as an insulator and, when the impulse is located at a given node, encourages most of the action current to pass through the relatively low resistance axonal cytoplasm to the next node of Ranvier. Thus, the threshold is reached quickly at the next node, and conduction occurs rapidly and reliably. As will be seen, this schema is altered in demyelinated axons.

The margin of reliability for conduction in a myelinated fiber can be expressed as its *safety factor*. The safety factor is the ratio between the amount of current *available* to stimulate a node of Ranvier and the amount of current *required* to stimulate the node. In normal myelinated fibers, the safety factor is approximately 5–6, providing for highly reliable conduction of action potentials. For reasons that will become apparent, the safety factor is diminished in demyelinated fibers.

MECHANISMS UNDERLYING ABNORMAL CONDUCTION IN DEMYELINATED FIBERS

In demyelinated fibers, the high-resistance, low-capacitance myelin sheath is damaged or lost (Fig. 1–6). Therefore, when an action potential approaches a demyelinated region, the density of action current (per square micron) is reduced due to capacitative and resistive shunting—or loss of current. The density of action current available to depolarize the axon membrane is thus decreased, resulting in reduction of the safety factor. If the safety factor is reduced but still has a value above 1, it will take longer for the axon to reach threshold and generate an action potential. As a result, the conduction velocity will be decreased. In more severely affected axons, the safety factor may fall below 1. Threshold will therefore not be reached at all, resulting in failure to propagate an action potential, i.e., conduction block.

As illustrated in Figure 1–6, the loss

of myelin over the previously myelinated internode leads to an important question concerning the functional organization of the internodal axon membrane. Is the demyelinated axon membrane, which was formerly internodal membrane, excitable? That is, can it conduct action potentials, or does the denuded axon membrane lack the capability for spike propagation? This question, while perhaps not of major relevance to conduction in normal myelinated fibers where the internodal axon membrane is covered by the insulating myelin sheath, is crucial to an understanding of conduction in demyelinated fibers, since, in these fibers, action current is shunted through the demyelinated internodal membrane.

A variety of approaches have been taken to answer this question. The available data indicate that there is a very high density of sodium channels in the axon membrane at the nodes of Ranvier, where they are required for the generation of the action currents in normal myelinated fibers. This is in contrast to a very low density of sodium channels (probably so low that the axon cannot support impulse conduction) in the axon membrane in the internodes. The result is an important one for neurological pathophysiology because it implies that demyelination not only removes the insulating myelin sheath from part of the fiber, causing loss of current, but also exposes essentially inexcitable membrane.

However, the situation is slightly more complex. There is evidence for a complementary distribution of sodium and potassium channels in mammalian myelinated fibers, with the sodium channels clustered in the axon membrane at the node of Ranvier and potassium channels located in the internodal axon membrane under the myelin. A schematic representation of this model of the myelinated fibers is presented in Figure 1–7. The sodium channels are represented by g_{Na} and the potassium channels by g_K in this dia-

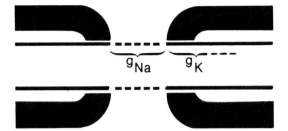

Fig. 1–7. Current working model of myelinated fiber. Sodium channels (g_{Na}) are clustered at node of Ranvier but are virtually absent from the internodal axon membrane, which is normally covered by myelin. Potassium channels (g_K) are present in low density or are absent at the node, but are present in the internodal axon membrane. Removal of the myelin sheath thus exposes inexcitable membrane. (From S. G. Waxman, Membranes, myelin, and the pathophysiology of multiple sclerosis. *New Eng. J. Med.* 306:1529–33, 1982.)

gram. Although there may be variations in the detailed architecture of fibers of different sizes or types, the concept that nodal and internodal axon membranes are structurally and functionally distinct is well established. The model shown in Figure 1–7 has important implications for the pathophysiology of conduction in demyelinated fibers. As indicated earlier, following the acute loss of myelin the density of sodium channels in the demyelinated area is probably too low to support impulse conduction. The demyelinated axon membrane is thus essentially electrically inexcitable. The presence of potassium channels in the demyelinated axon membrane will also tend to hold the demyelinated axon membrane close to its resting potential, further preventing conduction. Thus, the complex organization of the axonal membrane, which appears to be dictated by functional requirements in normal fibers, interferes with impulse conduction following acute loss of myelin.

The complex pattern of axon membrane architecture may also be important for the development of one type of symptomatic therapy for demyelinating diseases. It has been shown that conduction block in some experimentally demyelinated fibers can be relieved by treatment with pharmacological agents that block potassium channels. The relief of conduction block is presumably due to interference with the exposed (formerly internodal) potassium channels, which would otherwise tend to repolarize the axon and prevent the attainment of threshold. While study of these pharmacological agents has not progressed to the point of providing a practical clinical therapy that can be used in patients, it raises the possibility of designing symptomatic therapies based on an understanding of physiology and pathophysiology.

CONDUCTION ABNORMALTIES IN DEMYELINATED FIBERS

A spectrum of conduction abnormalities occurs in demyelinated fibers, depending in part on the severity of the demyelination. The abnormalities are represented schematically in Figure 1–8. In moderately demyelinated fibers, the conduction velocity is decreased (Fig. 1–8B). As a corollary to the reduction in conduction velocity, there can be *temporal dispersion* (Fig. 1–8C) of impulses (i.e., the loss of synchrony of impulses carried by fibers within a given nerve bundle or tract). This is a result of different degrees of conduc-

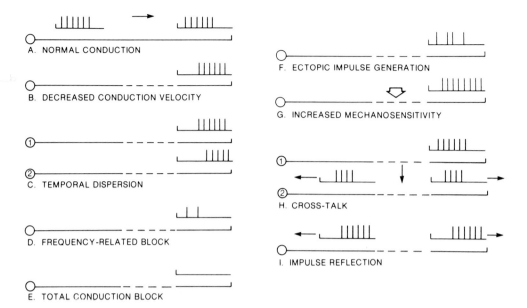

Fig. 1–8. Conduction abnormalities in demyelinated fibers. The cell body is represented by the circle to the left, and the axon by the line extending to the right. A region of demyelination is indicated by broken lines. The small insets to the right represent action potentials recorded after conduction along the entire fiber, including the demyelinated region. **A.** Normal conduction: Action potentials recorded near the cell body are shown on the left. These action potentials travel down the axon in the direction of the arrow, to be recorded again by another electrode farther down the axon. Both tracings begin at the same time. The time required for conduction down the axon is indicated in the trace on the right by the slightly longer interval between the beginning of the trace and the first action potential. **B.** Decreased conduction velocity in a partially demyelinated fiber is indicated by a long interval (latency) between the beginning of the trace and the first action potential. **C.** Temporal dispersion: Two axons (1 and 2) with different degrees of demyelination in the same nerve bundle or tract. Action potentials that start synchronously near the cell bodies of both fibers will be delayed by different amounts in the two fibers and will therefore no longer be synchronous when they reach the distal recording site. **D.** Frequency-related block: A high-frequency train of action potentials beginning near the cell body is partially blocked at the demyelinated zone, so that only a few action potentials are recorded distally. **E.** Total conduction block: No action potentials are recorded distally since none are conducted through the severely demyelinated region. **F.** Ectopic impulse generation: Action potentials generated at or near the site of demyelination are recorded distally. **G.** Increased mechanosensitivity: Pressure or stretch (open arrow) applied at the demyelinated zone generates action potentials. **H.** Cross-talk: Axons 1 and 2 are adjacent. Action potentials traveling down axon 1 activate axon 2 when they reach an abnormal zone. The impulses generated in axon 2 travel in both directions (Impulse reflection, **I**) from the site of cross-talk.

tion slowing, reflecting different degrees of myelin loss in the constituent fibers in the bundle or tract. This latter mechanism has been invoked as an explanation for the early loss of deep tendon reflexes and vibratory sensibility in patients with some peripheral neuropathies, in whom nerve conduction velocities (reflecting the conduction velocity of the population as a whole) are in the low-normal range. Presumably, the loss of temporal synchrony interferes with temporal summation at the central synapses mediating the monosynaptic reflex.

In more severely affected fibers, *conduction block* (Fig. 1–8D and 1–8E) can occur. This may be frequency related (Fig. 1–8D), with low-frequency impulse trains conducting relatively reliably, and high-frequency impulse trains failing to propagate. For example, every second or third impulse may fail to traverse a damaged region of the fiber. Alternatively, early impulses, but not later ones, in a high-frequency train may be conducted past the site of damage. In more severely affected fibers conduction is completely blocked; no information is transmitted beyond the site of damage (Fig. 1–8E).

Conduction block may produce clinical abnormalities that are more severe than those produced by a decrease in conduction velocity. For example, the visual evoked response (which provides an approximate measure of the conduction time from the retina along the optic pathways to the occipital cortex) can be prolonged by as much as 50 msec in some patients with multiple sclerosis, presumably as a result of decreased conduction velocity in the optic nerve. However, many patients with delayed visual evoked responses have little or no functionally apparent visual deficit. Apparently the delay in transmission of information from the retina to the visual cortex does not necessarily produce significant clinical abnormalities. On the other hand, conduction block in a significant number of fibers in the optic nerve or

any other tract will obviously produce clinical abnormalities.

Other abnormalities of impulse initiation and conduction can be viewed as "positive" abnormalities, in which hyperexcitability, rather than loss or depression of function, results in clinical signs or symptoms. Although several types of clinical phenomena can be accounted for by the hyperexcitability that occurs in or near demyelineated zones under certain circumstances, very little is known about the mechanisms by which hyperexcitability occurs. Abnormal (ectopic) impulse generation (Fig. 1–8F) may account for the dysesthesias experienced by some patients with demyelinating peripheral neuropathies or central demyelinating diseases. Increased mechanosensitivity (Fig. 1–8G) is present in demyelinated fibers and probably accounts for Tinel's sign (paresthesias elicited by percussion of a peripheral nerve) in the case of damaged peripheral nerve. It may also account for Lhermitte's sign, an electric-like sensation that is referred down the spine and into the limbs. This symptom occurs in patients with lesions in the cervical cord in response to flexion of the neck, which probably causes slight stretching of the cervical cord and mechanical stimulation of the dorsal columns. Finally, abnormal cross-talk (Fig. 1–8H) between fibers (which usually function relatively independently) may also occur in demyelinated fibers, as may reflection (backward conduction, Fig. 1–8I) of impulses from sites of demyelination.

EFFECTS OF EXOGENOUS FACTORS AND TEMPERATURE ON DEMYELINATED FIBERS

As noted earlier, the safety factor is approximately 5–6 in normal myelinated fibers. Thus, these fibers conduct impulses with a high degree of reliability. In demyelinated fibers, the safety factor falls. For those fibers in which the safety factor falls to about 1, conduction would be expected to occur in a labile and marginal manner. This, in fact, has been shown to be the case. For example, patients with multiple sclerosis often report that their neurological symptoms worsen when body temperature is raised (e.g., when in a hot bath, or when suffering from a febrile illness). This is due to the fact that, as temperature is raised, the kinetics of ionic channels are altered so that they open and close more rapidly, leading to a faster action potential, which generates less current at any given region of the axon, thereby further reducing the safety factor.

In addition to temperature, changes in metabolic status may alter the conduction properties of demyelinated fibers. For example, changes in acid-base balance, which can be produced by hyperventilation, or the introduction of intravenous bicarbonate or oral phosphate, can produce significant, although transient, changes in neurological status. These changes may reflect increased excitability due to lowered free calcium concentrations. While these findings have not yet provided a useful clinical therapy for demyelinating diseases, they illustrate the fact that demyelinated fibers are exquisitely sensitive to changes in temperature and the exogenous milieu. Thus the increased sensitivity of demyelinated fibers to changes in metabolic status or temperature may account for some of the clinical phenomenology and provides at least a partial explanation for the relatively rapid waxing and waning of symptoms that some patients with multiple sclerosis experience.

MECHANISMS OF RECOVERY OF CONDUCTION IN DEMYELINATED AXONS

An important question in neurological pathophysiology concerns the mechanism(s) of recovery of conduction in demyelinated axons. The clinical course of relapsing-remitting multiple sclerosis, for example, is punctuated by exacerbations in which neurological status worsens and remissions in which there is recovery of function. The mechanisms underlying the recovery of function that occur during remissions of multiple sclerosis are obviously important to an understanding of this disease and perhaps others as well.

Remyelination is one obvious mechanism for recovery of conduction following demyelination. This probably accounts, at least in part, for the recovery of patients with demyelinating peripheral neuropathies such as Guillain-Barré syndrome. It should be noted that, in remyelinated fibers, the nodes of Ranvier are more closely spaced than in normal fibers and thus are located in former internodal sites. Since the internodal axon membrane usually contains few sodium channels, the question arises as to whether the newly formed nodes function normally. There is evidence to suggest that the axon membrane at the newly formed remyelinated nodes reorganizes, developing a relatively high density of sodium channels similar to normal nodes of Ranvier. The newly formed nodes thus are capable of generating action potentials, although some degree of conduction slowing may occur if the distance between nodes in remyelinated axons is sufficiently reduced. However, as noted earlier, many clinically apparent deficits are the result of conduction block rather than conduction slowing. The recovery of impulse conduction, even at decreased velocities, can be of considerable clinical importance.

Remyelination occurs in the human peripheral nervous system, but little if any takes place after central nervous system demyelination. Nevertheless, in disorders such as multiple sclerosis there can be nearly complete recovery of function (the clinical remission) in the absence of a strict restoration of prepathological structure. A number of mechanisms have been proposed to explain this recovery. The possibility that recovery may partially be due to alterations in the levels of circulating factors (also termed "neuroelectric blocking factors") has been raised by a number of investigators. These factors are presumably related to antibodies directed against neurons, glial cells, or myelin. Such a hypothesis fits well with immunological theories of the etiology of demyelinating disease. However, most of the factors isolated to date affect synaptic activity rather than axonal conduction, and the specificity of such factors to the demyelinating diseases is not yet definitively established. It is also possible that resolution of edema may play a role in conduction recovery. However, the time course of remission suggests that in certain patients other factors are important. Conduction via alternative pathways, or synaptic alterations such as sprouting, may underlie recovery in some instances.

In other situations, such as total demyelination of the optic nerve in patients who recover vision, there must be recovery of conduction through demyelinated axons. Recent studies have, in fact, shown the development of continuous conduction (similar to that which occurs in nonmyelinated fibers) through demyelinated regions of some damaged fibers. This finding implies the capability for action potential electrogenesis, and thus the development of a density of sodium channels sufficient to support action potential propagation, in certain demyelinated areas. The question of whether this involves the redistribution of preexisting sodium channels, or the production of new ones, has not yet been answered. The introduction of new sodium channels would require their synthesis, probably more proximally in the cell body of the demyelinated axon. The mechanisms for synthesis of ionic channels and for their transport and insertion into appropriate parts of the nerve cell membrane are as yet unstudied.

Finally, it should be noted that the correlation between structure and function in the demyelinating diseases is often not precise. The clinical neurosciences tra-ditionally depend on the "localization approach," in which it is often possible, on the basis of the clinical presentation, to predict the anatomical site of the lesion with a high degree of precision. In demyelinating diseases such as multiple sclerosis, however, the clinicopathological correlations are much more complex. It is now well known that the number of demyelinated plaques present on pathological examination of the central nervous system in most patients with multiple sclerosis will be considerably greater than expected on the basis of the clinical examination. This apparent discrepancy between clinical findings and pathological results may, however, provide important clues for the pathophysiology and clinical study of demyelinating diseases. As indicated, the ensemble of clinical abnormalities produced by a given set of demyelinated plaques need not be fixed, but may vary considerably depending on factors such as temperature and metabolic status. Moreover, rearrangements at the level of the cell membrane, including alterations in ionic channel distribution and function, may play an important role in determining the degree of functional abnormality that results from demyelination.

GENERAL REFERENCES

Davis, F. A., and C. L. Schauf. Approaches to the development of pharmacological interventions in multiple sclerosis. In *Demyelinating Disease: Basic and Clinical Electrophysiology*, S. G. Waxman and J. M. Ritchie (eds.). New York, Raven Press, 1971, pp. 505–10.

Hodgkin, A. L. *The Conduction of the Nervous Impulse.* Springfield, Ill., Thomas, 1964.

McDonald, W. I. Pathophysiology in multiple sclerosis. *Brain* 97:179–96, 1974.

Rasminsky, M. Physiology of conduction in demyelinated axons. In *Physiology and Pathobiology of Axons*, S. G. Waxman (ed.). New York, Raven Press, 1978, pp. 361–76.

Rasminsky, M. Hyperexcitability of pathologically myelinated axons and positive symptoms in multiple sclerosis. In *Demyelinating Disease: Basic and Clinical Electrophysiology,* S. G. Waxman and J. M. Ritchie (eds.). New York, Raven Press, 1981, pp. 289–99.

Ritchie, J. M., and S. Y. Chiu. Distribution of sodium and potassium channels in mammalian myelinated nerve. In *Demyelinating Disease: Basic and Clinical Electrophysiology,* S. G. Waxman and J. M. Ritchie (eds.). New York, Raven Press, 1981, pp. 329–43.

Spencer, P. S., and H. J. Weinberg. Axonal specification of Schwann cell expression and myelination. In *Physiology and Pathobiology of Axons,* S. G. Waxman (ed.). New York, Raven Press, 1978, pp. 389–405.

Waxman, S. G. Membranes, myelin, and the pathophysiology of multiple sclerosis. *New Eng. J. Med.* 306:1529–33, 1982.

Waxman, S. G. Clinicopathological correlations in multiple sclerosis and related disease. In *Demyelinating Disease: Basic and Clinical Electrophysiology,* S. G. Waxman and J. M. Ritchie (eds.). New York, Raven Press, 1981, pp. 169–82.

Waxman, S. G., and M.V. L. Bennett. Relative conduction velocities of small myelinated and non-myelinated fibers in the central nervous system. *Nature New Biol.* 238:217–19, 1972.

Waxman, S. G., and R. E. Foster. Ionic channel distribution and heterogeneity of the axon membrane in myelinated fibers. *Brain Res. Rev.* 2:205–34, 1980.

2.

Peripheral Nerve

LESLIE J. DORFMAN and STEPHEN G. WAXMAN

The axons of peripheral nerves form the major afferent limb of sensory pathways leading to the central nervous system and the final common pathway for motor and autonomic effector mechanisms. Thus, the cardinal symptoms of peripheral nerve disease include sensory disturbances, muscle weakness, and autonomic dysfunction. The precise nature, extent, and severity of symptoms depend on the character of the disease process and on the alterations in the structure and function of peripheral nerve that it produces.

SPECIAL MORPHOLOGICAL AND PHYSIOLOGICAL FEATURES OF PERIPHERAL NERVE

Supporting elements

Peripheral nerve is enveloped with connective tissue at three levels (Fig. 2-1). The external surface of each major nerve trunk is surrounded by the epineurium, which consists primarily of fibroblasts and collagen and also contains a lymphatic capillary network. The epineurium overlies the perineurium, which most closely invests the external surface of the nerve bundle and its constituent fascicles. The perineurium, in turn, is continuous with endoneurium, which surrounds the individidual nerve fascicles (Fig. 2-1). The local intraneural microenvironment, as well as intraneural metabolism, is partially influenced by the properties of the endoneurium (see later discussion of endoneurial fluid pressure). The endoneurium is also important in nerve regeneration after nerve fiber damage. The distal segments of transected nerves degenerate, leaving behind the endoneurial tubes and the Schwann cell cylinders, which together help to guide regenerating axons to their appropriate distal connections. Diseases of connective tissue, such as collagen disorders and fascial inflammations, may injure nerve fibers by local extension of the inflammatory processes by or damage to epineurial or perineurial blood vessels.

Vasa nervorum

The blood supply to peripheral nerves usually originates from branches of the large regional arteries, which branch repeatedly and form anastomotic plexuses in the epineurium and perineurium. From

25

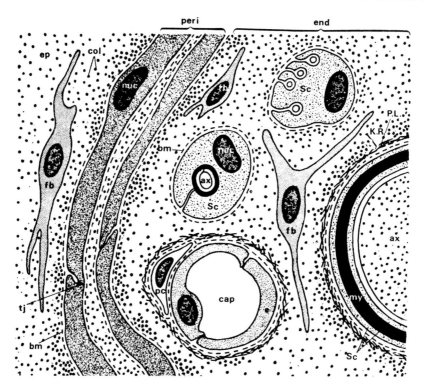

Fig. 2–1. Diagrammatic representation of a cross section of the mammalian peripheral nerve. ax, axon; my, myelin; Sc, Schwann cell; bm, basement membrane; pc, pericyte adjacent to blood vessel; cap, capillary; fb, fibroblasts; col, collagen; ep, epineurium; peri, perineurium. Note the tight junctions (tj) between perineurial cells. end, endoneurium. The sheath of Key and Retzius (K.R.), consisting of longitudinally oriented collagen surrounding the axon, and the sheath of Plenck and Laidlaw (P.L.), consisting of obliquely oriented collagen surrounding the axon, were referred to by earlier histologists. These two specialized sheaths constitute part of the endoneurium. (Reprinted with permission from E. G. Gray, The fine structure of nerve. *Comp. Biochem. Physiol.* 36:419–48, 1970.)

the perineurial plexus, smaller vessels course longitudinally within the interfascicular endoneurial septa. Despite the abundant collateral connectivity of the intrinsic nerve vasculature, local occlusion of the intraneural arterioles may lead to infarction of peripheral nerve, as occurs in diabetes mellitus and in diseases that produce arteritis.

Blood-nerve barrier

As in the central nervous system, there are barriers in the peripheral nerves that do not allow all of the components of plasma

to diffuse freely from the vasa nervorum into peripheral nerve tissue. The endoneurial vessels and the perineurium, in particular, are relatively impermeable to many proteins and ions, although there is marked species variability. It has been suggested that the vascular and perifascicular diffusion barrier may act to limit the spread of some disease-producing agents such as toxins, antibodies, and viruses.

Endoneurial pressure

Recent evidence suggests that just as the capillary endothelium of peripheral nerve is selectively permeable to different blood constituents, the endoneurium surrounding the smallest nerve fascicles also has limited permeability. In some disease states, particularly some intoxications, endoneurial fluid pressure may rise substantially. It has been suggested that this may lead in turn to secondary injury to axons and Schwann cell elements or may interfere with axoplasmic flow.

Axoplasmic transport

The peripheral axons of motor and sensory nerve fibers actively transport cytoplasmic materials both toward and away from the neuronal cell body. Rapid orthograde transport (from the soma to the terminals) of a wide variety of molecular species proceeds at a rate of approximately 400 mm per day in most mammalian nerves studied. This rapid transport is probably a mechanism for transmitting proteins and other complex molecules synthesized in or near the cell body along microtubules or neurofilaments—or both—to the metabolically active nerve terminal region (Fig. 2–2). An independent, slower, orthograde transport at the rate of 1–3 mm per day may be related to bulk flow of axoplasm. Retrograde transport (from periphery to soma) proceeds at an intermediate rate and is probably involved in the process by which growing nerve terminals "recognize" appropriate target connections. Retrograde transport may also be involved in chromatolysis of the neuronal soma after axonal injury and in the ascent of toxins such as tetanus to reach the central nervous system from the periphery. The degree to which disturbances of axoplasmic transport may play a role in the pathogenesis of peripheral nerve diseases is not known. There is as yet no clinically convenient way to measure axoplasmic transport.

Spinal roots

The beginning of the peripheral nerve is considered to be that point along the spinal root at which the axons lose their central myelin of oligodendroglial origin and acquire a peripheral myelin sheath from Schwann cells. In the clinical context, lesions of the spinal roots and the cauda equina may produce symptoms and signs very similar to more distal lesions. Therefore, root lesions (radiculopathies) and disorders of the cauda equina are often considered along with lesions of the peripheral nerves.

Axon populations

Peripheral nerve axons are of two general types: myelinated and unmyelinated (Fig. 2–3). The unmyelinated axons are not truly devoid of Schwann cell wrapping, but do not have a lamellated or compact myelin sheath and well-defined nodes of Ranvier and internodal regions; hence, they conduct impulses continuously, rather than by saltatory conduction, as discussed in Chapter 1. When the cross-sectional morphology of axons of peripheral nerves is examined, a trimodal population composed of large myelinated fibers, small myelinated fibers, and unmyelinated fibers becomes apparent. As might be expected from the relationship between fiber diameter and conduction velocity (Chap. 1), when a segment of mixed peripheral nerve is electrically excited in vitro, three distinct compound-action potential peaks are discernible, corresponding to the three fiber populations (Fig. 2–4). The largest myelinated fibers include the IA afferents from the muscle spindles, the sensory fibers that subserve light touch, proprioception, and vibration, and the alpha motor axons. The smaller myelinated fibers include the sensory fibers associated with sharp pain, temperature, and pressure, and the gamma motor fibers. The unmyelinated fibers include some pain afferents and the autonomic efferents to smooth muscle and glands.

Some peripheral nerve disorders differentially affect fibers according to their size. For example, in Friedreich's ataxia,

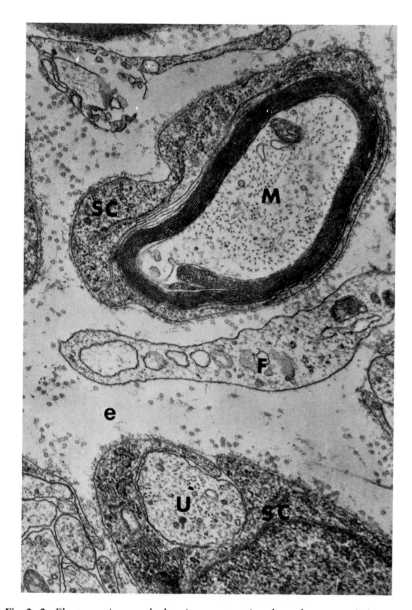

Fig. 2–2. Electron micrograph showing cross section through mouse sciatic nerve. A myelinated fiber (M), an unmyelinated fiber (U), and Schwann cells (Sc) are indicated. Note the cross sections of longitudinally oriented microtubules and neurofilaments within the axons. A fibroblast (F) is also present within the nerve. e, extracellular space. × 36,000

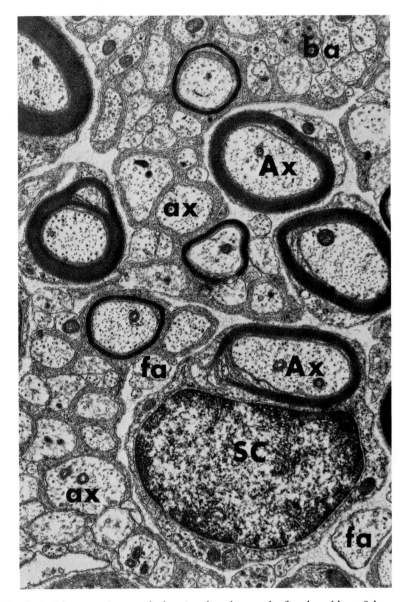

Fig. 2–3. Electron micrograph showing dorsal root of a five-day-old rat. Schwann cells (SC) form compact myelin around the larger-caliber axons (Ax). The smaller-caliber axons (ax) are often surrounded by Schwann cell processes. At this stage of development some axons (ba) are loosely bundled by Schwann cell processes while other axons (fa) remain free of Schwann cell investments. (Courtesy of Dr. T. Sims, Stanford University School of Medicine.)

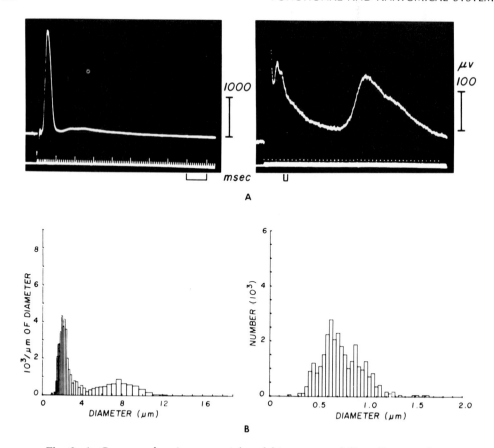

Fig. 2–4. Compound action potential and histograms of fiber diameters in a fascicular biopsy specimen of normal human sural nerve. **A.** Early components (left) of the compound action potential showing a large A-alpha peak corresponding to activity in large myelinated fibers, and a smaller A-delta peak corresponding to activity in small myelinated fibers. A very small, late C-fiber component representing unmyelinated fiber activity is evident in the trace on the right, which has a slower time base and higher amplification. **B.** Myelinated (left) and unmyelinated (right) fiber-diameter distributions from the same nerve biopsy. (Reproduced with permission from E. H. Lambert and P. J. Dyck, Compound action potentials of sural nerve in vitro in peripheral neuropathy. In *Peripheral Neuropathy*, P. J. Dyck, et al. (eds.). Philadelphia, Saunders, 1975, pp. 427–41.)

it is the largest fibers that undergo degeneration, leading to selective loss of vibratory and proprioceptive senses and of tendon reflexes. In contrast, in hereditary sensory neuropathy, it is the unmyelinated fibers that are involved earliest and to the greatest extent, producing disturbances of pain sensibility and of autonomic reactivity. In many generalized peripheral polyneuropathies, the pattern of affected modalities provides clues to preferential involvement of axons on the basis of caliber, and this in turn focuses attention on the appropriate diagnostic considerations.

ANATOMICAL ASPECTS OF PERIPHERAL NEUROPATHY

Mononeuropathy

When only a single major peripheral nerve trunk is affected by a pathophysiological process, the condition is referred to as a mononeuropathy. The most common causes of mononeuropathy include penetrating or compressive trauma and vascular occlusion. The common sites for compressive injuries to peripheral nerve include the ulnar nerve at the elbow, the median nerve in the carpal tunnel at the wrist, and the peroneal nerve at the knee. In each of these sites, the peripheral nerve is adjacent to a relatively rigid bony or ligamentous structure and is vulnerable to either an acute, severe compressive injury or to repeated episodes of milder intermittent compression that cumulatively damage the nerve.

The mildest of nerve compressions cause paresthesias, lasting only minutes, in the territory of the nerve (as in the familiar "limb falling asleep"). The pathophysiological substrate of this phenomenon is unknown but may be related to nerve ischemia. More severe or prolonged nerve compression produces local demyelination, with preferential involvement of the largest fibers, whch in turn leads to abnormalities of impulse conduction as discussed in the preceding chapter. Localized lesions that are largely demyelinative have a relatively good prognosis for recovery, provided the precipitating factors are removed. If the compressive injury is even more severe or prolonged, there may be damage to axons with secondary (Wallerian) degeneration of the distal axon segments. Recovery is likely to be much more protracted when this occurs because the proximal axonal stumps must regenerate at a rate that ordinarily does not exceed about 1 mm per day. The regenerating axons must also find their appropriate synaptic connections. The Schwann cell and endoneurial tubes often provide guidance, as mentioned earlier, but the accuracy of regeneration and reconnection is frequently less than perfect, particularly when the lesion is proximal in location. For example, the reinnervation of incorrect targets after facial nerve injury may result in inappropriate lacrimation ("crocodile tears") or to eyelid closure when the jaw is opened ("jaw–winking" synkinesis).

Monoradiculopathy

A lesion involving a single spinal nerve root is referred to as a monoradiculopathy, and it may share features with peripheral mononeuropathy. The most common cause of monoradiculopathy is compression of a spinal root by a herniated or ruptured fragment of degenerated intervertebral disk. The gradation of pathophysiologic events with severity of nerve injury is similar in the spinal root and in peripheral nerve. Symptoms include pain, paresthesia, hypesthesia, weakness, and hyporeflexia in the territory of the affected structure. Accurate anatomic localization of the involved nerve or root depends on precise knowledge of the dermatomal and myotomal innervation of the peripheral nervous system.

Mononeuropathy multiplex

When multiple major peripheral nerve trunks are involved (usually asymmetrically) by a disease process, the condition is often referred to as multiple mononeuropathy, or mononeuropathy multiplex. This is an uncommon disorder usually produced either by an arteritis or vasculitis involving the vasa nervorum, or by a chronic infection such as leprosy.

Polyneuropathy

Polyneuropathy is a symmetrical disorder of peripheral nerve function that, if sufficiently severe, involves all of the periph-eral nerves—though not necessarily to the same degree. The common causes of polyneuropathy include toxic, metabolic, and generalized inflammatory disorders, as well as some inherited conditions (Table 2–1). The clinical and pathological as-pects of polyneuropathy are discussed in the following sections.

Polyradiculoneuropathy

This is a term used to describe conditions such as the Guillian-Barré syndrome, a polyneuropathic disorder in which both the proximal segments of peripheral nerve and the spinal roots are often prominently in-volved.

CLINICAL FEATURES OF NEUROPATHY

Weakness and atrophy

When the motor fibers in peripheral nerve are affected by a disease process there will be weakness of the muscles innervated by the involved nerve. In the extreme case, the muscles may be paralyzed (plegic). Weakness may be comparable in degree whether the nerve injury is demyelinative or axonal in nature, i.e., whether the ax-ons are intact but demyelinated, or have undergone Wallerian degeneration. The lower motor neuron syndrome, character-ized by weakness in association with hy-potonia and hyporeflexia due to interrup-tion of the segmental spinal reflex arc, often accompanies peripheral nerve disease. This is to be distinguished from upper motor neuron weakness, which is associated with hypertonia and hyperreflexia (Chap. 9).

When the peripheral motor nerve fi-bers become demyelinated the affected muscles frequently undergo atrophy as a result of disuse. Morphologically, such muscles exhibit reduction of fiber caliber, particularly of the type II fibers (Chap. 4).

However, the muscle fibers retain their sarcolemmal integrity and regenerative capacity. When the motor axons have de-generated, muscle atrophy is much more severe and associated with a predictable sequence of events in the denervated mus-cle fibers. Within several days to several weeks after degeneration of the motor axon terminals, acetylcholine receptors, which normally are present primarily in the neu-romuscular junction, proliferate over the entire surface of the muscle membrane. The resting potential of the muscle fibers falls and they become hypersensitive to acetyl-choline. Shortly thereafter, the denervated muscle fibers develop spontaneous electri-cal activity (fibrillations), which can be detected in the electromyographic exami-nation. It is not yet certain whether the sequence of denervation changes in mus-cle fibers results from a decrease in the normal neuromuscular electrical activity, or whether muscle fibers require some "trophic" substance(s) ordinarily pro-vided by the intact motor axon. Dener-vated muscle fibers progressively atrophy over many months and may disappear after about one year if not reinnervated, after which time restoration of function is usu-ally not possible.

Sensory loss

Injury to sensory nerve fibers produces impairment of sensation in the area of the affected nerve. The modalities affected de-pend in part on the severity of the patho-physiologic process and its predilection for selectively involving fibers according to their size, as discussed earlier. When the disturbance of sensory function is severe, the affected body parts become virtually anesthetic and therefore subject to re-peated injuries because the protective pain mechanisms are lost. Under these circum-stances, the involved body parts may be-come progressively mutilated by a cycle of repeated trauma and secondary infection. This is commonly seen in leprosy, heredi-

Table 2–1. Etiologic classification of peripheral neuropathies.

A. Toxic	B. Metabolic	C. Genetic	D. Infectious

1. Drugs
  a. Isoniazid
  b. Hydralazine
  c. Nitrofurantoin
  d. Vincristine
  e. Disulfiram
  f. Imipramine
  g. Thalidomide
  h. Phenytoin
  i. Stilbamidine
2. Heavy Metals
  a. Lead
  b. Arsenic
  c. Mercury
  d. Thallium
  e. Gold
3. Organic Compounds
  a. Organophosphates
  b. Trichlorethylene
  c. Carbon disulfide
  d. Acrylamide
  e. Aldrin and dieldrin
  f. Hexocarbons
	1. Nutritional
	  a. Alcoholism
	  b. Vitamin deficiency
	    1) Thiamine
	    2) Pantothenic acid
	    3) Pyridoxine
	    4) Niacin
	    5) Vitamin B_{12}
	  c. Malabsorption
	  d. Postgastrectomy
	2. Uremia
	3. Porphyria
	4. Hypoglycemia
	5. Diabetes mellitus
	6. Hypothyroidism
	7. Dysproteinemias
	  a. Macroglobulinemia
	  b. Myeloma
	  c. Cryoglobulinemia
		Dominant
		1. Charcot-Marie-Tooth peroneal
		  muscular atrophy
		  a. Hypertrophic form
		  b. Neuronal form
		2. Amyloidosis
		3. Hereditary sensory neuropathy
		Recessive
		1. Hypertrophic neuropathy
		  (Dejerine-Sottas)
		2. Refsum's disease
		3. Abetalipoproteinemia (Bassen-
		  Kornzweig)
		4. Analphalipoproteinemia
		  (Tangier)
		5. Hereditary sensory neuropathy
		6. Metachromatic leukodystrophy
		7. Globoid cell leukodystrophy
		  (Krabbe)
			1. Leprosy
			2. Diphtheria
			3. Herpes zoster
			4. Sarcoidosis (?)
			
			E. Ischemic
			1. Vasculitides
			2. Peripheral vascular insuffi-
			  ciency (arteriosclerosis)
			
			F. Immune
			1. Idiopathic polyneuritis of
			  Guillain-Barré (?)
			2. Serum sickness neuritis
			3. Infectious mononucleosis (?)
			4. Recurrent polyneuritis
			
			**G. Neoplastic: Tumor Implants or
			  Remote Effects**
			1. Carcinoma or sarcoma
			2. Lymphoma
			3. Primary tumors of peripheral
			  nerves
			
			H. Traumatic

Modified from Asbury and Johnson, 1978.

tary sensory neuropathy, and can also occur in severe diabetic polyneuropathy.

Trophic disturbances

Impairment of autonomic fiber function in peripheral nerve leads to a sequence of changes that include loss of vasomotor tone in the skin and deeper tissues, leading to cutaneous erythema of the affected limb and disturbances of local thermoregulation. Another frequent aspect of autonomic impairment is abnormality of sweating, which may be either excessive or deficient in the affected regions. Longstanding autonomic dysfunction may lead to atrophic changes in the integument and nails, and eventually even in the bones and subcutaneous tissues.

Positive symptoms

The symptoms discussed in the preceding paragraphs all reflect loss or diminution of normal function in peripheral nerve elements. Diseases of peripheral nerve can, however, produce positive symptoms, including pain, paresthesias (spontaneous somesthetic sensations, usually in the form of prickling or tingling feelings) and dysesthesias (abnormal qualities of sensation in response to somesthetic stimuli). The origin of these symptoms, particularly the pain and paresthesias, is not known. Some evidence suggests that they may represent spontaneous activity arising in damaged nerve fibers. Dysesthesia may also represent abnormal cross-talk between neighboring axons in the vicinity of a nerve lesion (Chap. 1). It is worth noting that there is probably no such thing as true "hyperesthesia," which properly means an excess amount of normal sensation. It is not uncommon in nerve disease for a stimulus to elicit a strong or intense sensation, but this is always abnormal in character and more correctly referred to as hyperpathia.

The pain associated with peripheral nerve lesions may be very severe and de-

bilitating. This is particularly true, for example, in the syndrome of causalgia, which consists of pain and autonomic dysfunction in the territory of a partially injured nerve (most commonly the median), and in the "phantom limb" pain that sometimes follows an amputation. Measures that may be employed to control such discomfort are discussed in the section on therapy and in Chapter 5.

CLINICAL FEATURES OF POLYNEUROPATHY

Polyneuropathy is characterized by its symmetry, typical distribution of involvement, and nature of progression. While a polyneuropathy may have some minor asymmetrical features, particularly at its onset, typically the disorder becomes, and continues to be, nearly symmetrical once the symptoms are well established. Major asymmetrical or focal features should therefore prompt consideration of other pathophysiological processes.

Early and predominant involvement of the distal body parts is the cardinal anatomic feature of polyneuropathy. Sensory symptoms commonly begin in the toes or sometimes in the fingertips. As the disease progresses, the symptoms tend to ascend the legs and arms, giving rise at some point to the "stocking-and-glove" distribution of sensory impairment. With further worsening, involvement of more proximal parts of the limbs becomes apparent, and ultimately the trunk and head may also be involved (Fig. 2–5). The fact that the toes are the most frequent site of first involvement is thought to be related to the extreme length of the involved axons. The dorsal root ganglion cells that subserve sensation in the toes have bipolar axons extending from the toes to the gracile nuclei at the cervicomedullary junction near the foramen magnum. It has been suggested that these large neurons normally maintain a high metabolic rate of activity in order to sustain the large cell volume

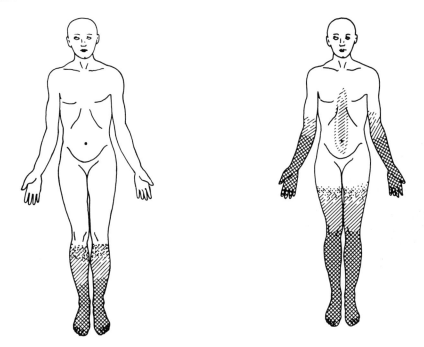

Fig. 2–5. Topography of sensory impairment in a patient with mild alcoholic-nutritional polyneuropathy (left), and in a case of more severe diabetic polyneuropathy (right). Single cross-hatching indicates areas where pinprick sensibility is impaired but not lost; double cross-hatching denotes absence of pinprick sensation; the stippled regions correspond to zones of hyperpathia. Note the predilection for symmetrical involvement of distal body parts.

represented by these long processes. Therefore, a modest metabolic perturbation may interfere with the function of these elements and result in failure to maintain the most distal axon ramifications. An alternative interpretation is that the long axons are more likely to be selectively vulnerable to multifocal processes that randomly affect nerve fibers and their associated Schwann cells. When there is a prominent motor component to a peripheral polyneuropathy, it too usually affects distal regions of innervation first. For example, the extensor digitorum brevis muscle in the foot often becomes atrophic before other muscles.

A few polyneuropathic disorders, for reasons that are not known, stand in marked contrast to the general rule of distal-to-proximal gradient of involvement. These include heavy metal neuropathies, in which the extensor muscles of the forearm are often involved early; the Guillain-Barré syndrome, in which proximal rather than distal weakness is frequently an early sign; and porphyric polyneuropathy, in which there may be proximal sensory loss in a "bathing trunk" pattern over the torso.

FUNCTIONAL CLASSIFICATION OF POLYNEUROPATHY

Sensorimotor polyneuropathy

The majority of peripheral polyneuropathies involve both motor and sensory elements to comparable degrees. Examples include alcoholic/nutritional polyneuropathy and uremic polyneuropathy, in which motor signs and symptoms usually accompany sensory disturbances.

Predominantly motor polyneuropathy

It is uncommon for a polyneuropathy to involve exclusively either motor or sensory fibers. However, in some disorders, the motor involvement far exceeds the relatively minor sensory disturbance. Examples of this situation include heavy metal neuropathies such as that produced by chronic lead intoxication, the Guillain-Barré syndrome, diphtheritic neuropathy, and some of the hereditary polyneuropathies. In most of these disorders, some degree of sensory involvement can be demonstrated by careful clinical examination, by clinical electrophysiological studies of sensory nerve fibers, or by morphological examination of biopsied sensory nerves. The spinal muscular atrophies are a group of degenerative disorders, usually not classified with the polyneuropathies, in which the involvement is virtually limited to the anterior horn cells of the spinal cord and their peripheral axonal processes.

Predominantly sensory polyneuropathies

While sensory signs and symptoms predominate in some types of polyneuropathy, it is also often possible to demonstrate lesser degrees of motor involvement by electromyographic examination or by muscle biopsy. A common example of predominantly sensory polyneuropathy is the ubiquitous diabetic polyneuropathy. A few hereditary conditions, such as Friedreich's ataxia and hereditary sensory neuropathy, are characterized by degeneration of dorsal root ganglion cells and their axons (both peripheral and central) with sparing of motor function.

Predominantly autonomic polyneuropathy

Disorders in which autonomic features predominate are the least common of the functionally selective polyneuropathies. Examples include amyloid polyneuropa-

thy and some hereditary system atrophies with peripheral autonomic involvement such as the Riley-Day syndrome (familial dysautonomia), which is sometimes also associated with congenital insensitivity to pain due to absence or reduction in the number of small peripheral nerve fibers. When severe, these disorders produce symptoms of impaired autonomic function. These include severe orthostatic hypotension, disturbances of micturition and gastrointestinal motility, impotence, and abnormalities of pupillary reactivity.

PATHOPHYSIOLOGICAL CLASSIFICATION OF POLYNEUROPATHY

Demyelinative polyneuropathy

When a disease process selectively involves peripheral nerve myelin or its parent Schwann cell, the condition is referred to as a demyelinative polyneuropathy. The nerve axons generally tend to maintain their gross histological integrity in such disorders. Therefore, muscles do not become denervated or severely atrophic, as discussed earlier. Demyelinative polyneuropathies tend to be more rapidly progressive in their onset than axonal polyneuropathies. For example, the Guillain-Barré syndrome usually reaches its peak in a matter of days or at most a few weeks. Once the demyelinative process has stopped, the recovery phase is often relatively rapid and the restoration of function more complete than in diseases that damage the axons.

As discussed in the preceding chapter, the properties of impulse conduction in demyelinated nerve are abnormal. Patients with demyelinative polyneuropathy usually exhibit slowing of peripheral nerve conduction velocity and impairment of ability to transmit nerve signals at high frequency. These changes usually occur in the absence of electromyographic evidence of muscle denervation. Although patients with CNS demyelinating diseases, such as multiple sclerosis, frequently exhibit marked transient worsening of symptoms when body temperature rises, it is not known why corresponding phenomena are rare in peripheral demyelinative polyneuropathies.

Neuronal polyneuropathy

A neuronal or perikaryonal disorder is one in which the abnormality is primarily found in the neuronal cell bodies. The neuron and its processes undergo degeneration, producing secondary changes in the myelin and Schwann cells. Examples of neuronal polyneuropathy include the spinal muscular atrophies, the hereditary sensory neuropathies, and the neuronal form of Charcot-Marie-Tooth disease (hereditary motor and sensory polyneuropathy).

If the disease process is not too advanced and some nerve axons survive, nerve conduction velocities may be normal or nearly so. However, the electromyographic examination will show evidence of denervation in the affected muscles. Recovery, to the extent that it is possible, occurs through compensatory mechanisms arising in surviving neurons, such as sprouting with subsequent innervation of previously denervated structures.

Axonal polyneuropathy

Axonal polyneuropathy refers to the idea that some polyneuropathies may be manifestations of disease primarily affecting the peripheral nerve axons, as opposed to the neuronal perikarya or the myelin. Uremic polyneuropathy is thought to be such a disorder. Certain toxic polyneuropathies may also fall into this category, particularly those—such as vinca alkaloid neuropathy—in which there seems to be a primary interference with axoplasmic transport. Whether these disorders are true axonal polyneuropathies, or whether they represent neuronal polyneuropathies in which the axonal manifestations are secondary to involvement of the cell bodies, is still undetermined.

Distal or "dying-back" axonopathy

There is evidence that in some neuropathies caused by exogenous toxins, such as acrylamide or *n*-hexane, the brunt of the disorder occurs in the distal parts of axons, i.e., those parts located farthest from the cell bodies. The term *distal axonopathy* has been proposed since both peripheral and central axons seem to be involved. Interestingly, there may also be some selectivity with respect to fiber type as well as length. In some toxic neuropathies, for example, the distal axonal regions innervating Pacinian corpuscles and muscle spindles are preferentially involved.

SPECIAL PROCEDURES IN THE DIAGNOSIS OF NEUROPATHY

Clinical Examination

Accurate diagnosis of peripheral nerve disorders requires precise knowledge of neuroanatomy and the range of clinical expression of disease in order to first differentiate central from peripheral diseases, and then to localize peripheral disorders to spinal root(s), plexus(es), or peripheral nerve(s). In addition to the standard features of the clinical neurological examination, some special aspects of physical diagnosis may be of particular value in patients with peripheral neuropathy. Inspection of the integument can reveal atrophy of the skin, hair, and nails (suggesting autonomic dysfunction), areas of anhidrosis or hyperhidrosis corresponding to sweat gland dysfunction in the territory of diseased nerve(s), or evidence of muscle atrophy and fasciculation, indicative of axonal or neuronal dysfunction. Clues to the presence of hereditary nerve disorders may also be evident in the skin, such as café-au-lait spots in von Recklinghausen's neurofibromatosis.

Palpation of muscle and nerve is infrequently practiced, but is often of great value. Muscle atrophy and fibrosis can be best appreciated on palpation, as can muscle cramps, a common feature of many peripheral nerve disorders. Enlarged or hypertrophic peripheral nerves may be encountered in cases of chronic demyelinative polyneuropathy, amyloid polyneuropathy, and leprosy. Enlarged nerves can often be detected by palpating the ulnar nerve at the elbow, the superficial sensory branch of the radial nerve at the wrist, the peroneal nerve at the head of the fibula or the superficial greater auricular nerve in the neck. Nerve tumors, such as neurofibromata, may frequently be appreciated as localized areas of nerve enlargement.

Percussion of a peripheral nerve, if sufficiently vigorous, may elicit paresthesias in the cutaneous territory of the nerve, referred to as Tinel's sign. In demyelinative neuropathy, Tinel's sign can often be elicited by very slight percussion over an area of nerve abnormality, reflecting the increased mechanosensitivity of demyelinated nerve (Chap. 1). This sign is sometimes helpful in localizing nerve lesions and in following the regeneration of peripheral nerve after transection.

Clinical electrophysiology

The measurement of nerve conduction velocity is of great value in the diagnosis, localization, and quantitation of peripheral nerve dysfunction. Methods in wide clinical application include measurement of maximal motor and sensory conduction velocities, spinal reflex latencies, and spinal and cerebral somatosensory evoked potentials. Conduction velocity is measured by applying an electrical pulse percutaneously to a specific peripheral nerve and recording the response at a known dis-

tance either from the nerve itself, or from a muscle it innervates. As discussed earlier and in the preceding chapter, the most marked abnormality of nerve conduction velocity is encountered in demyelinating disorders.

Electromyography (EMG) is an examination of the electrical activity of muscle, usually by means of an intramuscular needle electrode (Chap. 4). From the presence or absence of abnormal spontaneous activity in the resting muscle and from examination of the properties of motor unit action potentials, it is possible to distinguish neurogenic from myopathic weakness, to ascertain the presence of denervation, and to detect evidence of reinnervation.

Nerve and muscle biopsy

Histological and biochemical analysis of biopsied muscle and nerve tissue is sometimes of value in the diagnosis of peripheral neuromuscular disorders. Examination of muscle may provide evidence of denervation and reinnervation (Chap. 4). Examination of biopsied nerve may permit differentiation of axonal and demyelinative neuropathy and can provide morphological and/or biochemical clues to specific diagnoses such as amyloidosis, arteritis, and certain leukodystrophies.

PRINCIPLES OF THERAPY IN NEUROPATHY

Removal of the offending agent

Prevention of additional trauma often constitutes the major form of treatment in cases of traumatic injury to peripheral nerves. This is frequently the case in the common occupational traumatic mononeuropathies, including crossed-leg palsy (foot drop caused by peroneal nerve injury at the knee) related to trauma produced by crossing one leg over the other, Saturday-night palsy (wrist drop caused by radial nerve injury in the upper arm) often caused by sleeping on the arm after excessive alcohol ingestion, and tardy ulnar palsy (weak hand caused by compression at the elbow) related to habitual leaning on the elbows. If the nerve is entrapped by adjacent anatomical structures it may be necessary to relieve the entrapment surgically as in section of the transverse carpal ligament for carpal tunnel syndrome (median nerve at the wrist), or transposition of the ulnar nerve out of the ulnar groove at the elbow. If the trauma has been chronic and severe, and the nerve has become secondarily scarred and fibrotic, there may possibly be merit in freeing the fascicles of nerve by performing internal neurolysis.

In cases of peripheral polyneuropathy of toxic or metabolic origin, treatment of the disease requires removal of the neurotoxic agent. In this context, metabolic polyneuropathies—such as those associated with diabetes and uremia—are frequently considered to reflect the effects of endogenous toxins, although in most cases the specific neurotoxic agent is unknown. In both cases the toxic activity must be removed, either by ceasing exposure to the external agent, or by correcting the underlying metabolic abnormality.

Regeneration

If nerve damage has been mainly demyelinative in nature, recovery is usually relatively prompt (i.e., within weeks to months) and complete. Recovery must occur by other mechanisms if axons have been damaged. Axon regrowth is slow even under optimal circumstances, with the maximal rate in peripheral nerve approximating 1mm per day. Central nervous system axons do not exhibit regenerative capacities comparable to those of peripheral axons, a distinction currently under intense study. The ability of regenerating axons to reestablish appropriate functional end-organ connectivity is also associated with a substantial degree of un-

certainty. Factors associated with less favorable prognosis include a long regenerative path, discontinuity of the supportive connective tissue elements (as in a nerve that is severed rather than compressed), and the presence of scar tissues or neuroma formation. In cases of incomplete axonal damage to peripheral nerve, some degree of muscle recovery may occur by peripheral sprouting of undamaged motor axons, which reinnervate muscle fibers that have lost their original neural supply. This creates a situation in which muscles have fewer motor units, each containing more muscle fibers than normal, and the fibers are closely grouped together within the muscle. The factors limiting the collateral reinnervative capacity of motor axons are not fully understood.

Pain control

Some of the most severe chronic pain disorders are those associated with peripheral nerve lesions. Examples include trigeminal neuralgia, postherpetic neuralgia, phantom limb pain, and causalgic pain associated with partial nerve injuries. Diabetic and alcoholic polyneuropathies often cause a severe hyperpathia or chronic neuropathic pain syndrome. One reasonable working hypothesis is that some of these painful manifestations result from abnormal excitability of damaged peripheral nerve membrane (Chap. 1). Alternatively, it is possible that there is a resetting of some central mechanism that, as a result of a primary peripheral nerve insult, contributes to the pain syndrome (Chap. 5). There is evidence for abnormal generation of impulses in demyelinated nerve fibers and in nerve fibers that have formed a neuroma. Thus, at least a significant part of the mechanism underlying pain in the disorders of peripheral nerve probably reflects dysfunction of the peripheral axon.

One form of treatment that is frequently used with modest success is the administration of anticonvulsant agents such as diphenylhydantoin or carbamaze-pine, which tend to decrease the excitability of nerve cell membranes. Another approach is to stimulate the large myelinated fibers in the affected nerve through the skin. This and other approaches to pain management are considered in Chapter 5.

GENERAL REFERENCES

Asbury, A. K., and P. C. Johnson. *Pathology of Peripheral Nerve*. Philadelphia, Saunders, 1978.

Dyck, P. J., P. K. Thomas, E. H. Lambert, and R. Bunge (eds.). *Peripheral Neuropathy*. Philadelphia, Saunders, 1984.

Landon, D. N. (ed.). *The Peripheral Nerve*. New York, Wiley, 1976.

Mitchell, S. W. *Injuries of Nerves and their Consequences*. New York, Lippincott, 1872. Reprint. New York, Dover, 1975.

Omer, G. E., and M. Spinner (eds.). *Management of Peripheral Nerve Problems*. Philadelphia, Saunders, 1980.

Sumner, A. J. (ed.). *The Physiology of Peripheral Nerve Disease*. Philadelphia, Saunders, 1980.

Waxman, S. G. (ed.). *Physiology and Pathobiology of Axons*. New York, Raven Press, 1978.

3.

Neuromuscular Junction

ALAN L. PEARLMAN

The neuromuscular junction continues to be the subject of intensive study, in large measure because it is one of the most accessible synapses in the nervous system and is thus highly suited for working out the basic mechanisms of synaptic transmission. As a result, a great deal has been learned about the synthesis, storage, and release of synaptic transmitter from the presynaptic terminal, and about the interaction of the transmitter with the postsynaptic receptor. These studies have provided an important basis for analyzing synaptic function in the central nervous system and have brought us very close to a complete understanding of the pathogenesis of one of the major diseases affecting the human neuromuscular junction, myasthenia gravis. This chapter will review selected aspects of the structure and function of the neuromuscular junction and will then consider how these are altered in various disease states.

THE NEUROMUSCULAR JUNCTION

The axons of individual motor neurons in the brainstem and spinal cord divide intramuscularly to provide a fine terminal branch to each of the 10–500 muscle fibers in its motor unit. As this branch approaches the muscle fiber it loses its myelin sheath and forms an expanded terminal that is closely applied to a specialized region of the muscle membrane called the *end-plate* region (Fig. 3–1). Each muscle fiber has only one end-plate, innervated by one axon. The axon terminal contains mitochondria and the enzyme *choline acetyltransferase,* which is necessary for synthesis of the transmitter, *acetylcholine.* The terminal also contains small, membrane-closed sacs called *synaptic vesicles.* There is good evidence that these vesicles contain acetylcholine and that transmitter release is accomplished by a process *(exocytosis)* that involves the fusion of vesicles with presynaptic membrane. The presynaptic membrane contains many discreet areas of specialization that are thought to be the sites of active transmitter secretion. Synaptic vesicles collect in double rows at these *active zones* (Fig. 3–1). The released molecules of acetylcholine diffuse across the narrow (40–50 nm) synaptic cleft, passing through a collagenous structure, the *basal lamina,* which does not impede diffusion significantly.

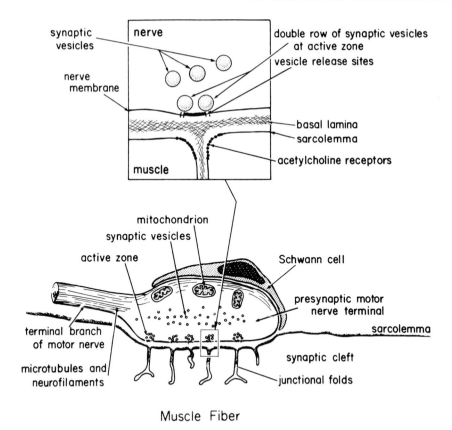

Fig. 3–1. A schematic representation of a mammalian neuromuscular junction. The inset shows a presynaptic active zone with adjacent synaptic vesicles, and the postsynaptic junctional folds with clusters of acetylcholine receptors on their crests. (Modified from R. P. Lisak and R. L. Barchi, *Myasthenia Gravis.* Vol. 11 of *Major Problems in Neurology.* Philadelphia, Saunders, 1982.)

Transmitter release from the presynaptic terminal occurs both spontaneously and as a result of invasion of the axon terminal by an action potential. The spontaneous release of acetylcholine leads to tiny depolarizations of the postsynaptic membrane known as *miniature end-plate potentials.* Careful analysis of miniature end-plate potentials has demonstrated that acetylcholine is released from the presynaptic terminal in multimolecular packets, or quanta, of fixed size. The *quantum* is the fundamental unit of transmitter release; each quantum probably corresponds to the contents of a single synaptic vesicle, which has been estimated to be

between 10,000 and 50,000 molecules of acetylcholine.

Action potentials traveling down the axon of the motor neuron invade the axon terminal, causing a depolarization of the terminal membrane. As a result of this depolarization, voltage-dependent calcium channels are opened and calcium enters the nerve terminal. Calcium entry produces the simultaneous release of many quanta of acetylcholine, each identical to the quanta released spontaneously. The way in which calcium causes transmitter release is not fully understood, but it probably acts to promote the fusion of synaptic vesicles with the presynaptic membrane. In any case, calcium entry is essential for the release of the approximately 300–400 quanta that enter the synaptic cleft following the invasion of the terminal by a single action potential. Reducing the concentration of calcium in the extracellular fluid reduces the number of quanta released by a given presynaptic membrane depolarization, and the replacement of calcium by magnesium or manganese also reduces transmitter release. It should be stressed that it is the number of quanta released that is calcium dependent, not the number of acetylcholine molecules present in each multimolecular packet.

Just across the synaptic cleft from each presynaptic active zone, the postsynaptic membrane contains a fold, and there are concentrations of particles evident on the lips of these folds that correspond to acetylcholine receptors. It is the concentration of acetylcholine receptors in the membrane of the end-plate region that provides its exquisite sensitivity to acetylcholine; the muscle membrane just a few microns away contains many fewer receptors and is about 100 times less sensitive to acetylcholine. Following denervation, the entire muscle fiber becomes much more sensitive to acetylcholine because new extra junctional receptors are inserted into the membrane.

Both the anatomical localization and the biochemical characterization of the acetylcholine receptor have been facilitated greatly by the discovery of a series of related snake neurotoxins, including alpha-bungarotoxin and alpha-cobratoxin. These toxins bind tightly to the acetylcholine receptor of mammalian skeletal muscle and can be radioactively labeled without significantly altering their affinity for the receptor. They also bind to the acetylcholine receptors that are present in enormous concentrations in the electric organs of eels and rays. These sources have provided the large quantities of receptors necessary for isolation and characterization of the receptor. Although this char-

acterization is not complete, it appears that each receptor is a molecule of about 250,000 molecular weight, and comprising five polypeptide subunits. Each receptor probably contains two binding sites for acetylcholine. Although the mammalian acetylcholine receptor has been harder to isolate, most evidence indicates that it is both structurally and antigenically similar to those of the eel and ray.

The interaction between acetylcholine and its receptor produces a conductance change in the postsynaptic membrane, markedly increasing the membrane's permeability to both sodium and potassium ions. Ions flowing through the channels opened by the transmitter-receptor interaction produce a local depolarization in the end-plate region called the *end-plate potential* that brings the muscle fiber membrane to threshold, firing an action potential that spreads quickly along the muscle fiber and leads to contraction (see Chap. 4).

The number of quanta released from the presynaptic terminal by the invasion of a single action potential is several times greater than is required to produce an end-plate potential that will lead to an action potential in the muscle membrane. Normally, the current flow during an end-plate potential is about four times that required to produce an action potential; the reserve current is called the *safety factor* for neuromuscular transmission. Repetitive activity in the nerve produces two phenomena that will be of importance when we consider the disorders of the neuromuscular junction in the next section. The first of these, called *facilitation,* is evident when two or three action potentials arrive in the nerve terminal in rapid succession. The number of quanta released after the second and third is larger than was released after the first and produces a larger postsynaptic depolarization. Facilitation is thought to be due to an accumulation of calcium ions inside the nerve terminal, thus facilitating the release of quanta. If repetitive stimulation of the nerve is continued at a rate similar to that which might occur during normal exertion, the number of quanta released by each impulse is rapidly reduced to about 30% of the quanta released during a single response. This phenomenon, called *synaptic depression,* is probably the result of decreased availability of synaptic vesicles immediately adjacent to the active zone of the presynaptic membrane. Although the number of quanta released during the period of depression is markedly reduced, it is still quite sufficient for the production of an adequate postsynaptic response in a normal neuromuscular junction but may not be sufficient in the disorders of the neuromuscular junction to be considered in the next section.

The action of acetylcholine on the postsynaptic membrane is brief. It is terminated by the action of an enzyme, *acetylcholinesterase,* that splits the molecule into choline and acetate. If acetylcholinesterase is inhibited, nerve-released acetylcholine produces a larger and longer synaptic potential. This prolongation occurs, not because the opening of individual ionic gates is prolonged, but rather because acetylcholine molecules remain in the synaptic cleft for longer periods and thus are able to bind repeatedly to receptors instead of binding to only one receptor and then undergoing hydrolysis as would normally occur. Inhibition of acetylcholinesterase permits diffusion of active acetylcholine molecules laterally in the cleft, enlarging the postsynaptic area over which a given quantum is effective, thereby producing potentiation of adjacent quanta. *Cholinesterase inhibitors* function by binding to the active site of the enzyme. The reversible inhibitors, such as edrophonium and pyridostigmine, are useful in the diagnosis and treatment of myasthenia gravis. The irreversible inhibitors (organophosphate insecticides and certain nerve gases) bind to the enzyme covalently. The resultant overactivity of acetylcholine produces first hyperexcitability and then desensitization of the postsynaptic receptors, which can lead to paralysis and death.

After the acetylcholine molecule is split by the action of acetylcholinesterase, the choline molecules are taken up by a specific uptake mechanism in the presynaptic terminal, and used in the production of new acetylcholine. Acetylcholine is synthesized in the cytoplasm of nerve terminals by the cytoplasmic enzyme choline acetyltransferase from choline and acetylcoenzyme A. Choline acetyltransferase and the synaptic vesicles are synthesized in the neuronal cell body and transported down the axon. There is also good evidence for a mechanism that recycles vesicles within the nerve terminal itself. Little is known of the actual mechanism for incorporating cytoplasmic acetylcholine into vesicles, although synthesis and incorporation are stimulated by neuronal activity, increased neuronal activity and transmitter release producing increased transmitter synthesis. The mechanism by which activity is linked to transmitter synthesis is poorly understood. It does not seem to be simply a response of choline acetylase to decreasing levels of acetylcholine, since the purified enzyme shows little sensitivity to acetylcholine concentration. Acetylcholine synthesis may be decreased or blocked experimentally by hemicholinium, an agent that blocks the uptake of choline by the nerve terminal.

As this brief review is meant to indicate, there are many steps in the process of synaptic transmission at the neuromuscular junction, and thus many ways in which the process can be disrupted. The next section will consider several clinical disorders affecting the neuromuscular junction and will attempt to delineate the stage at which normal functioning is altered by the pathological process.

MYASTHENIA GRAVIS

The primary clinical feature of myasthenia gravis is motor weakness that worsens with exercise and improves with rest. The eye muscles are affected early in the disease in over half of the cases and are affected at some stage in more than 90%. Myasthenia gravis is therefore an important diagnostic consideration in patients with diplopia and ptosis (Chap. 8). Weakness of the limb musculature is usually more pronounced proximally than distally and only rarely occurs in the absence of involvement of muscles innervated by cranial nerves. It produces symptoms that are common to most of the myopathies, including difficulty in climbing stairs, arising from a chair, or lifting. Involvement of the bulbar musculature produces nasal speech and difficulty in chewing and swallowing. Involvement of pharyngeal and respiratory musculature can lead to aspiration and respiratory failure, two major causes of death from the disease.

Myasthenia gravis occurs over a wide range of ages, from early infancy onward, but is most common in the second and third decade (when it affects women more frequently than men) and in late middle age (when it affects more men than women). There is an increased prevalence of the major histocompatibility antigen HLA-B8 in the younger group of patients. Studies of identical and fraternal twins and of other familial instances of the disease also indicate that there are genetic influences in the pathogenesis of the disease, but that other factors must be involved as well.

Several early clinical observations have proven to be quite important in providing clues to the pathogenesis of the disease. The first is that children born of myasthenic mothers often have transient myasthenia lasting a few days or weeks, suggesting the transplacental transfer of a serum factor, perhaps an antibody. Second, a small number of patients with myasthenia gravis have thymomas, and many patients have evidence of lymphoid hyperplasia in the thymus, including an increased number of germinal centers.

These observations, along with the more-than-chance association of myasthenia gravis with autoimmune diseases such as hyperthyroidism, lupus erythematosis, and rheumatoid arthritis, led to the speculation that the immune system is playing a role in the pathogenesis of myasthenia, a speculation that has been strongly supported by current experimental and clinical evidence.

Pathophysiology

Electromyographic (EMG) studies of patients with myasthenia and in vitro studies of muscle and nerve obtained by biopsy from these patients have both pointed to a disorder of the neuromuscular junction. These studies demonstrated normal electrical activity in the nerve and normal responses of the muscle to direct electrical stimulation. The EMG of involved muscle often shows a normal response to single stimuli, since in the rested state the end-plate potential, although small, is still large enough to produce activation of muscle. As indicated earlier, repetitive nerve stimulation rapidly reduces the number of quanta released by each impulse and thus reduces the safety factor for transmission. In the normal neuromuscular junction this does not produce a failure of transmission since the safety factor is normally several times larger than necessary. But the small end-plate potential of the myasthenic neuromuscular junction reduces the safety factor; with repetitive stimulation the end-plate potential falls below threshold for activation of postsynaptic muscle membrane. As transmission fails at individual neuromuscular junctions, the action potential recorded by an EMG electrode, which is the summed activity of many muscle fibers, is reduced in amplitude (Fig. 3–2). Prolonged repetitive stimulation or exercise produces a pronounced reduction in the size of end-plate potentials and EMG recorded responses from the muscle that is characteristic of myasthenia gravis and

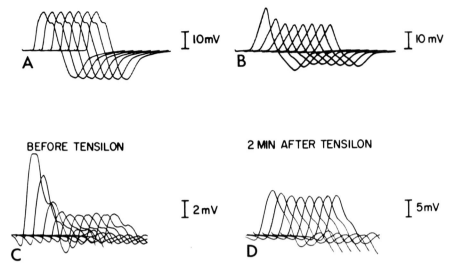

BEFORE TENSILON   2 MIN AFTER TENSILON

Fig. 3–2. Action potentials recorded with a surface EMG electrode from the abductor digiti minimi muscle during repetitive stimulation of the ulnar nerve at the rate of three per second. A. Normal; no change in the electrical response. B. 46-year-old male with myasthenia gravis. Stimuli at the same rate produce a 40% decrement of the electrical response. C. 19-year-old female with severe myasthenia gravis. There is a pronounced decrement in the response that is abolished (D) by the intravenous administration of a cholinesterase inhibitor, edrophonium (Tensilon). Note that the amplification was reduced for the recording in D. (From R. P. Lisak and R. L. Barchi, *Myasthenia Gravis*. Vol. 11 of *Major Problems in Neurology*. Philadelphia, Saunders, 1982.)

corresponds to the clinical phenomenon of weakness that follows exertion.

Studies of biopsy specimens from myasthenic patients have shown that miniature end-plate potentials occur with normal frequency, but with markedly decreased amplitudes. End-plate potentials elicited by nerve stimulation are smaller than normal, but contain the normal number of acetylcholine quanta. These observations led to the conclusion that transmitter-release mechanisms are normal, but that either the number of acetylcholine molecules in a packet is reduced, *or* the postsynaptic muscle membrane is less than normally responsive to transmitter. The former possibility would suggest a deficit in the synthesis or packaging of acetylcholine in the presynaptic terminal, whereas the latter might come about by a block of postsynaptic receptor sites or a

reduction in their number. Although the pendulum of opinion has swung back and forth over the years between presynaptic and postsynaptic localizations for the defect in myasthenia gravis, the evidence is now overwhelmingly in favor of a postsynaptic defect.

One of the major pieces of evidence that supported a presynaptic defect in myasthenia was the difficulty in demonstrating the physiological phenomenon of the disease by the experimental application of curare, which was known to block postsynaptic receptors. This problem was overcome by the demonstration that another agent that binds to and blocks receptors, (i.e., alpha-cobratoxin, derived from the venom of the cobra) is capable of reproducing many of the electrophysiological features characteristic of myasthenia. These include decremental responses to stimulation at a relatively slow rate (three per sec), markedly reduced end-plate potentials after prolonged repetitive stimulation (postactivation exhaustion), and reduced amplitude of miniature end-plate potentials. Further evidence for a postsynaptic defect in myasthenia came from electron microscopic studies of the myasthenic end-plate, which demonstrated a marked reduction in postsynaptic folds and a widening of the synaptic cleft (Fig. 3–3). Quantitative determinations with another snake-derived neurotoxin, alpha-bungarotoxin, labeled with horseradish peroxidase or radioactive iodine, demonstrated that the number of acetylcholine receptors in human myasthenic muscle is markedly reduced (Fig. 3–3). The reduction of the number of receptors, the widening of the synaptic cleft, and the distortion of the geometry of the postsynaptic membrane all make it less likely that a given molecule of acetylcholine will reach a receptor before it is destroyed by cholinesterase. The end-place potential is therefore smaller than normal, even though the amount of acetylcholine released from the presynaptic terminal is normal.

Pursuit of the prospect suggested by various clinical observations that myasthenia gravis is an immune disorder was greatly facilitated by the availability of relatively pure preparations of acetylcholine receptors from electric eels and rays, which have a large number of acetylcholine receptors in their electric organs. Inoculation of rabbits with purified receptors produces circulating antibodies to receptor protein and also produces a syndrome in the rabbit that resembles myasthenia gravis. The purified receptor preparations were then used to demonstrate that humans with myasthenia have circulating antibodies against acetylcholine receptors. In addition, immunoglobulins (IgG) from patients with myasthenia produce a myasthenic picture in mice that in many ways replicates the human syndrome. Such mice have the EMG findings typical of myas-

thenia and also have small miniature end-plate potentials and a reduced number of receptor sites in the endplate region.

Although the antibodies present in the serum of patients with myasthenia gravis bind to the receptor (Fig. 3–4), most do not bind to the acetylcholine binding site itself, but to an adjacent part of the receptor molecule. Thus the reduced responsiveness of the end-plate is not due to competition between the antibody and acetylcholine for receptor sites, but rather to a reduced number of receptors. At present, the best evidence indicates that the decrease in the number of receptors comes about because there is an antibody-mediated increase in the normal rate of receptor degradation, with no compensatory increase in receptor synthesis.

The percentage of patients with demonstrable antibodies to the acetylcholine receptor varies depending on the source of the receptor preparation used in the assay; 70%–90% of patients have demonstrable serum antibodies to the receptor when the preparation comes from mammalian muscle, but the percentrage is lower when the source is the eel. Only about 50% of patients whose disease is restricted to the eye muscle have demonstrable antibodies. There is no direct correlation between the level of serum antibody and the activity or severity of the disease, and no fully satisfactory explanation for the lack of correlation. Nor is it understood why 10%–30% of patients with systemic myasthenia have no detectable antibodies. But the most critical unanswered question in this disease, as in other autoimmune disorders, is why certain individuals develop antibodies to their own acetylcholine receptors.

Treatment

The treatment of myasthenia gravis is directed at both the altered synaptic physiology and the autoimmune disorder. Treatment of the disease involves choices among several drugs and procedures, and

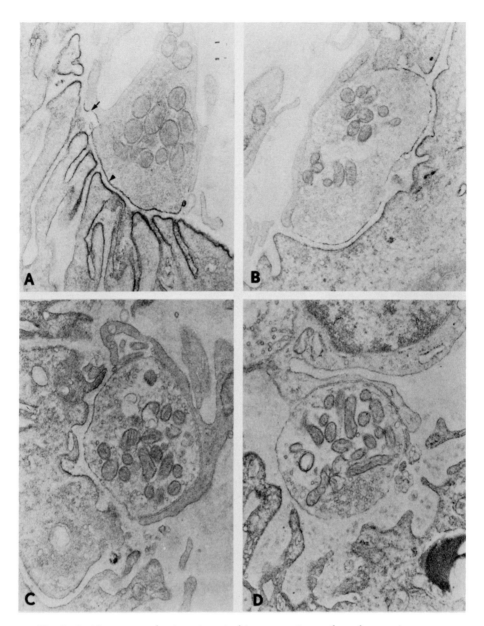

Fig. 3–3. Neuromuscular junctions in biopsy specimens from human intercostal muscles. **A.** Nonmyasthenic control. The presynaptic nerve ending contains numerous synaptic vesicles and mitochondria. The dark material on the crests of the postsynaptic folds indicates the acetylcholine receptors that have been tagged with alpha-bungarotoxin labeled with horseradish peroxidase. The presynaptic membrane (arrowhead) and Schwann cell membrane (arrow) adjacent to the synaptic cleft are faintly labeled with peroxidase, which is probably an artifact. **B, C,** and **D** are from patients with moderately severe myasthenia gravis. Acetylcholine receptors are markedly reduced in **B** and **C,** and absent in **D.** The synaptic cleft is widened and the postsynaptic folds are simplified in all three cases. (From A. G. Engel, J. M. Lindstrom, E. H. Lambert, and V. A. Lennon, Ultrastructural localization of the acetylcholine receptor in myasthenia gravis and in its experimental autoimmune model. *Neurology* 27:307–15, 1977)

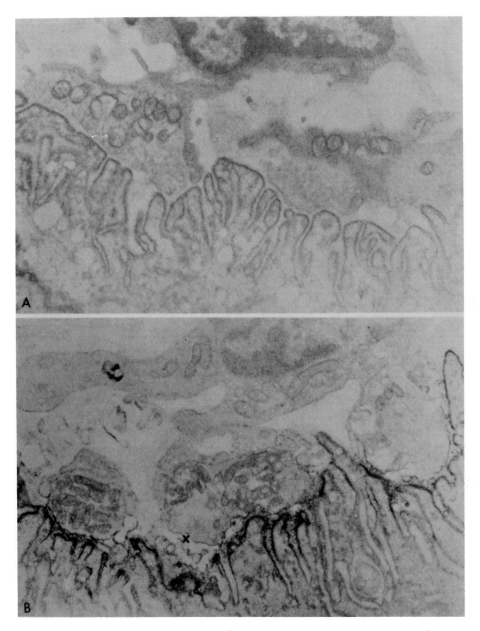

Fig. 3–4. Neuromuscular junctions from a nonmyasthenic control (**A**) and a patient with mild myasthenia gravis (**B**). The dark material on the crests of the postsynaptic folds in **B** marks the presence of antibodies (IgG) that have been stained with peroxidase-labeled staphylococcal protein A. The postsynaptic folds are intact except at X, where the synaptic space is widened and contains IgG deposits. No IgG deposits are present in **A**. [From A. G. Engel, E. H. Lambert, and F. M. Howard, Immune complexes (IgG and C3) at the motor end-plate in myasthenia gravis. *Mayo Clin. Proc.* 52:267–80, 1977.]

the choices must take into account such factors as the severity of illness, the patient's age, and the response to prior treatment. There is a great deal of diversity of opinion on these issues, which are beyond the purposes of this chapter. Although modern methods of therapy have greatly improved the outlook for patients with the disease, none provides a cure; most patients must continue to take some form of medication. We will consider each of the types of therapy briefly, concentrating on the relationship between the mode of action of the drug or procedure and the pathophysiology of the disease.

Cholinesterase inhibitors: As indicated earlier, inhibition of cholinesterase produces a larger and longer end-plate potential by making more of the acetylcholine release from the presynaptic terminal available to the reduced number of receptors and by prolonging its action. Depending on how severely the end-plate is affected by the disease, this enhancement of the abnormally small synaptic potential can produce a depolarization large enough to trigger an action potential in the muscle, and thus overcome the defect in synaptic transmission. This form of treatment attempts to circumvent the underlying reduction in the number of receptors rather than correct it, so that therapy often becomes less effective as the disease progresses. The drugs must be carefully regulated, since an excess of acetylcholine can produce desensitization block of the receptors, with resultant weakness *(cholinergic crisis)*. In addition, since the cholinesterarase at the neuromuscular junction does not appear to be significantly different from that at the other cholinergic synapses, the action of acetylcholine at the nicotinic cholinergic synapses of the autonomic ganglia and the muscarinic cholinergic synapses on smooth muscle will also be enhanced by cholinesterase inhibitors, producing troublesome side effects such as diarrhea and tachycardia.

The most effective cholinesterase inhibitors, pyridostigmine (Mestinon) and neostigmine (Prostigmin), bind reversibly to the esterase and are broken down relatively slowly. Edrophonium (Tensilon) has a very short duration of action and is therefore useful in making the diagnosis of myasthenia gravis by producing rapid improvement in obvious muscle weakness such as ptosis, or in the EMG-recorded responses to repetitive stimulation (Fig. 3–2). Although diplopia and ptosis are often markedly improved by edrophonium, they frequently respond poorly or not at all to oral cholinesterase inhibitors, especially in those cases where the disease is restricted to the eye muscles.

Corticosteroids: These have suppressive actions at many levels of the immune system and are commonly used in the treatment of myasthenia gravis. For reasons that are not yet clear, there is often some worsening of the disease in the first several days of therapy, sometimes severe enough to require tracheostomy and artificial respiration. Although a large number of patients eventually experience moderate to marked improvement, many require long-term daily or alternate-day therapy, with a significant incidence of steroid-induced side effects. Chronic administration of steroids produces a decrease in levels of serum antibodies to acetylcholine receptors, but since clinical improvement can occur at a time when there has been no significant decrease in antibodies, this cannot be the sole mode of steroid action.

Cytotoxic immunosuppressive drugs (azathioprine and cyclophosphamide): These agents have been used alone and in conjunction with steroids or plasmapheresis in some centers. They have been shown to produce decreased levels of antibodies to acetylcholine receptors and clinical improvement, but are not widely used because of their bone-marrow suppressive effects.

Plasmapheresis: This method was introduced relatively recently, so its role in the management of the disease is still evolving. It produces a reduction in the level of serum antibodies to receptors, along with clinical improvement, in many patients. Although the improvement may be dramatic, it is usually temporary unless the patient undergoes repeated courses of treatment. Plasmapheresis therefore has a role in the management of acute and subacute worsenings, but its usefulness in the long-term management of the disease is less clear.

Thymectomy: This procedure was instituted as a treatment for myasthenia gravis many years ago based on the observations of lymphoid hyperplasia and thymomas in the glands of patients with the disease. Although some controversy remains as to its efficacy, the best studies indicate a higher rate of improvement and remission in patients who underwent thymectomy compared to those who did not. Interestingly, there is now general agreement that although the operation is necessary in patients with thymoma to prevent the intrathoracic spread of the tumor, it does not alter the course of the myasthenia in these patients. It has not been clearly demonstrated that thymectomy reduces the levels of antibodies to acetylcholine receptors, although some studies indicate that it does. Thymectomy does not appear to have its effect by producing a state of generalized immunosuppression, or by removing a significant source of production of the antibody against the acetylcholine receptor. It may be effective because it alters some immunologic control mechanism that affects the production of antibodies to receptor, or because it eliminates a trigger to antibody production such as the antigens shared with muscle that the thymus contains. There is also some evidence that the thymus contains acetylcholine receptors, which could be acting as a trigger to the production of the antibodies that result in the clinical manifestations.

Drugs that adversely affect myas- *thenia gravis:* Several patients with myasthenia gravis were first diagnosed when they had a very prolonged recovery after the administration of drugs that block the acetylcholine receptors during surgery. These drugs include curare-like agents (gallamine and pancuronium) and those that produce depolarization block (succinylcholine). Myasthenics are also sensitive to the antibiotics that reduce the safety factor for neuromuscular transmission by decreasing the release of acetylcholine. These are primarily the aminoglycosides (colistin, polymyxin, streptomycin, kanamycin, gentamicin, neomycin, etc.) and in some instances bacitracin and the tetracyclines. These drugs should therefore be avoided except when the myasthenic patient has a severe infection that can only be treated by one of these agents, and the conditions are appropriate for very close observation. In addition, myasthenics are adversely affected by quinidine and procainamide, and the quinine in tonic water has also been reported to cause a worsening of symptoms. Penicillamine, which is used in the treatment of Wilson's disease and rheumatoid arthritis, occasionally produces myasthenia gravis, apparently by inducing the production of antibodies to the acetylcholine receptor rather than by a pharmacologic effect on the neuromuscular junction.

THE EATON-LAMBERT SYNDROME

The Eaton-Lambert syndrome, also known as the myasthenic syndrome or the pseudomyasthenic syndrome, resembles myasthenia gravis, but differs in several important ways. The clinical syndrome is characterized by muscle weakness that is seldom severe, affecting primarily the proximal limb musculature and the trunk. Involvement of the muscles of the eyes, face, and pharynx is much less common than in myasthenia gravis, but does occur and occasionally is the presenting manifestation. The weakness is "myasthenic" in the sense that it worsens with prolonged exercise, but careful testing will demonstrate an improvement in strength after brief exercise, another feature distinguishing it from myasthenia gravis. Since the cholinergic synapses of the autonomic system are also involved, dry mouth, blurred vision, impotence, and decreased sweating are frequent manifestations of the syndrome. Tendon reflexes are often diminished or absent.

The Eaton-Lambert syndrome occurs in two groups of patients. The largest group (70%–80%) has some type of malignancy, most commonly an oat-cell carcinoma of the lung. The syndrome may occur months before the malignancy is detected, and sometimes improves when the tumor is treated. Patients in the second group have no malignancy, but many have an associated autoimmune disorder such as rheumatoid arthritis, pernicious anemia, or thyroiditis. A large proportion of these patients have the major histocompatibility antigens HLA-B8 and DR3, and about half also have organ-specific gastric and/or thyroid autoantibodies. The first group contains a larger proportion of men, while the second group has more women and also includes some children.

Pathophysiology

As in myasthenia gravis, the neuromuscular junction was implicated as the site of the abnormality in the Eaton-Lambert syndrome when no abnormality could be found in the responses of the motor nerve or muscle to direct electrical stimulation. The EMG features that characterize this syndrome include small electrical responses from the muscle to single stimuli delivered to the nerve, and a marked *increase* in the response after the nerve is stimulated repetitively at about 50 per second. An increase in response amplitude can also be demonstrated after brief periods of voluntary contraction of the muscle (Fig. 3–5). Analysis of the neuromuscular junction in biopsy specimens from patients with the syndrome demonstrates that the postsynaptic membrane is normally responsive to acetylcholine and that miniature end-plate potentials are normal in amplitude. End-plate potentials evoked by single stimuli to the nerve are small, indicating that a reduced number of quanta are being released from the presynaptic terminal. Recent freeze-fracture electron microscopic observations of the end-plate region in biopsy specimens have demonstrated a disruption of the orderly arrangement of the release sites in the presynaptic active zones, with a reduction in the small particles that are thought to represent sites of exocytosis of transmitter.

The defect in transmitter release in the Eaton-Lambert syndrome is similar to that seen when the normal neuromuscular junction is subjected to reduced concentrations of extracellular calcium. Repetitive stimulation produces a rapid increase in the abnormal end-plate potential, presumably by producing the same facilitation seen in the normal neuromuscular junction. As indicated earlier, this facilitation is thought to be due to an accumulation of intracellular calcium in the presynaptic terminal, which facilitates transmitter release.

The occurrence of the Eaton-Lambert syndrome in patients with autoimmune diseases led to attempts to transfer the disorder passively to mice by repeated injections of IgG from patients with the syndrome. Although the mice did not become weak, the action potential elicited from their muscles by nerve stimulation was smaller than normal, and there was a decrease in the number of quanta released as determined by measurements of the end-plate potential at the neuromuscular junction. As in the patients, there was no reduction in the number of alpha-bungarotoxin binding sites.

Thus the current evidence indicates that there is a defect in the release of acetylcholine from the nerve terminals in the

Before Exercise   After Exercise

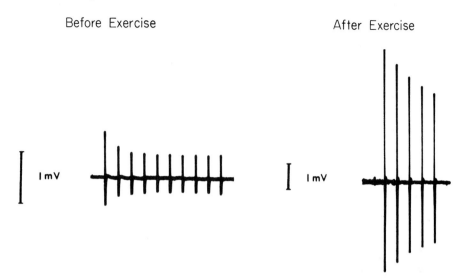

Fig. 3–5. Eaton-Lambert syndrome. Muscle action potentials recorded with an EMG electrode from the abductor digiti minimi muscle during repetitive stimulation of the ulnar nerve at the wrist at the rate of three per second. The record at the left was taken just before a maximum voluntary contraction of the muscle, and the record on the right was taken immediately after. The improvement after exercise is the characteristic finding in the Eaton-Lambert syndrome. [Modified from N. M. F. Murray and J. Newsom-Davis, Treatment with oral 4-aminopyridine in disorders of neuromuscular transmission. *Neurology* 31:265–71, 1981.]

Eaton-Lambert syndrome and suggests that there may be an IgG autoantibody to some component of the nerve terminal that is responsible. This hypothesis is supported by the observation that patients with the syndrome improve with immunosuppressive therapy (see next section). It has been suggested that those patients who have oat-cell carcinoma may be producing an antibody to some tumor antigen that cross-reacts with the nerve terminals. This hypothesis is supported by the fact that the oat cells are thought to be of neuroectodermal origin; they have many biochemical markers of neurons, and recordings from the cells in tissue culture indicate that they have voltage-dependent calcium channels. It is also possible that the tumor itself might be secreting a polypeptide that produces the abnormality in transmitter release, although most efforts to reproduce the syndrome by injecting tumor extracts have not been successful.

Treatment

Drugs that increase the safety factor for neuromuscular transmission have been used with varying degrees of success in patients with the Eaton-Lambert syndrome. Cholinesterase inhibitors are minimally effective. Guanidine and 4-aminopyridine, which increase the number of quanta released, are more effective but have a high rate of toxic side effects. Plasmapheresis does not produce the relatively rapid recovery that frequently occurs in myasthenia gravis, but it does produce some degree of improvement after 2–3 weeks of repeated administration. As in myasthenia, the improvement usually is not sustained unless the patient is also treated with immunosuppressive therapy. As indicated earlier, these observations have been taken as evidence for the presence of an autoantibody to some component of the presynaptic terminal involved in transmitter release. The delay in recovery with plasmapheresis suggests that the component involved has a relatively slow turnover rate.

BOTULISM

Poisoning by the exotoxin of *Clostridium botulinum* occurs infrequently, but it presents a very dramatic clinical picture that calls for rapid diagnosis and treatment. Botulism usually occurs as the result of eating home-canned foods that have not been properly sterilized prior to canning. Occasional cases also arise from clostridial wound infections. Botulism in infants between the ages of 1 and 38 weeks apparently results from toxin produced in the gastrointestinal tract. The toxin has not been recovered from food sources in these cases, but has been found in stool samples, along with the spores and organisms of *C. botulinum*.

The toxin is one of the most potent known; the dose fatal to humans has been estimated to be 0.05 mg. The toxin is relatively heat labile, and thus destroyed if the food is heated before ingestion. Seven immunologically distinct strains of *C. botulinum* have been identified; types A, B, and E are most frequently involved in human disease in the United States. The toxin is primarily absorbed in the stomach and upper small bowel, but toxin reaching the lower small bowel and colon may be slowly absorbed and account for the delayed onset and prolonged nature of symptoms in some patients.

The clinical syndrome of botulism varies from one that is mild and does not require medical attention to one that is extremely severe and leads to death in less than 24 hours. The syndrome usually begins within 12 to 36 hours after ingesting the toxin, but may be delayed for several days. The first symptoms are usually nausea and vomiting, with associated dryness of the mouth. Neurological manifestations often begin concurrently, but are sometimes delayed. Blurred vision and diplopia are early symptoms, the former as a result of the paralysis of the muscles of accommodation and the pupillary constrictors, and the latter as a result of involvement of extraocular muscles. Dilated, sluggishly reacting pupils are characteristic. As the paralysis extends, weakness of the face becomes evident, as does weakness of the tongue and pharynx, leading to dysarthria and dysphagia. These symptoms are often followed by weakness of the muscles of respiration and the proximal limb musculature. Abdominal distension with absent bowel sounds and urinary retention are also common manifestations. Respiratory failure, either as a result of upper airway obstruction or involvement of the respiratory musculature, may occur very quickly. Together with pulmonary infections, it is the principle cause of death from botulism.

Pathophysiology

Because of the availability of the pathogenic agent, botulism was one of the first diseases of neuromuscular transmission to be studied experimentally. *In vitro* studies demonstrated a failure of transmission at the neuromuscular junction, even though the nerve showed normal excitability and conduction, and the muscle also responded to direct electrical stimulation and contracted. The presynaptic terminal was implicated as the site of action of the toxin when it was shown that the postsynaptic membrane depolarized normally to iontophoretically applied acetylcholine. Since a presynaptic defect could involve an abnormality in transmitter synthesis, storage, or release, a great deal of effort has gone into attempts to determine which of these is the case. Most experimental evidence indicates that an abnormality in synthesis or storage of acetylcholine is not the primary effect of botulinum toxin, but that the abnormality is in transmitter release. Miniature end-plate potentials, the postsynaptic depolarizations that reflect the release of single quanta of acetylcholine, occur after poisoning of the neuromuscular junction with botulinum toxin, but are markedly reduced in frequency. The number of quanta released following the invasion of the nerve terminal by an action potential is also reduced, yielding postsynaptic potentials that are too small to reach threshold for an action potential in the muscle. Morphological evidence demonstrates decreased fusion of synaptic vesicles to the presynaptic membrane, a process that requires calcium. Calcium influx does not appear to be altered by the toxin, but the toxin does seem to decrease the sensitivity of the release mechanism to calcium ions, since the defect can be partially overcome by agents that increase calcium in the nerve terminal.

Treatment

The treatment of botulism is primarily directed at support of the patient and attempts to counteract the toxin. Respiratory failure is the common cause of death from botulism; tracheostomy and mechanical ventilation may well be necessary. When the clinical impression strongly favors botulism, antitoxin against types A, B, and E should be administered after appropriate skin tests for sensitivity are carried out. Cathartics and enemas are also administered in an attempt to eliminate unabsorbed toxin from the gut. Guanidine hydrochloride has been used as an adjunct to therapy because it promotes acetylcholine release. Its efficacy in botulism is not dramatic, however, and many cases do not respond significantly. Thus, once antitoxin has been administered, therapy consists mainly of intensive patient support during the many days or weeks that may be required for recovery.

GENERAL REFERENCES

Cherington, M. Botulism: Ten-year experience. *Arch. Neurol.* 30:432–37, 1974.

Drachman, D. B. The biology of myasthenia gravis. *Ann. Rev. Neurosci.* 4:195–226, 1981.

Engel, A. G., and G. Fumagalli. Mechanisms of acetylcholine receptor loss from the neuromuscular junction. In *Receptors, Antibodies and Disease*. Ciba Foundation Symposium 90. London, Pitman, 1982, pp. 197–224.

Grob, D. (ed.). Myasthenia gravis: pathophysiology and management. *Ann. N.Y. Acad. Sci.* 377:1–898, 1981.

Gunderson, C. B. The effects of botulinum toxin on the synthesis, storage and release of acetylcholine. *Prog. Neurobiol.* 14:99–119, 1980.

Gutman, L., and L. Pratt. Pathophysiologic aspects of human botulism. *Arch. Neuro.* 33:175–9, 1976.

Lambert, E. H., and D. Elmquist. Quantal components of end-plate potentials in the myasthenic syndrome. *Ann. N.Y. Acad. Sci.* 183:183–99, 1971.

Lang, B., J. Newsom-Davis, D. Way, A. Vincent, and N. Murray. Autoimmune aetiology for myasthenic (Eaton-Lambert) syndrome. *Lancet* 2:224–6, 1981.

Lennon, V. A., E. H. Lambert, S. Wittingham, and V. Fairbanks. Autoimmunity in the Lambert-Eaton myasthenic syndrome. *Muscle and Nerve* 5:521–5, 1982.

Lindstrom, J. M. Structure of the acetylcholine receptor and specificities of antibodies to it in myasthenia gravis. In *Receptors, Antibodies and Disease*. Ciba Foundation Symposium 90. London, Pitman, 1982, pp. 178–96.

Lisak, R. P., and R. L. Barchi. *Myasthenia Gravis*. Vol. 11 of *Major Problems in Neurology*. Philadelphia, Saunders, 1982.

4.

Muscle

JAMES E. CARROLL and MICHAEL H. BROOKE

PATHOPHYSIOLOGY OF MUSCLE

Muscle is the body's effector system; it is the only organ capable of mechanical work. Force is generated in muscle when the electrical signal in the muscle membrane activates a complex series of contractile proteins. The energy that muscle requires to do its work is generated by the metabolism of carbohydrates and fat. The processes of muscle membrane excitation, excitation-contraction coupling, force generation, and energy metabolism are the subjects of brief reviews in the first part of this chapter. The second part outlines the features of some of the major categories of muscle disease and relates these features to normal muscle function where such relationships are understood.

Muscle contraction

Excitation of the muscle membrane occurs after the nerve impulse travels along the peripheral nerve terminal to cause the release of acetylcholine. Acetylcholine diffuses across the synaptic cleft, binds to receptors on the postsynaptic side, and produces a depolarization that initiates an action potential in the muscle membrane

(Chap. 3). In the resting state, the intracellular potential of muscle, like that of nerve (Chap. 1), is negative with regard to the extracellular space because of differences in the concentration of sodium, potassium, and chloride ions on the two sides of the cell membrane. A sodium-potassium pump in the membrane maintains a high intracellular potassium concentration and pumps out the sodium that leaks into the cell. There are also large, nondiffusible anions that cannot pass out of the cell through the membrane. Chloride ions are in higher concentration outside the cell than inside. The movement of potassium and chloride ions along their concentration gradients (potassium outward and chloride inward) tends to leave the muscle with a net intracellular negative charge. If the large anions were diffusible, they would tend to diffuse outward and counteract this phenomenon. Similarly, but for the sodium-potassium pump, sodium would tend to diffuse into the cell and also eliminate the negative potential. When the membrane is depolarized, the sodium conductance increases, sodium moves into the cell, and the intracellular potential moves toward the equilibrium potential for so-

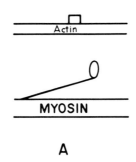

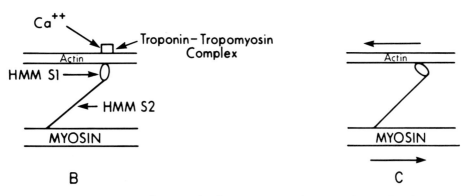

Fig. 4–1. A. In the absence of calcium, actin and myosin interaction is re-pressed by the troponin-tropomyosin complex. B. Calcium binding to troponin-tropomyosin complex allows binding of the HMM S_1 fragment to actin. C. The change in angles between myosin fragments applies the force for contraction.

dium. The action potential is terminated by the reduction in sodium conductance and the resurgence of potassium conduct-ance. The presence of a chloride "leak" into the cell also shunts the sodium cur-rents. Propagation of the action potential occurs at a conduction velocity of about 1 per second over the muscle surface. This electrical activity is transferred via the transverse tubules, or T system, into inter-nal portions of the muscle fibers. The im-pulse then connects with the sarcoplasmic reticulum, allowing release of calcium.

Muscle contraction (or shortening) occurs because of the interaction between actin and myosin, resulting in a forceful sliding action of the parallel filaments. Ac-tin comprises the thin filaments of skeletal muscle. It is composed of globular sub-units 80 Å in diameter, which are ar-ranged in a double helical structure. The molecular weight is 47,000. Myosin forms the thick filaments with a molecular weight of about 500,000 and a diameter of 150 Å. Myosin is composed of a double α-helix of two heavy chains and a three or four light chains. The heavy-chain fragments are known as heavy meromyosin (HMM) and the light-chain fragments as light mero-myosin (LMM). The globular portions (HMM S_1) of the protruding heavy chains contain the sites that combine with actin and hydrolyze ATP. The interaction of ac-tin and myosin results from their inherent affinity and does not require ATP. This natural affinity or interaction between ac-tin and myosin is controlled by the tro-ponin-tropomyosin system, which func-tions as repressor of the interaction of actin and myosin (Fig. 4–1). Tropomyosin is an

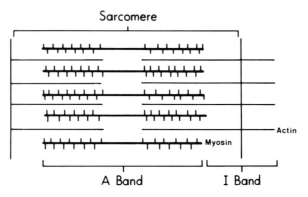

Fig. 4–2. Sarcomere with crossbridges unconnected.

α-helical protein of two polypeptide chains associated with actin. Troponin is anchored to tropomyosin. Tropomyosin mediates the Ca^{2+} message from troponin to actin. If the troponin-tropomyosin complex is present, actin is unable to combine with myosin, and the ATPase activity of myosin is not stimulated. When calcium is released from the sarcoplasmic reticulum and its concentration exceeds 10^{-6}M, the combination of actin and myosin is permitted by the binding of Ca^{2+} to troponin, with calcium acting as a derepressor of troponin. Myosin ATPase is thus activated for ATP hydrolysis.

The crossbridges between actin and myosin are arranged in a helical manner. The functional unit of contraction is the sarcomere (Fig. 4–2). Actin and myosin become cross-linked only on excitation, and the variation in sarcomere length is based on the degree of overlap of actin and myosin. The tension generated is proportional to the number of crossbridges thus formed. One molecule of ATP is split by myosin ATPase at each crossbridge per cycle. Hydrolysis of ATP results in dissociation of the link between actin and myosin, so that reattachment occurs at another site. Observations with electron microscopy and x-ray diffraction show that the polarity of the crossbridges is arranged so that all of the crossbridges in

half of the A band have the same polarity. The actin filaments in each half of a sarcomere are thus oriented to pull toward the center of the A band. As the sarcomere and I band shorten, the distance between actin and myosin increases, requiring the myosin attachment to be flexible. The actin connection is rigid. Therefore, a flexible hinge is required in myosin and the bending is thought to occur at two places: (1) the connection between the HMM S1 and S2 fragment, and (2) between the HMM S1 fragment and the LMM fragment. This allows the globular portion of the S1 fragment to attach over a wide range of angles. The driving force of contraction is the interaction between actin and the S1 portion of myosin. The change in the orientation of the attached bridges gives rise to the sliding force (Fig. 4–1).

Energy generation

Contracting muscle uses about 1 mmole of ATP per gram per minute. Only about 5 μmol are present per gram of muscle, supplying energy for less than 0.5 second of contraction. Therefore muscle requires a mechanism for rapid generation of ATP. It stores approximately four to six times as much phosphocreatine as ATP. Phosphocreatine provides a ready source of ATP in the presence of ADP, inorganic phosphate, and creatine kinase, yielding creatine plus ATP. But this amount of ATP and phosphocreatine can sustain activity for only a few seconds. The energy demands of muscle then must be met by carbohydrates and fat, and to a much lesser degree by amino acids. Most of the oxidative energy metabolism in resting muscle is supplied by fatty acid oxidation. The proportion of energy supplied by glycogenolysis and fatty acid oxidative metabolism during exercise is determined by the duration and intensity of exercise along with the fitness of the subject. During prolonged exercise, free fatty acids are mobilized by catecholamines, and the blood flow to muscle increases. These factors serve to increase the availability of fatty acids to muscle. Intramuscular triglycerides are also a source of fatty acids. Exercise of increasing duration utilizes increasing amounts of fatty acids as long as the intensity of exercise does not exceed 60%–70% of the individual's maximum capacity. In excess of that level, increasing amounts of glycogen are burned. Subjects who are trained for endurance exercise tend to rely more on fatty acids than those who are untrained. Shorter periods of exercise require a high proportion of carbohydrate substrates.

Glycogenolysis proceeds by the pathway shown in Figure 4–3. ATP is first formed when 1,3-diphosphoglycerate is converted to a 3-phosphoglycerate. Pyruvate that is eventually formed is either oxidized by pyruvate dehydrogenase and the Kreb's cycle or metabolized to lactate by lactate dehydrogenase.

Fatty acids supply energy by the pathway shown in Figure 4–4. Carnitine is required as a carrier for the fatty acid moiety across the mitochondrial membrane. Carnitine is not synthesized in muscle, and its uptake requires an active transport system. β-oxidation for saturated fatty acids begins with acyl CoA dehydrogenase. Unsaturated fatty acids utilize additional enzymes for oxidation. Oleic acid requires enoyl-CoA isomerase, and linoleic acid requires both the isomerase and 3-hydroxy fatty acyl-CoA epimerase.

The energy transformation occurring in the oxidative consumption of the various substrates results in the formation of large amounts of ATP. The process takes place through a series of electron transfers with oxygen being the final electron acceptor (Fig. 4–5).

Several types of laboratory evaluations are important in the assessment and categorization of muscle disease. These include electromyography, muscle biopsy with histological and histochemical examination, and exercise testing.

Electromyography

The motor unit of skeletal muscle is made up of all of the muscle fibers innervated by a single motor neuron. The summed electrical activity of the fibers that comprise a motor unit is recorded in the electromyogram (EMG) as the motor unit potential (Fig. 4–10A). The motor unit potential is defined by its shape, amplitude, and duration. The shape of the potential depends on the position of the electrode in relation to the action potentials that propagate along the muscle fibers. In normal muscle at rest, very little electrical activity can be detected. Insertion of the EMG needle results in brief activation of the muscle. As the subject gradually contracts the muscle under study with increasing force, more motor unit potentials begin to discharge since the tension generated by a muscle is proportional to the number of motor units activated. As the tension in the muscle is increased further, the resulting electrical activity becomes so complex that individual motor units can no longer be detected. This phenomenon as seen on the oscilloscope is referred to as an "interference pattern."

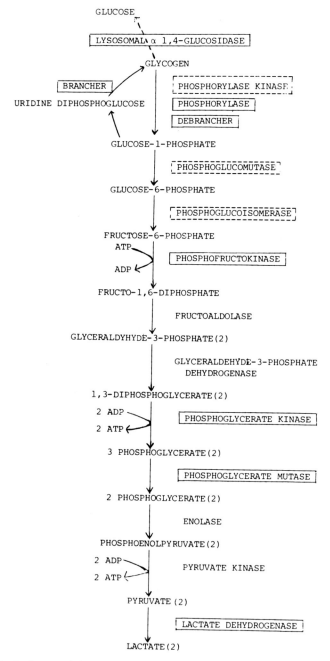

Fig. 4–3. Pathway of glycogen breakdown. Known enzymatic defects are noted in blocks, and less well documented defects are in dashed lines.

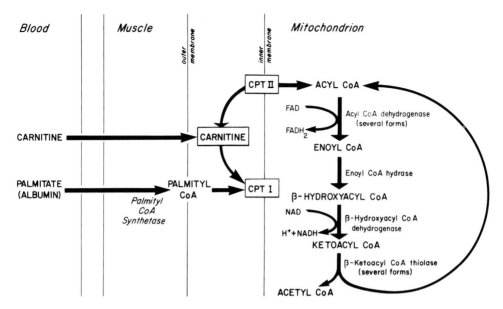

Fig. 4–4. Fatty acid entry into mitochondria and β-oxidation. Acyl-CoA dehydrogenase and β-ketoacyl-CoA thiolase probably have several isoenzymes. Known defects are noted in the blocks.

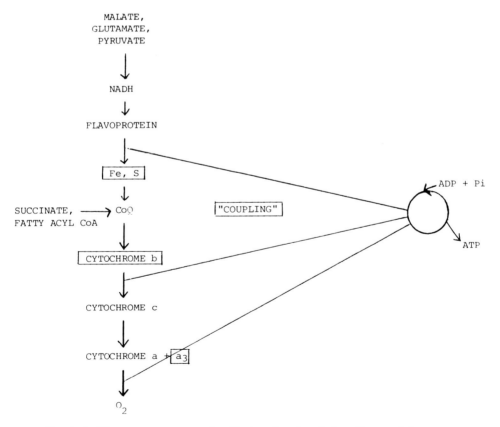

Fig. 4–5. Electron transport and oxidative phosphorylation. Known defects are in boxes. (Fe, S indicates nonheme iron sulfur centers)

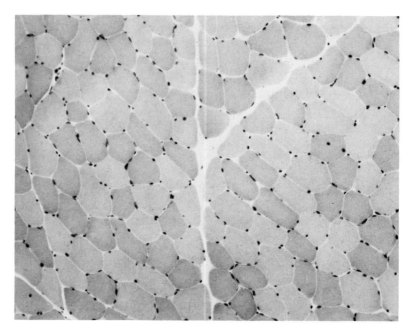

Fig. 4–6. Modified Gomori trichrome of normal muscle. All fibers are about the same size. Minimal connective tissue is present. ×138

Histochemistry

The examination of skeletal muscle obtained by muscle biopsy is usually carried out with a series of histochemical stains. The most common of these are the hematoxylin-eosin and trichrome stains, which are used for the morphological examination of structures in skeletal muscle, including the shape and size of the fibers, the nuclei, fibrous tissue, and the presence or absence of cellular infiltrates (Fig. 4–6). Other groups of stains are used for the assessment of oxidative enzyme activity. These stains, such as NADH-tetrazolium reductase and succinate dehydrogenase, stain more intensely, according to the activity of the oxidative enzyme systems present (Fig. 4–7). In addition, these stains allow evaluation of the structure of the network between the individual myofibrils. The ATPase reactions produce different intensities of staining for the various fiber types, depending on variations

in incubation pH. With these stains (Fig. 4–8), skeletal muscle fibers can be characterized as type 1 or type 2. Type 1 fibers are high in oxidative activity and low in glycolytic activity, whereas type 2 fibers are low in oxidative activity and high in glycolytic activity. Incubation of the ATPase stain at pH 4.6 results in the further differentiation of type 2 fibers into groups A and B. Type 2A fibers have greater oxidative activity than 2B fibers, whereas 2B fibers have greater glycolytic activity.

The correlation between histochemical fiber types and muscle contractile properties is not precise, but several generalizations may be helpful. Type 1 fibers (red) are slow-twitch fibers with a relatively high resistance to fatigue. Type 2 fibers (white) are fast-twitch fibers and have less resistance to fatigue. A single anterior horn cell supplies many muscle fibers of the same fiber type. Eye muscles characteristically have only 5–10 muscle fibers

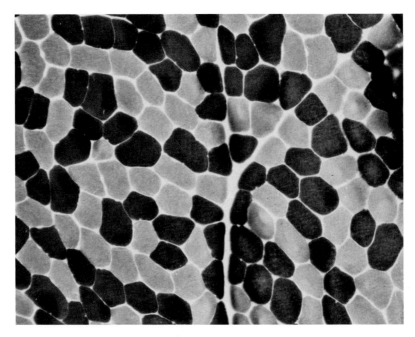

Fig. 4–7. NADH-tetrazolium reductase reaction of normal adult muscle. Fibers with greater oxidative activity stain more darkly. × 138

supplied by one anterior horn cell; larger postural muscle may have several hundred fibers innervated by a common axon. The muscle fibers innervated by an individual alpha motor neuron are either type 1 or type 2 fibers, not both.

Exercise testing

As mentioned earlier, the substrate utilized by muscle during exercise is determined in part by the kind of exercise. Exercise of high intensity relies more on the use of glycogen; longer exercise of submaximal intensity tends to rely more on fatty acid oxidation. Thus, various tests for the assessment of muscle energy and muscle substrate utilization are based on these physiologic principles. Forearm exercise of high intensity over a brief period is used to examine the breakdown of glycogen. Blood collected from the antecubital vein of the exercising forearm normally shows a marked rise in lactate. Although the ef-

fects of glycogenolysis are most easily observed under ischemic conditions, they are also evident without ischemia. Prolonged exercise (usually about 90 minutes) at submaximal intensity is performed with a bicycle ergometer to assess the subject's ability to oxidize fatty acids. The subject's maximal exercise capacity is determined by maximal ergometric testing. The importance of fatty acid oxidation can be enhanced by fasting the subject before the exercise test. During prolonged exercise blood fatty acids normally rise and are thus more available to skeletal muscle.

DISORDERS OF BRAIN, SPINAL CORD, AND PERIPHERAL NERVE

Diseases of the upper motor neuron (Chap. 9) usually do not affect skeletal muscle directly. The changes that do occur are consistent with disuse. Disuse from any cause, for example, lack of movement because of an upper motor neuron lesion or a restric-

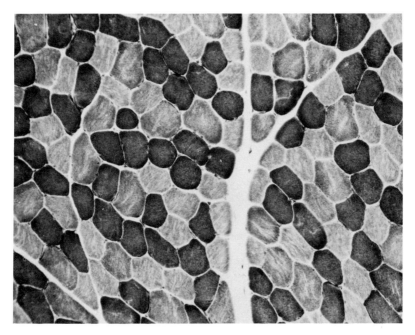

Fig. 4–8. pH 9.4 ATPase reaction of normal adult muscle. Type 1 fibers are light. × 138

tive device around the limb such as a cast, results in atrophy of type 2 muscle fibers. Stretch or contraction is the primary stimulus for incorporation of protein and the maintenance of muscle mass; muscle that fails to contract will atrophy and weaken. Since type 2 muscle fibers are thought to subserve voluntary movements, this may be the reason they are more subject to disuse atrophy.

Disorders of the anterior horn cell and peripheral nerve result in denervation of skeletal muscle. The histologic changes that occur in denervated muscle include atrophy of the affected fibers. Neighboring normal axons sprout to reinnervate denervated fibers, resulting in groups of fibers of the same histochemical type (Fig. 4–9). Electromyographic changes include fibrillations and fasciculations (Fig. 4–10 B, C) along with decreased numbers of motor units. Fasciculations are visible contractions of entire motor units that occur as a result of spontaneous discharges arising in the damaged motor neuron. The motor unit potentials may be increased in amplitude and duration because surviving motor units contain more muscle fibers than normal as a result of sprouting and reinnervation.

Cramps are a common disturbance of muscle, affecting all individuals at times. They consist of painful, involuntary contractions of muscle that may be induced by exertion or even minimal movements. They may also occur in some denervating diseases of muscle such as amyotrophic lateral sclerosis and peripheral neuropathies. Electromyography of a cramp shows that it is electrically active and that the activity is stopped by nerve blockade. The cause of cramps is essentially unknown.

DISEASES OF MUSCLE

Many disorders of skeletal muscle are thought to arise from a defect or a disease of the muscle itself rather than of its in-

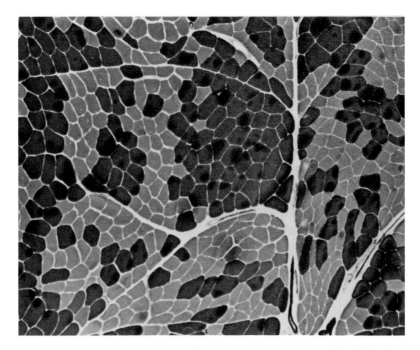

Fig. 4–9. pH 9.4 ATPase reaction showing type grouping, produced by denervation and reinnervation.

nervation. These can be classified on the basis of their clinical and pathological features. The major classes include disorders with myotonia, periodic paralyses, muscular dystrophies, congenital myopathies, inflammatory diseases of muscle, and diseases affecting muscle substrate utilization.

Disorders with myotonia

Myotonia is an involuntary contraction of muscle produced by mechanical stimulation of muscle or by a preceding voluntary contraction. The muscle also fails to relax in the usual manner. The excitability of the fibers is so altered that they tend to fire

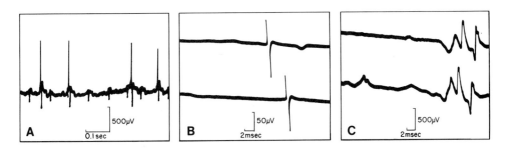

Fig. 4–10. A. Single motor unit action potentials. Normal amplitude ranges from 300 μV to 5 mV, and total duration from 3 to 16 msec. B. Fibrillation potentials. Duration ranges from 1 to 5 msec and amplitude from 20 to 300 μV. C. Fasciculation potentials. Wave may be diphasic, triphasic, or polyphasic. Duration and amplitude are in same ranges as single motor unit potentials. (Courtesy of Margaret H. Clare.)

repetitively to stimuli that are normally subthreshold. The involuntary contraction is not abolished by peripheral nerve section or curare, since the abnormality arises in the muscle itself. Myotonia occurs most commonly in myotonic dystrophy, but it is also present in myotonia congenita, paramyotonia, acid maltase deficiency, and debrancher deficiency. Myotonia can be reproduced experimentally by diazacholesterol and certain carboxylic acids.

All forms of myotonia share common electromyographic abnormalities. There are bursts of repetitive depolarization of the muscle membranes, which follow either a mechanical stimulus (such as the movement of an electromyographic needle) or voluntary contraction. The action potentials wax and wane in amplitude and frequency gradually diminishes. When this EMG pattern is reproduced through a loudspeaker, the sound is of a dive bomber or of a motorcycle engine being revved up. Although the electrical phenomena are similar in all forms of myotonia, the other findings may be quite different.

Myotonia can be produced experimentally with 20,25-diazacholesterol, which blocks endogenous synthesis of cholesterol by inhibiting $\Delta 2,4$-reductase. As a result, desmosterol accumulates in membranes. The substitution of desmosterol for cholesterol in the sarcolemmal membrane results in a decrease in membrane chloride conductance and thus in increased excitability and myotonia. The aromatic monocarboxylic acids (e.g., clofibrate) also produce myotonia by attaching to the chloride channel.

Myotonic dystrophy is an autosomal dominant disorder affecting many organ systems in addition to skeletal muscle. Patients with this illness often have cataracts, cardiac conduction defects, endocrine dysfunction, and mental retardation. In addition to the myotonia, there may also be considerable atrophy and weakness of the distal musculature. As the disorder slowly progresses, it also involves more proximal muscles. As muscles become weak, they lose myotonia. The disease is quite variable in severity; the examination of families with one severely involved member may disclose others who have not sought medical attention. The appearance of the patient with myotonic dystrophy is usually characteristic. In the male, there may be frontal balding and testicular atrophy. Atrophy of the temporalis and masseter muscles imparts a "hatchet-faced" appearance. Atrophy and weakness of the anterior neck muscles also occur early. As in other mytonic disorders, myotonia is elicited by firmly tapping the muscle belly. The specific defect is unknown, but electrochemical manifestations consist of reduced resting membrane potentials and increased membrane resistance due to decreased chloride conductance.

Myotonia congenita occurs in both autosomal dominant and autosomal recessive forms. It affects only skeletal muscle. The patients characteristically have bulky muscles and mild weakness. The myotonia and weakness may improve after a "warm-up" period. The autosomal recessive forms tend to be more severe with more weakness. Histology of skeletal muscle in these patients shows nearly complete absence of 2B fibers. The cause of this is unknown.

Myotnia congenita is thought to be due to a reduction in the resting membrane permeability to chloride. In this disorder, the resting membrane potential is not altered, so that depolarizations are required to initiate action potentials. Since there is a reduction in membrane conductance to chloride, the membrane is deprived of the normal chloride conductance, which helps to effect repolarization. Repolarization of the membrane occurs less effectively because the depolarization that occurs with each action potential as a result of increased sodium conductance can be counterbalanced only by an increased potassium conductance.

Paramyotonia congenita is characterized by marked worsening on exposure to cold and attacks of weakness with cold. In contrast to most other myotonias, the myotonia of paramyotonia worsens with exercise. It is also more frequently marked in the face, tongue, and bulbar muscles than are other types of myotonia.

Myotonia is also sometimes seen in the different varieties of periodic paralysis, but is most commonly encountered in the hyperkalemic form.

Periodic paralyses

Periodic paralysis is associated with abnormal shifts in muscle potassium. All the forms of periodic paralysis are either autosomal dominant diseases or sporadic in occurrence. It has been suggested that the electrical silence of the paralytic attack is associated with a continued fall in membrane potential and an eventual depolarizing block.

Hypokalemic periodic paralysis typically occurs on arising, frequently after consuming a high-carbohydrate meal the night before. This clinical observation is analogous to the provocative test for hypokalemic periodic paralysis, i.e., using insulin and glucose to drive potassium into the cell. This form usually first occurs at 7–10 years of age and may improve later in life.

Hyperkalemic periodic paralyaisis tends to cause attacks of shorter duration that frequently follow a rest period after exercise. In contrast to the hypokalemic form, attacks may sometimes be prevented by high-carbohydrate meals. Myotonia frequently occurs in this disorder. A decreased resting membrane potential has been found both during and between attacks. The onset may be in infancy. A normokalemic form may also exist.

Muscular dystrophies

Duchenne muscular dystrophy is an X-linked recessive disorder of relatively homogeneous clinical expression. In most cases no abnormality is apparent during the first year of life, but as the children begin walking they develop a waddle. Affected boys usually begin to show signs of weakness at about 3–4 years of age. The typical clinical picture includes proximal muscle weakness and hypertrophy of proximal muscles. This weakness is progressive, so that most patients become unable to walk by 8 to 12 years of age. Once the patient becomes confined to a wheelchair, he often develops progressive kyphoscoliosis and contractures of the joints. Though current methods of care, including bracing and improved care for respiratory infections, have improved longevity, death usually occurs from respiratory failure between 18 and 24 years of age.

Three abnormal laboratory findings are helpful in making the diagnosis. Creatine kinase is enormously elevated in patients with Duchenne dystrophy. This elevation is thought to result from leakage of the muscle enzyme through abnormal "holes" in the sarcolemmal membrane. The EMG shows an early interference pattern and small, brief, polyphasic potentials. The full interference pattern occurs early because more units must be recruited to accomplish a minimal amount of work. Although the number of motor units is probably normal, each individual unit contains many "sick" fibers. Consequently, more units must be used for any given task; hence the "early" interference pattern. The large number of "sick" fibers are thought to be responsible for the brief, small, polyphasic potentials. As more and more of the fibers deteriorate, the amplitude of the action potential is reduced, the duration becomes shorter, and the smooth contours of the motor unit potential degenerate to a jagged, polyphasic (four or more phases) pattern. The muscle biopsy demonstrates degenerating fibers, excessive fibrosis, variation in fiber size, and numerous hypercontracted fibers (Fig. 4-11).

Many theories have been advanced as to the cause of this disorder. It has been suggested that the disease is caused by de-

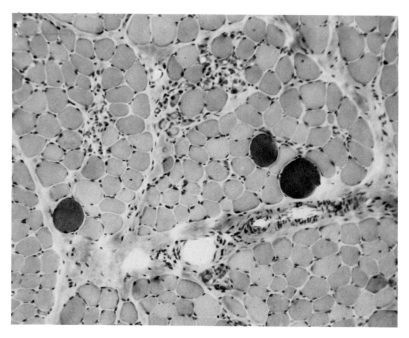

Fig. 4–11. Modified Gomori trichrome stain from patient with Duchenne muscular dystrophy. Some fibers are undergoing necrosis. Three hypercontracted fibers are shown. Connective tissue is increased. ×138

fective or altered innervation of the muscle, or by decreased blood flow to the muscle. Both of these hypotheses seem unlikely at the present time. The defect is currently thought to lie in the muscle membrane, but the genesis of this defect is unknown. This notion has arisen because of excessive amounts of creatine kinase that appear to leak into the blood, along with the observation of apparent structural defects in the muscle membrane. However, this abnormality has not been reproduced in cultured Duchenne muscle. The most widely confirmed defect has been dysfunction of the sarcoplasmic reticulum; isolated sarcoplasmic reticulum from Duchenne patients has shown defective calcium accumulation. Many groups have attempted to demonstrate a generalized abnormality of membranes using the red blood cell as a model. However, most of these studies are matched by studies of the same function from other groups that show no abnormality.

Limb girdle dystrophy is a term applied to a number of disorders that are usually first noted in adolescence or early adulthood. The patients present with proximal muscle weakness that is slowly progressive. They frequently complain of difficulty in arising from a chair, going up stairs, and in getting out of a car. The predominant symptoms are those of muscle weakness, the legs often being more severely involved than the shoulders. Previously, many different diseases were considered in this group. As specific etiologies are uncovered, this group is being whittled down to a remaining disease (or perhaps still a group of diseases) with muscle biopsies that show the usual signs of dystrophy. These consist of degenerating fibers with internal nuclei, fibrosis, and many fibers undergoing splitting. There is more disruption of the intermyofibrillar network than in Duchenne dystrophy. The EMG findings are similar to those in Duchenne dystrophy. Creatine kinase is usually quite elevated, but not so much as in Duchenne dystrophy.

Facioscapulohumeral dystrophy is usually inherited as an autosomal dominant disorder. The course of the disease is quite variable; some individuals are severely affected whereas others have barely detectable signs. Characteristically the disease affects the muscles of the face, shoulders, and upper arms. Other muscles, such as the anterior tibial group, may also be affected. If the disease progresses, the more proximal muscles become weak. Usually the disorder begins early in adult life and is so slowly progressive that it does not shorten life. A form of the disorder may present in infancy with hearing loss, retinal abnormalities, and more severe weakness. EMG findings are those of a dystrophy, though not as marked. Creatine kinase elevations are often mild. Muscle biopsy findings range from minimal abnormalities to more obvious changes that include hypertrophic type 2 fibers, fibrosis, and inflammation.

Congenital myopathies

Structurally specific congenital myopathies begin in infancy. Much of the literature on the subject refers to these infants as "the floppy child." The weakness is usually not as severe as that seen in many other neuromuscular disorders such as the spinal muscular atrophies. The progress of the disease is generally rather slow. Categorization of the disorders is based on the unusual structural features seen in muscle biopsies. The best known of these disorders are *central core disease* and *nemaline myopathy.* In central core disease, there are central regions within the muscle fibers that are abnormal, although the peripheral portions of the fibers remain normal. The abnormality usually consists of an absence of mitochondria in the central portions of the fiber. The central regions of the fibers do not take up oxidative enzyme stains. In nemaline myopathy, there are numerous rod-like bodies that are thought to consist of α-actinin, a myofibrillar protein.

There are other disorders that probably fall into this category of congenital myopathies, but in which characteristic structural features are not evident. These children tend to have a predominance of type 1 fibers on muscle biopsy and a rather mild clinical course.

Inflammatory diseases of muscle

Like any other tissue, muscle can demonstrate inflammation from a variety of infectious processes. However, most inflammatory diseases affecting muscle are probably autoimmune. These include *dermatomyositis,* which involves skin along with muscle, and *polymyositis,* which primarily affects muscle alone. Autoimmune disorders such as lupus erythematosis and other collagen-vascular disorders may also secondarily affect muscle.

Inflammatory diseases of muscle occur sporadically. Dermatomyositis is the characteristic form in childhood. Symptoms include irritability, low-grade fever, an erythematous rash that covers the face and extensor surfaces of the limbs, and progressive proximal weakness. Polymyositis is the more common form in the adult, although skin involvement may also occur. The onset of the disease is usually insidious, but may on occasion be much more rapid. Muscle pain occurs in about half of the patients, but this is not necessary for the diagnosis. Facial and bulbar muscles are usually not involved, although swallowing problems are common.

The EMG shows signs of muscle irritability with fibrillations and spontaneous, high-frequency discharges. There may also be brief, small action potentials, as are seen in other myopathies. The creatine kinase is often elevated. The muscle biopsy may show a perivascular inflammatory response. The most characteristic finding is atrophy around the periphery of the muscle fascicles, referred to as perifascicular atrophy. This is most commonly seen in dermatomyositis and is thought to be related to a reduction in blood flow to these areas of the muscle.

Most evidence suggests that myositis is secondary to an abnormality of the immune system, attacking muscle and its blood vessels. Blood flow, as measured by isotopic techniques, is reduced in the abnormal muscle, confirming the involvement of the blood vessels. As noted earlier, many patients with myositis have an associated collagen-vascular disorder. Muscle antibodies have been detected in patients with myositis, but they are not specific since they are sometimes seen in normal controls as well. An animal model of the disease has been produced by injecting a muscle extract in conjunction with Freund's adjuvant. In this model, the disease was transferred to other animals by infusion of washed lymphocytes. Lymphocytes from patients with polymyositis have been shown to be toxic to muscle; the degree of this toxicity may parallel the activity of the disease. Other investigators have suggested that humoral factors may be responsible for the muscle damage. It is not known what initiates the autoimmune reaction. Perhaps the immune system represents a final common pathway for a number of inducing factors, ranging from viral infections to autosensitization.

DISORDERS OF ENERGY SUPPLY

Glycogen utilization disorders

Knowledge about the diseases caused by defects in energy utilization is increasing rapidly. Disorders of glycogen utilization segregate into two different clinical syndromes. The first category conforms to the pattern of the most typical of these disorders, *McArdle's disease* or *muscle phosphorylase deficiency*. These patients experience pain and contractures after brief,

strenuous exercise. Following exercise, the muscle becomes contracted, hard, and painful, and the EMG is electrically silent. Later in life, progressive muscular weakness may occur, particularly involving the proximal muscles. Patients with this disorder usually modify their lives to avoid exercise. The symptoms occur because the muscles are not able to utilize gylcogen as an energy substrate. Sometimes the phenomenon of "second wind" is prominent in patients with McArdle's disease. This occurs if the patient slows down or rests for a while at the onset of fatigue and then immediately starts exercising again. He is then often able to continue with the exercise for long periods of time. The recovery is thought to be due to increased blood flow to the muscle with increased mobilization of free fatty acids. These fatty acids provide an alternate energy source for the production of ATP, bypassing the glycolytic pathway. When the forearm is exercised and blood collected from the antecubital vein, blood lactate does not rise in these patients as it does in normal individuals. These patients may also develop myogloburinuria, another symptom of an energy crisis in muscle. Other defects with a similar clinical syndrome include those of *phosphofructokinase, phosphoglycerate kinase, phosphoglycerate mutase,* and *lactate dehydrogenase* (Fig. 4–3).

The second category of glycogen breakdown diseases exhibits proximal weakness as the dominant symptom. *Acid maltase deficiency (α1,4-glucosidase deficiency)* (Fig. 4–3) results in the accumulation of membrane-bound glycogen and vacuolar myopathy. This pathway functions peripherally to the main flow of glycogen to pyruvate. Excessive amounts of glycogen are stored in lysosomes, which rupture, spilling hydrolytic enzymes into the muscle cytosol. Patients with this disorder experience progressive weakness with loss of muscle mass. Acid maltase deficiency may arise at any age, but is more common in infancy, when it affects skeletal muscle, heart, and liver (Pompe's disease). A similar disease may also occur in older children or even in adults. In this form only skeletal muscle is affected, and the clinical picture resembles muscular dystrophy.

Debrancher enzyme deficiency (Fig. 4–3), said to be one of the more common glycogen storage diseases, also results in slowly progressive proximal muscle weakness and vacuolar myopathy. Liver dysfunction dominates the clinical picture early in life, while weakness may develop in adults. Blood lactate does not rise after ischemic exercise. Exercise intolerance and cramps are usually not significant symptoms.

Although the typical form of phosphorylase deficiency presents with muscle pain and myoglobinuria, an infantile form is now known with severe, progressive proximal weakness. The condition resembles spinal muscle atrophy clinically. The phosphorylase protein appeared to be absent in one patient.

Brancher deficiency (Fig. 4–3) is usually manifested by severe liver dysfunction in infancy. The patients may also have hypotonia and weakness. Polysaccharides with longer outer chains and few branching points accumulate in tissue.

Lipid utilization disorders

Diseases of lipid utilization have thus far not been as well characterized as the glycogen utilization diseases. Since the original descriptions of carnitine deficiency and carnitine palmityl transferase (CPT) deficiency in 1973, no other specific deficiency diseases have been described in this pathway. Although these defects are contiguous in the metabolic pathway (Fig. 4–4), they have very different manifestations. *Carnitine deficiency* results in lipid storage (Fig. 4–12) and proximal weakness in the form in which the defect is restricted to skeletal muscle. In subjects with generalized carnitine deficiency, other organs such as liver and heart may be affected. These patients may experience episodes of metabolic encephalopathy with acidosis and hypoglycemia and often die prematurely. The best evidence regarding the cause of carnitine deficiency indicates that the tissue either fails to take up or to hold the carnitine in a normal fashion. Earlier suggestions that a generalized form of the disease results from a failure of synthesis of carnitine have thus far not been proven. In addition, more and more patients with carnitine deficiency arising from other causes are being discovered. These causes include exclusive intake of soy formula in infants (a diet deficient in carnitine), renal dialysis, and malnutrition with liver disease. Although adults normally synthesize carnitine from lysine and methionine, infants may not have this capacity. In patients with "secondary" carnitine deficiency, the clinical picture is usually less distinctive.

CPT deficiency, on the other hand, is characterized by well-preserved strength and difficulty only after prolonged exercise. These patients are more homogeneous clinically; muscle biopsies are frequently histologically normal.

There are other diseases that result in lipid storage, but for the most part the biochemistry of these disorders is undefined. Since patients with CPT deficiency frequently do not have excessive lipid storage in muscle, the possibility remains that other diseases of lipid utilization may likewise exist without lipid storage.

Mitochondrial disorders

Disorders of mitochondrial function also result in myopathy. These are a heterogeneous group of disorders and their classification is still uncertain. Patients with these diseases may have severely decreased exercise tolerance with lactic acidemia on exercise. Because the mitochondria are abnormal in many tissues in addition to skeletal muscle, they may suffer from a

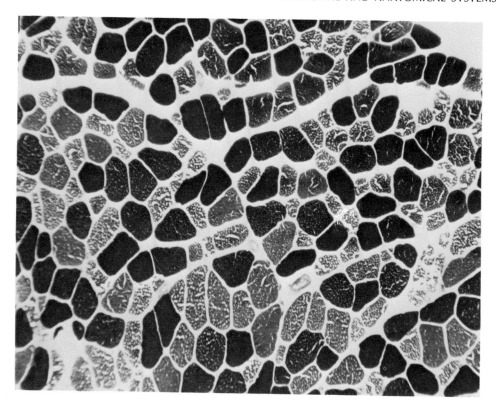

Fig. 4–12. pH 9.4 ATPase stain from patient with muscle carnitine deficiency. Holes in type 1 fibers (light) are filled with lipid. ×125

variety of problems, including small stature, encephalopathy, and cardiac malfunction. This group of diseases originally came to light with the observation of structurally abnormal mitochondria in muscle, sometimes seen as the "ragged red fiber" by light microscopy of muscle stained with the trichrome stain. Perhaps the main reason these disorders are so poorly understood is that the respiratory chain in skeletal muscle is difficult to study. Preparation of mitochondria for polarographic studies requires comparatively large amounts of muscle, and few laboratories have adequate samples from pathologic material. Very few of the described defects have been demonstrated by more than one laboratory.

The prototype of the mitochondrial myopathies is *Luft's syndrome,* characterized by loosely coupled oxidative phosphorylation. The few patients with this condition who have been described have increased oxygen utilization at rest. They also have the other features of hypermetabolism, including increased caloric intake and heat intolerance. Although loose coupling is frequently mentioned in patients with mitochondrial abnormalities, this term is often used inappropriately. Its use should be restricted to patients who have increased oxygen consumption at rest, which is defined in polarographic studies as increased oxygen consumption in the absence of ADP.

Other disorders in the group of mitochondrial myopathies have been demonstrated. These affect the loci shown in Figure 4–5. In contrast to Luft's syndrome, patients with these disorders demonstrate exercise intolerance but not hypermetabolism.

Provocative studies of disorders of muscle energy supply may help elucidate the various categories of these diseases. Forearm exercise studies are designed to pick out those conditions in which there is failure in the breakdown of glycogen to lactate. The absence of a rise in serum lactate points to a glycogen storage or utilization disease. Prolonged exercise is used to make defects of fatty acid oxidation more obvious. This occurs since the normal response to prolonged exercise is to rely more on fatty acids as the duration of exercise increases. Patients with this group of disorders often have abnormalities with prolonged exercise including excessive fatigue, pain, and increased elevation of myoglobin and creatine kinase. Fasting also stresses patients who have defects in fatty acid utilization, since during fasting fatty acids normally rise while glycogen is depleted. If a subject is unable to use fatty acids, then an energy crisis arises that produces muscle pain near the end of the fast. Other abnormalities that have been described include increased elevation of fatty acids, abnormalities in ketone bodies, and low blood glucose. Subjects with mitochondrial myopathies or respiratory chain defects develop extremely elevated blood lactate concentrations with bicycle exercise. Tests such as these can be used to detect patients with poorly understood defects who should be studied further.

GENERAL REFERENCES

Brooke, M. H., and K. K. Kaiser. Muscle fiber types. How many and what kind? *Arch. Neurol.* 23:369–79, 1970.

DiMauro, S. Metabolic myopathies. In *Handbook of Clinical Neurology*, vol. 4, P. J. Vinken and G. W. Bruyn (eds.). Amsterdam, North Holland, 1978, pp. 175–235.

Dubowitz, V., and M. H. Brooke. *Muscle biopsy: A modern approach.* Saunders, London, 1973.

Goldberg, A. L., and H. M. Goodman. Effects of disuse and denervation on amino acid transport by skeletal muscle. *Am. J. Physiol.* 216:1116–19, 1969.

Huxley, H. E. The mechanism of muscular contraction. *Science* 164:1356–66, 1969.

Layzer, R. B., and L. P. Rowland. Cramps. *New Eng. J. Med.* 285:31–40, 1971.

Lipicky, R. J., J. H. Bryant, and J. H. Salmon. Cable parameters, sodium, potassium, chloride, and water content, and potassium efflux in isolated external intercostal muscle of normal volunteers and patents with myotonic congenita. *J. Clin. Invest.* 50:2091–103, 1971.

Munsat, T. L., and R. T. Scheife. Myotonia. In *Clinical Neuropharmacology*, vol. 4, H. L. Klawans (ed.). New York, Raven Press, 1979, pp. 83–107.

Rowland, L. P. Biochemistry of muscle membranes in Duchenne muscular dystrophy. *Muscle and Nerve* 3:3–20, 1980.

Walton, J. N. (ed.). *Disorders of voluntary muscle.* Edinburgh, Churchill Livingston, 1974.

5.

The Somatosensory System and Pain

DAVID B. CLIFFORD

A primary goal of physicians is to relieve pain and suffering. Despite the importance of this objective, until recently our understanding of the mechanisms of pain was rudimentary. In the last 20 years, however, experimental investigations have provided a wealth of new information on the anatomy and synaptic pharmacology of pain, affording new insight into puzzling clinical features and suggesting new avenues for the treatment of pain.

SOMATOSENSORY SYSTEMS

Survival demands that organisms be able to sense and interact in a meaningful way with their environment. Sampling of the environment is done in many ways, which constistute sensory experiences. The brain must transform sensory phenomena to neural activity that reliably transmits the information of importance.

The principal sensory modalities are sight, sound, smell, taste, and touch. Somatic sensation includes touch-pressure sensation, position sense and sense of movement, temperature, and pain. Pain, or nociception, is the submodality of somatic sensation that we will consider in

greatest detail. However, many of the general concepts of sensory processing apply equally to pain and to other sensations since all sensory systems must be able to detect events, determine their characteristics, and localize and quantify them.

Afferent pain systems

All sensory stimulation must first be transformed into neural events, or action potentials. The process by which this is accomplished is called transduction. During transduction sensory stimulation triggers changes in the properties of neuronal membranes that lead to a generator potential. If the generator potential reaches a certain threshold, it initiates action potentials in the nerve endings. Receptors have developed that achieve transduction of *specific* modalities to neural impulses. The eye is a dramatic example of specialization, in which transduction of photic energy to neural information is performed by photoreceptors, aided by a vast neural system for orienting the eye, focusing, controlling the amount of illumination, and interpreting the patterns sensed. In the somatosensory system various specializations have evolved for interpretation of sensory events for the brain. Muscle and tendon stretch are measured by muscle spindles and Golgi tendon organs. Merkle cells in the skin seem to play a role in fine touch. Various encapsulated nerve endings including Pacinian corpuscles, Meissner corpuscles, and Krause end bulbs play a part in reception of vibration, fine touch, and pressure, respectively.

Nociception is associated with free nerve endings, the anatomy and physiology of which are incompletely understood. It is clear that even in these free nerve endings there is a degree of specialization. There are at least three different types of nociceptors. Mechanical nociceptors are most effectively stimulated by sharp objects, though mechanical stimulation sufficient to threaten tissue damage will also cause them to fire. Heat nociceptors are activated by elevation of the temperature above 45° C, a temperature that causes tissue damage if applied over prolonged periods. Mixed or polymodal nociceptors are less specific and respond to any modality of stimulus that threatens to damage tissue.

Electrophysiologic analysis indicates that free nerve endings have differential sensitivity to mechanical, thermal, or chemical stimuli. In some free nerve endings, deformation of the nerve membrane causes a generator potential. In others, the mechanisms that control conductance of the membrane are markedly temperature sensitive. Still other free nerve endings respond primarily to local chemicals such as bradykinin, prostaglandins, serotonin, substance P, or even elevated potassium concentrations. These chemical stimuli cause a generator potential and, eventually, action potentials in the afferent primary neurons. Sometimes several of these systems work synergistically, increasing the likelihood that the generation potential will reach threshold for action potential generation.

Peripheral nerves are bundles of axons of various sizes, the larger and more heavily myelinated conducting much faster than the small unmyelinated fiber (see Chap. 1). Conduction velocities of cutaneous nerve fibers range from less than 2.5 m per second to about 100 m per second. There are three to five times as many small axons as large ones in cutaneous nerves, so most of the fibers have relatively slow conduction velocities. Many of the specialized structures of sensation, such as the Pacinian corpuscles, are associated with large fibers whereas nociception and temperature sensation are primarily associated with unmyelinated (C fibers) and sparsely myelinated (A-delta) fibers.

Small myelinated and unmyelinated nerves are involved with the sensation of pain, which has both fast and slow components. Fast pain is a rather well localized, brief, and often sharp sensation that is carried by the faster conducting A-delta fibers. Slow pain consists of the prolonged, diffuse, poorly localized sickening sensation that is carried by the slower conducting C-fiber system. This type of pain often signifies tissue damage and implies a more serious clinical problem than that associated with sharp, well-localized pain.

Once an action potential is generated in the afferent primary neuron the interpretation of the stimulus by the brain will be substantially defined by the modality specificity of that neuron. This concept is referred to as a labeled line code. An example of this general concept of somatosensory physiology is the experience of paradoxical cold. There are discrete patches of skin innervated by free nerve endings that discharge with punctate cold stimuli. However, painful hot stimuli nonspecifically cause activity in these same fibers. The interpretation of the noxious hot stimulus is a cold sensation when it is applied focally to a cold receptor.

Since action potentials are all-or-none events, other means must be provided to indicate the intensity of the stimulus. This is done in at least two ways. As the magnitude of the stimulus increases, the rate of firing increases and the population of neurons brought to threshold increases. Thus, increasing intensity is encoded for the brain by the frequency of firing and size of the receptor population that responds to the stimulus. A large stimulus will result in rapid firing of a large population of nociceptive neurons.

Localization of the stimulus is made possible by precise mapping of the body in the brain. Stimulation of the surface area that activates an afferent fiber defines that fiber's receptive field. Thus, activity within a specific afferent indicates not only the kind of sensory stimulus but also the location on the body surface. In areas where very precise localization is important, such as the finger tips, receptive fields are very small, providing precise localization. Where exact localization is of little advantage (such as on the back) the receptive fields are large. Sensory afferents are grouped by receptive field, and a type of isotopic representation of the body surface is maintained in all somatosensory relays up to and including cortex. By contrast, receptive fields are poorly maintained in the nociceptive system. Often the localization of pain depends on activity in parallel systems such as touch or pressure to assist in localization. The diffuse nature of localization of pain explains why this sensation often extends far beyond an actual trauma zone.

Afferent somatosensory information is transmitted rostrally by two major systems (Fig. 5–1). The larger A-beta (Aβ) fibers have direct projections into the dorsal part of the cord forming the dorsal columns. These carry the sensations of touch-pressure, vibration, and position sense-kinesthesia ipsilaterally to the lower medulla, where they synapse in dorsal column nuclei. Projections from here cross to the contralateral side forming the medial lemniscus, which ascends to the ventral posterior thalamus. This system is called the dorsal column-medial lemniscal system. The other major afferent system is the anterolateral or spinothalamic system, which transmits pain, thermal, and crude touch sensations. This system is often subdivided into neospinothalamic and paleospinothalamic. Both of these pathways consist of second-order neurons, resulting from synapses of primary afferents in the dorsal horn of the spinal cord. The former provides more direct afferents to thalamus, while the latter consists of diffuse afferents to brainstem.

The dorsal horn of the spinal cord can be divided into six anatomically distinct layers (Fig. 5–2). It is now evident that there is functional significance to these divisions and that there is considerable modification of the afferent information by the dorsal horn interactions. The superficial layer (lamina I) contains marginal cells that contribute to the contralateral anterolateral tract, which projects directly to thalamus. "Fast pain," which is relatively well localized, may result from activity of this system. The majority of the anterolateral system is a paleospinothalamic system that has its origin in the nucleus proprius (lamina V) and responds to stimuli of all the cutaneous afferent types. These neurons project to the reticular substance of the brainstem and to the thalamus. It is believed that these fibers are important in poorly localized, chronic pain. It is important to realize that most of the anterolateral tract projections are to the brainstem rather than to the thalamus, as the term *spinothalamic* would suggest. Though the projections to brainstem include numerous regions, one of particular importance is the periaqueductal gray matter. This in turn has reciprocal projections with the periventricular region, hypothalamus, and the limbic system. This area would seem to be a nodal area for interaction of emotional, behavioral, and autonomic responses to pain (see Chap. 10).

The thalamic terminations of the nociceptive pathways are segregated for the neospinothalamic and paleospinothalamic tracts. Neospinothalamic termina-

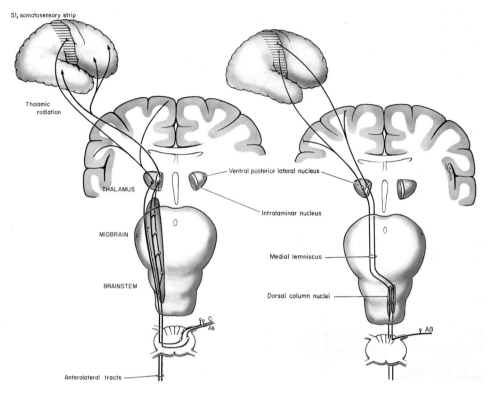

Fig. 5–1. The major ascending somatosensory systems in the spinal cord are called the anterolateral-spinothalamic "pain-temperature" system (left), and the dorsal column–medial lemniscal "touch-pressure" system (right). Pain pathways can be further subdivided into fast, well-localized pain carried peripherally by A delta fibers and ending in specific thalamocortical projections. Slow, poorly localized pain originates in unmyelinated C fibers, which synapse on projections ending mainly in brainstem and midbrain reticular formations and intralaminar thalamic nuclei. Projections of pain sensation from these nuclei to cortex are probably diffuse (arrows). Projections to the sensory strip of cortex of dorsal column sensation (right) is specific for modality and somatotopic place.

tions are intermingled with those of the medial lemniscus fibers in the ventral posterior thalamus. The receptive fields of the thalamic terminations are very large, such that localization of painful stimuli must be accomplished by association with the surrounding mechanoreceptors. This is an example of *parallel processing* refining the interpretation of afferent information. Some paleospinothalamic fibers terminate in intralaminar nuclei of the thalamus.

The role of the cerebral cortex in nociception is not well defined. Large cortical ablations of somatosensory regions of the postcentral gyrus do not abolish pain

sensation on a long-term basis. However, when frontal lobotomies were performed for treatment of psychiatric disease, diminished suffering from chronic pain was sometimes noted. In addition, cingulotomies have been reported to interrupt the sensation of pain. Recent anatomic studies in cats suggest that the nucleus submedius of the thalamus receives nociceptive afferents from the marginal zone of the dorsal horn and projects to the orbital aspect of the prefrontal cortex. Although the functional significance of this finding remains to be evaluated, it does suggest that there are cortical regions of particular

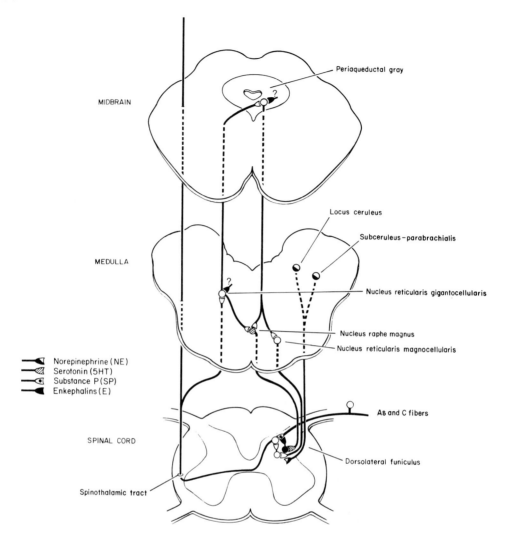

Fig. 5–2. The dorsal root entry zone of the spinal cord contains complex neuronal interactions that modify afferent pain sensation. Afferent fibers end on projection neurons in Rexed layers I and V and on modulatory interneurons in Rexed II (substantia gelatinosa). The dorsolateral fasciculus contains peripheral afferents that ascend for a few segments, as well as descending fibers that interact in these dorsal gray zones to modulate pain sensation (see Fig. 5–2). (Modified from Basbaum and Fields, 1978.)

importance for processing nociceptive inputs.

DESCENDING PAIN SYSTEMS

Until the past decade, it was hard to understand the variability of the experience of pain from moment to moment, culture to culture, and between different individuals. While the extreme variability of the pain experience was well recognized, it could not be explained by differences in the afferent system. One interpretation was that there was a very strong descending cortical influence on pain sensation and perception. Some believed this made animal experimentation impossible. Advances in two areas of research over the past decade have changed this picture and have modified our understanding of modulation of the pain experience. First, it has been found that stimulation of certain areas of the brain can block pain sensation, a phenomenon called stimulus-produced analgesia. Second, a group of endogenous opioid-like substances has been isolated from brain that may act as central neurotransmitters in modulating, or even blocking, pain sensation.

Stimulus-produced analgesia results in profound behavioral analgesia in humans and experimental animals. It may be produced by electrical stimulation in focal areas of the brain including the periaqueductal gray, periventricular gray, and the nucleus raphe magnus of the medulla. The onset of analgesia is delayed for a few minutes, then extends for a variable period after cessation of the stimulus. The degree of analgesia is sometimes sufficient to perform abdominal surgery in experimental animals, and it is sometimes unilateral. These observations strongly suggest that there is a neuronal system for analgesia.

Opiates have long been used for analgesia. In recent years it has been possible to describe the distribution of high-affinity binding for these potent analgesics. Interestingly, they showed binding in many of the same areas involved in stimulus-produced analgesia. The discovery of high-affinity binding suggested the possibility of endogenous substances to interact at these sites. This led to the discovery of endogenous opiates, termed endorphins. The first two discovered were pentapeptides that were identical except for their last amino acid substitution. They are known as Met-enkephalin and Leu-enkephalin. These were followed by the description of a substantial collection of endogenous peptides with affinity to opiate binding sites. Most of these are biochemically related and derive from three families of precursor peptides. Proopiomelanocortin is found in the pituitary and median eminence and is the precursor for ACTH and β-endorphin. Proenkephalin A, the precursor for met-enkephalin and leu-enkephalin, and proenkephalin B, the precursor for neoendorphins and dynorphins, have a wide distribution in spinal cord, brainstem, and limbic system. It is thought that each family of peptides has a high affinity for one receptor.

An increasing amount of experimental evidence points toward an intrinsic, descending pain-inhibiting system (Fig. 5–3). The periaqueductal region appears to be a major link in that system. Stimulation at this site, or injection of opioids, results in marked analgesia. Of particular note is that systemic injections of naloxone, an opioid antagonist, block both the opioid- and stimulation-produced analgesia. At least one of the projections of this area is to the nucleus raphe magnus of the medulla. This is a group of serotinergic neurons that appear to play a very significant role in intrinsic analgesia. Stimulation at nucleus raphe magnus also produces analgesia. One projection from cells in this area is via the dorsolateral fasciculus of the spinal cord to the dorsal horn of the cord. Transverse lesions of dorsolateral fasciculus block the analgesic actions produced by stimulation or injections of opioids. The raphe projection appears to synapse on opioid interneurons located in the substantia gelatinosa of the dorsal horn of the cord. These neurons are believed to have presynaptic actions on the primary afferent nociceptive fibers (Fig. 5–2), resulting in decreased afferent nociceptive input. Section of the dorsal root results in decreased opioid receptors, without substantially decreasing the opioid content of the dorsal horn of the spinal cord. This kind of observation, however, does not exclude the possibility of postsynaptic actions of the opioids in the dorsal horn. It should also be emphasized that the opioid interneurons are only one of a large group of neu-

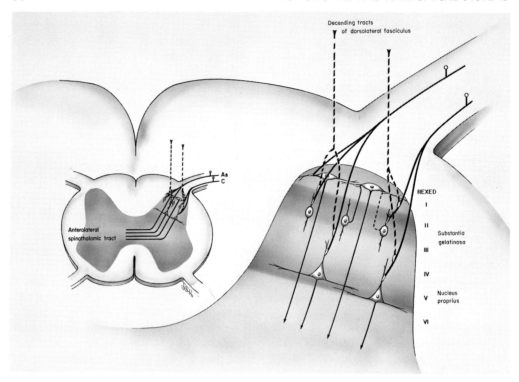

Fig. 5–3. The major descending systems that modulate pain originate in the periaqueductal gray, medullary raphe (serotonin system), and locus ceruleus (norepinephrine). Interactions take place at these two levels, as well as in the dorsal root entry zone of spinal cord. Opioid compounds such as the enkephalins play a role at each site.

rons that modulate activity at the level of the dorsal horn. Among other neurotransmitter candidates implicated in modulation of afferent activity are GABA, glycine, norepinephrine, acetylcholine, vasopressin, oxytocin, and angiotensin II.

There are probably several descending control systems. Of note, stimulus-produced analgesia is not completely blocked by naloxone, suggesting there is a system that is not dependent on opiates. Two candidates include the reticular formation of the medulla and the adrenergic projections from locus ceruleus and the subceruleus-parabrachial regions of the dorsolateral pons (Fig. 5–3). Further, it is very likely that there are hormonal systems modulating pain, some of which may be related to the opioid system (possibly β-

endorphin), whereas others are probably independent of the opioid system.

An important issue is the control system for determining activity in descending pain systems. Since naloxone does not cause pain by itself, it is assumed that tonic inhibition of the afferent system by endogenous opiates is not necessary. It has been suggested that afferent pain signals, a large number of which are transmitted to the reticular substance of the medulla (Fig. 5–1) may be involved in the activation of the opioid system. There is evidence that in the presence of pain, naloxone increases the pain, suggesting that the endogenous opioid system is activated by pain. Thus, it seems likely that the intrinsic analgesic system provides a negative feedback for the afferent pain system.

PHARMACOLOGY OF PAIN

Treatment of pain is one of the physician's most compelling responsibilities, but the modes of therapy are actually quite limited. The best hope of success comes with therapies that correct the abnormal causes of pain. For example, the pain of angina pectoris is more effectively treated by increasing the blood supply to the heart or decreasing its oxygen requirements, not by analgesics. Nitroglycerin is more effective than aspirin for angina. Unfortunately, all too often the cause of pain is unknown, or the pathophysiology cannot be immediately remedied. In these instances, analgesics are required. Currently three major classes of drugs are available: opioids and antidepressants, which act centrally, and the peripherally acting analgesic, antipyretic, anti-inflammatory drugs, like aspirin and other nonsteroidal anti-inflammatory agents.

Central analgesics: opioids and antidepressants

The discovery of stereospecific, saturable, high-affinity, opioid-binding sites in the brain has provided an anatomical basis for understanding the action of opioids. These binding sites occur in various areas of the nervous system including the spinal cord, midbrain, hypothalamus, striatum, thalamus, and in various parts of the limbic system. The areas most likely related to analgesia include the spinal receptors in the substantia gelatinosa and the brainstem and mesencephalic periaqueductal gray matter. Local injections of opioids at either of these sites in experimental animals inhibit pain responses. In addition, focal injections of the specific opioid antagonist naloxone in the periaqueductal gray substantially reverse the analgesic effects of systemic morphine. For these reasons it is believed that the major component of systemic opioid analgesia originates in the midbrain. In addition, the rostral connections from this region to the limbic system and hypothalamus may modulate and decrease the emotional and autonomic responses to pain, which are often so debilitating.

Opioids are far from specific analgesics, and thus fall short of being ideal drugs. In fact, the diversity of side effects, including drowsiness, respiratory depression, decreased bowel motility, nausea, vomiting, and autonomic alterations, is explained by the presence of opioid-binding sites in many areas of the brain. Pharmacologic studies have revealed the presence of multiple, stereospecific opioid-binding sites. These seem to be related to different actions of the drugs. The mu(μ) receptor is thought to be the type primarily involved in supraspinal analgesia, respiratory depression, euphoria, and physical dependence. The kappa (κ) receptor seems to be involved in spinal analgesia, miosis, and sedation, whereas the sigma(σ) receptor may be involved in dysphoria, hallucinations, and respiratory and vasomotor stimulation. A fourth type, which has higher affinity for the enkephalins, has been called the delta (δ) receptor. There is strong evidence that μ and δ sites are distinct, since they have different binding properties, affinities, biochemical mechanisms, and distribution. The σ sites also differ from the others and may relate more to such hallucinogens as phencyclidine than to the opioid series. The presence of these differing sites suggests that modification of the chemical structure of opioids might confer some pharmacologic specificity and reduce the side effects.

Opioids have other drawbacks aside from the direct, unwanted effects. Increasing doses of morphine and other analgesic opioids are required to achieve the same pharmacologic effect over time. The mechanism by which such tolerance develops is not yet well defined, but it seems likely to relate to modulation of receptor properties or receptor numbers. When chronic use of these drugs is suddenly stopped, or direct antagonists are given, a characteristic withdrawal syndrome occurs. This reveals a state of physical dependence that develops with opioids. Unfortunately, it has not been possible to separate useful analgesic action from tolerance and physical dependence, but this remains an important goal in opioid pharmacology.

Tricyclic antidepressant drugs are also effective in relieving pain. Controlled studies have indicated that they modify the pain experience independent of their antidepressant actions. It seems quite plausible that their actions on serotinergic and/or noradrenergic pathways may be crucial in this action. There is growing evidence for an integral role for serotinergic neurons in the endogenous pain system (Fig. 5–3). The known action of tricyclic antidepressant drugs in blocking the reuptake of serotonin and norepinephrine would be expected to augment the action of these neurotransmitters centrally. Recent studies support a direct central action of antidepressants in the augmentation of opioid-induced analgesia by presynaptic serotinergic mechanisms.

Peripheral analgesics: anti-inflammatory analgesic drugs

The most commonly used analgesic is aspirin. Despite its widespread use, an understanding of the mechanism of action of aspirin and related anti-inflammatory drugs is incomplete. It was not until the recent work on the prostaglandins that our current notions of these analgesics were formulated. Prostaglandins can be produced by any cell in the body, but they are not stored. When cells are damaged or inflammation occurs, prostaglandins become synthesized. The unifying action of aspirin, acetominophen, and a host of nonsteroidal, anti-inflammatory drugs is the inhibition of biosynthesis and release of prostaglandins. This is the reason for the shared properties of analgesia, anti-in-

flammatory action, and antipyretic action of these agents. Prostaglandins appear to be one of a group of factors active in the inflammatory response. Intradermal injections of prostaglandin E in relatively high concentrations cause pain and local inflammation. However, in the concentrations actually present in inflamed tissue it is likely that the prostaglandins serve to amplify the effects of other agents, or to sensitize nociceptive nerve terminals. In the presence of low levels of prostaglandin E, the effects of mechanical or chemical stimuli are augmented, such that stimuli that are not painful under control conditions are perceived as painful. Clinically this phenomenon is called hyperalgesia.

Aspirin-like drugs act peripherally against inflammatory diseases and are particularly effective against arthritic pain, minor trauma, and headaches. By contrast, they are relatively ineffective for other pains, particularly those that appear to be initiated within the nervous system (neuropathic pain, discussed later). A hypothalamic action of salicylates probably accounts for its antipyretic activity.

THE PHENOMENOLOGY OF PAIN

New information on pain pathways and central opioids has provided a framework for interpreting clinical phenomena that have puzzled clinicians for centuries. The placebo effect, stimulation-produced analgesia, stress analgesia, congenital insensitivity to pain, central pain syndrome, and phantom limb pain are among the phenomena we shall consider.

Placebo

One of the most perplexing aspects of pain phenomena is the extreme variability in the response to painful stimuli. This has meant that all clinical drug studies must be rigorously controlled by the administration of an inactive substance in the same way as the proposed analgesic drug. A routine finding in such studies is that pain is relieved by inactive substances (the placebo) in a third of subjects. Unfortunately, for years it was not recognized how common the placebo effect is, and inactive substances were administered diagnostically to indicate the absence of "real" pain. In fact, the placbo response occurs frequently in people who have real pain (e.g., dental extractions), and if anything, it occurs less often in patients found to be malingering. The mechanism of the placebo response was unknown until the recent evidence for the intrinsic analgesia systems was recognized. Now it is thought that the placebo response is mediated by the central opioid system. The evidence for this is based primarily on the finding that naloxone can block placebo-induced analgesia. Furthermore, opioid cross-tolerance may develop with placebo, reinforcing the relation of this phenomenon with opioids. One of the important lessons to be drawn from the recent advances in our understanding of pain is respect for the placebo as a means of activating the descending limb of the pain system.

Stimulation-produced analgesia

While electrical stimulation of nerve endings is one means of activating the afferent pain signal, certain types of electrical stimulation of nervous tissue may actually produce analgesia. Transcutaneous electrical stimulation is one example. This method derives from a theory proposed by Melzack and Wall in the mid-1960s that suggested that large sensory afferents inhibited pain transmission cells of the dorsal horn of the spinal cord. Although the specifics of this "gate theory" have not been experimentally demonstrated, it suggests that the painless stimulation of peripheral nerves with low-intensity, high-frequency inputs should produce analgesia. This seems to be the case, although the clinical efficacy of such stimulation over long periods has proved to be disappointing. It

seems likely that the analgesia produced in this way results from a segmental, spinal mechanism rather than from supraspinal, descending pathways.

Acupuncture analgesia is a method of stimulus-produced analgesia that remains controversial. Some evidence suggests that electroacupuncture (a modification of the traditional Chinese system) activates the central analgesia system. Low-frequency, high-intensity electroacupuncture analgesia is inhibited by naloxone. Recent studies have further suggested that electroacupuncture analgesia in mice is mediated via serotinergic systems. Inhibitors of serotinergic metabolism, or serotinergic receptor blockers, inhibit electroacupuncture analgesia, whereas metabolic precursors augment it. Such data suggest that the effect of acupuncture may be largely accounted for by a combination of placebo effect and augmentation of endogenous pain-inhibiting systems.

Central stimulation is another means of producing analgesia with electrical stimuli. As discussed, the recognition of this phenomenon has been instrumental in the development of the concept of intrinsic analgesia systems. Clinically, it has been possible to produce relief of pain with either medial or lateral diencephalic stimulation. This approach has been helpful in selected patients with chronic pain, such as that caused by cancer, but its applicability is limited. It also appears that this approach might be particularly helpful for treatment of some of the central pain syndromes resulting from deafferentation (discussed later).

Congenital insensitivity to pain

The absence of pain is no blessing. A small group of patients who do not perceive pain at all commonly suffer serious burns, infections, multiple fractures, and deformed joints as a result of trauma. These maladies are witness to the utility of the pain experience for survival. Relatively few patients with this condition have been extensively studied. In some it is believed that endogenous opiates played a role in the diminished pain response since naloxone resulted in augmentation of evoked potentials from stimulation of tooth pulp, and in a lowering of avoidance response thresholds. Other patients with insensitivity to pain appear to have a congenital lack of nociceptive receptors, or impaired transmission in afferent systems of peripheral or central pathways.

Stress-induced analgesia

Although the consequences of an inability to recognize pain are obvious, it is not so clear what functional purpose the intrinsic analgesic system serves. A plausible clue to this mystery lies in the phenomenon of stress-induced analgesia. Many have observed soldiers experience painful wounds during battle, but not notice it until some time later. A similar lack of response to pain can occur in athletes during the excitement of sporting contests.

The current understanding of stress induced analgesia from animal experiments suggests that a complex system is operable. The response varies considerably depending on the type of stress. One interesting observation is that removal of the pituitary blocks some forms of stress analgesia. It is known that opioid peptide β-endorphin is released from the pituitary in conjunction with adrenocorticotropin (ACTH) during stress, and its action may mediate analgesia. One might expect that this would be a naloxone-sensitive analgesia, however, and this is not generally the case. At present it appears that there is a separate, hormone-related endogenous analgesia system that can be activated apart from the neural-opiate system under certain conditions.

Nonirritative, ablative pain syndrome

One of the perplexing aspects of clinical pain syndromes has been the extreme pain that follows certain neurologic injuries. Sensations of pain arise with several ablative lesions. Some arise with injury to peripheral nerves and loss of peripheral afferents. Peripheral neuropathies, including diabetic and amyloid neuropathies, are characteristically associated with pain. The syphilitic syndrome of tabes dorsalis, in which dorsal columns and dorsal roots are damaged, produces prominent "lightning" pains. People who have lost a limb frequently experience severe pain, termed phantom limb pain. The pathophysiology of this is unknown, but the central somatotopic representation of pain for the lost extremity, combined with the loss of normal afferent information to activate the endogenous analgesic system(s), gives a framework in which to consider this phenomenon. Iatrogenic peripheral lesions also are known to produce a very unpleasant sensation. For example, tic douloureux is a severe neuropathic pain in the distribution of the trigeminal nerve that at times is treated by surgical ablation of the trigeminal ganglia. The procedure sometimes gives rise to anesthesia dolorosa— the paradoxical occurrence of severe pain in the presence of anesthesia.

Another type of lesion that can give rise to pain follows infarction in certain brain areas. The most common condition causing this syndrome is a stroke in the thalamus. Less commonly it occurs following brainstem or cord lesions. The contralateral pain resulting from such damage is severe, persistent, and very hard to treat. As there is no evidence in most of these patients for ongoing, irritative lesions, it is presumed that the symptoms represent an alteration in the critical balance of afferent and efferent pain systems. The fact that the pain often takes the form of a hyperpathia supports the concept that the recognition of pain is intact (afferent pathway), but the normal negative feedback from the descending systems is lost. This is thought to result in the exacerbation and prolongation of the sensation.

Pain resulting from central lesions is often quite resistent to treatment. Peripherally acting analgesics have no value, since there is no peripheral inflammation to act upon. If there is a disturbance in the descending tracts that contributes to central pain, then neither opioid analgesics nor central stimulation would be expected to work well. In general, the clinical approach to these troublesome syndromes has been to use tricyclic antidepressant agents or anticonvulsants, which are sometimes effective.

GENERAL REFERENCES

Basbaum, A. I., and H. L. Fields. Endogenous pain control mechanisms: review and hypothesis. *Ann. Neurol.* 4:451–62, 1978.

Botney, M., and H. L. Fields. Amitriptyline potentiates morphine analgesia by a direct action on the central nervous system. *Ann. Neurol.* 13:160–4, 1983.

Emmers, R. *Pain: A Spike-Interval Coded Message in the Brain*. New York, Raven Press, 1981.

Fields. H. L. Pain II: new approaches to management. *Ann. Neurol.* 9:101–6, 1981.

Ignelzi, R. J., and J. H. Atkinson. Pain and its modulation. *Neurosurgery* 6:577–83, 584–9, 1980.

Kelly, D. D. Somatic sensory system IV: central representations of pain and analgesia. In *Principles of Neural Science*, E. R. Kandel and J. H. Schwartz (eds.). Elsevier North-Holland, New York, 1981

Snyder, S. H., and S. R. Childers. Opiate receptors and opioid peptides. *Ann. Rev. Neurosci.* 2:35–64, 1979.

Wamsley, J. K., M. A. Zarbin, W. S. Young, and M. J. Kuhar. Distribution of opiate receptors in the monkey brain: an autoradiographic study. *Neurosci.* 7:595–613, 1982.

Willis, W. D., and R. E. Coggeshall. *Sensory Mechanism of the Spinal Cord*. New York, Plenum Press, 1978.

Yaksh, T. L., and D. L. Hammond. Peripheral and central substrates involved in the rostral transmission of nociceptive information. *Pain* 13:1–85, 1982.

6.

Auditory System

JUDITH L. LAUTER

There are three general aspects of the design of the auditory system that are important for a consideration of auditory pathophysiology. First, only the end-organ (within the cochlea) and first-order axons in the very short (5 mm) peripheral nerve lie outside the central nervous system. In addition, both of these components are encased within the petrous ("rock-like") portion of the temporal bone and are thus protected from insults such as those that can affect the lengthy optic nerve and the longer somatosensory fibers that lie outside the CNS.

Second, lesions affecting central auditory pathways in the brainstem almost always result in damage to adjacent structures as well. Such lesions cause a complex and often catastrophic clinical picture in which auditory dysfunction is a very minor part. Third, each ear projects bilaterally to all portions of the auditory system above the lower brainstem. As a result, damage to the central auditory structures rarely results in deficits that can be localized to one ear or the other. This situation is very unlike the clear contralateral deficit that occurs with unilateral damage to somatosensory or visual systems. Like visual

system deficits that develop slowly, some auditory deficits can be compensated for in day-to-day sensory behavior and are only demonstrable with appropriate diagnostic testing.

A battery of audiometric tests is required to define the nature of an auditory disorder and to establish its effects on an individual's ability to function in everyday communication. Both behavioral and physiological tests are available for discovering disorders of the peripheral hearing system (outer, middle, and inner ear, and the VIIIth nerve) and the auditory central nervous system. These tests can be used to examine such disorders as deficits in sensitivity (ability to detect sounds), deficits in recognition ability, and problems involving different types of auditory distortion such as tinnitus (ringing in the ears) or recruitment (abnormal increase in loudness of sounds).

However, auditory testing is currently in a state of development. Physiological tests of hearing have been created on the basis of knowledge about the physics of sound and the physiology of the auditory system. These tests are designed to be applicable, as much as possible, without the conscious participation of the patients. In contrast, behavioral tests have been developed largely as a result of trial and error. Tests in use today generally are limited to sounds and tasks that are either very simple (e.g., detection of pure tones) or very complex (e.g., repetition of sentences). Not surprisingly, such tests have proven to be most useful for examining the results of lesions at the extremes of the auditory system: the end organ and auditory nerve, and the auditory association cortex. Thus, most of what is known about the pathophysiology of hearing relates to function of the peripheral mechanism, somewhat less to cerebral auditory processes, and little, if at all, to disruptions involving components of the auditory system in between. In our survey of auditory disorders we will present the disadvantages of test design limitations and illustrate the need for tests serving as diagnostic tools for systematic examination of the entire auditory system from outer ear into association cortex.

ANATOMY AND FUNCTION

The auditory stimulus

Sounds are characterized by four physical dimensions. The first three are frequency, amplitude, and duration. A fourth dimension relates to the manner in which sounds change with time (e.g., phase, waveform temporal patterns, and frequency and amplitude modulation). Figure 6–1 shows waveforms (as might be seen on an oscilloscope) demonstrating these dimensions for different types of sounds. Panels A and B show tones differing in frequency and amplitude, respectively. Panel C shows tones that have been temporally shaped with rise and fall times. Panels D–H show waveforms of other types of tones and of some speech sounds. Sound complexity can be either spectral or temporal. A pure tone that is steady state (no changes over time) is both spectrally (only one frequency) and temporally simple. Two different steady-

state pure tones played simultaneously represent an increase in spectral complexity (two frequencies), but are temporally as simple as the single tone. Similarly, the same tone played twice in succession is temporally more complex, yet spectrally as simple as the single tone. Figure 6–2 illustrates samples of another representation of sounds, the spectrogram. Spectrograms are useful for visualizing the two types of sound complexity because they are created by a device that performs a spectral analysis (shown on the vertical dimension) of sound characteristics over time (the horizontal dimension). The intensity in each frequency band is indicated by the darkness of the tracing. This figure presents spectrograms of sounds representing a range of complexity from a pure tone to a spoken syllable. As discussed later, some neurons in auditory pathways respond only to specific spectral and temporal patterns.

Figure 6–3 illustrates the frequency-by-intensity auditory space used for describing normal auditory function, with indicated values for detection threshold and threshold of pain, as well as the range of intensity (shaded region) at different frequencies required for accurate auditory perception of speech. Current measurements of hearing use the parameter UCL (uncomfortable listening level) instead of pain to mark the ceiling of the effective hearing range. This diagram of auditory space is used as a reference in testing to evaluate the effect of hearing loss on auditory sensitivity and the ability to identify speech sounds.

The periphery

As an anatomical and functional system, the auditory pathways begin at the *outer ear,* which consists of the pinna and the external acoustic meatus (see Fig. 6–4A). These structures play a major role in the spectral shaping (filtering) of sounds that enter the ear. Pathology affecting the outer ear (congenital absence of the pinna, canal

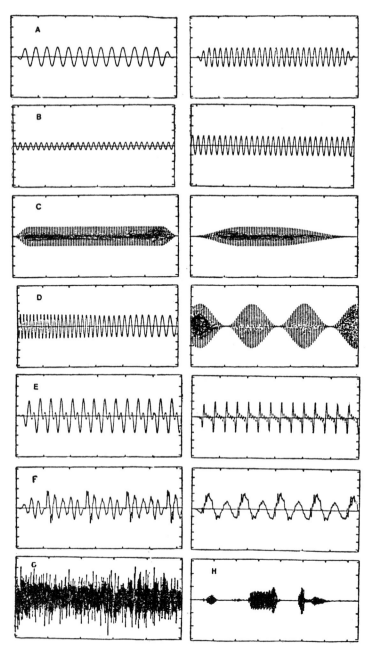

Fig. 6–1. Waveforms of a variety of sounds. A. Two pure tones differing in frequency (500 Hz on the left, 1,000 Hz on the right). B. Two tones of the same frequency, differing in intensity. C. Two tones differing in temporal shaping: rise and fall times of 10 msec on the left, versus a rise time of 25 msec, flat time of 35 msec, fall time of 30 msec on the right. D. Two tones that change over time: a frequency-modulated (FM) tone on the left and an amplitude-modulated (AM) tone on the right. E. Two complex tones: on the left with a fundamental frequency of 500 Hz and a second harmonic at 1,000 Hz; on the right the same fundamental, but two harmonics, one at 1,000 and another at 1,500 Hz. F. Two vowels spoken by a male talker, /a/ on the left and /i/ on the right. G. The waveform of white noise (equal energy at all frequencies). H. The waveform of a multisyllabic word, "confidence," filtered to highlight the peaks of energy associated with each syllable.

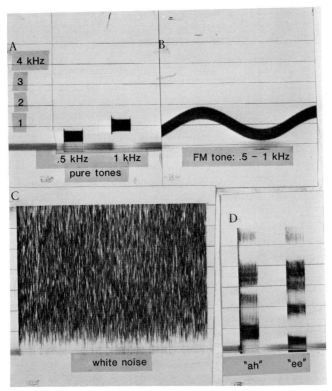

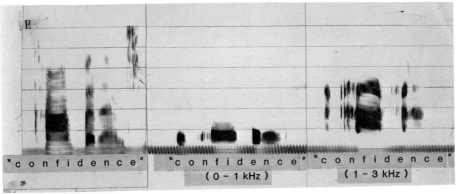

Fig. 6–2. Spectrograms of a sample of sounds. Frequency (marked in 1,000-Hz steps) is on the ordinate, time along the abscissa. These tracings were made with a spectrograph using a bank of 300-Hz-wide filters ("broad-band spectrogram"). **A.** Two pure tones, 500 Hz and 1,000 Hz. **B.** Spectrogram of a tone modulated between frequencies of 0.5 and 1.0 kHz. **C.** The spectrogram of white noise. **D.** Two vowels spoken by a male talker, "ah," and "ee." **E.** Versions of the word "confidence"—first the full spectrogram, then two tracings showing the effects of filtering the utterance, first including only energy below 1,000 Hz, then only energy between 1,000 Hz and 3,000 Hz.

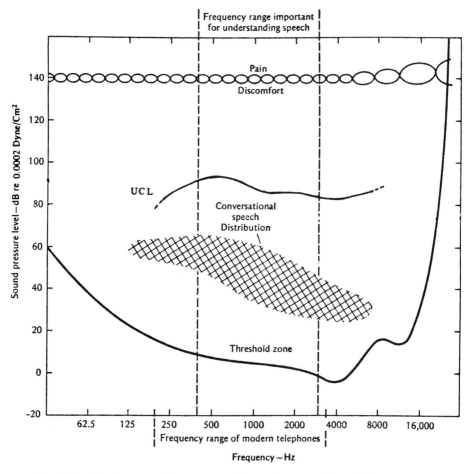

Fig. 6–3. The human auditory range, shown in terms of sound frequency as a function of intensity. Extremes of the range are indicated (detection threshold and ceiling of pain/discomfort), as well as the region of sounds used in speech. Modern descriptions of the range use "uncomfortable listening level" (UCL) instead of a pain ceiling, and include a "most comfortable listening level" (MCL) as well (cf. Fig. 6–9B). The ordinate is a scale in decibels, a ratio scale of sound pressure referred to a physical baseline of 10^{-16} W/cm². The dB scale is related to (but not the same as) a scale of perceived sound loudness. The abscissa is a frequency scale, measured in cycles per second (Hertz). (Modified from Davis and Silverman, 1970, p. 28.)

atresia, etc.) can have demonstrable effects on hearing.

The *middle ear* contains the next group of auditory structures, including the tympanic membrane, the middle-ear cavity with its associated mastoid air-cell complex and the Eustachian tube, and the middle-ear ossicles (malleus, incus, and stapes). The stapedius muscle attached to the stapes is part of a system involved in the acoustic reflex. The reflex involves a sensorimotor loop from the cochlear nuclei to the superior olivary complex within the brainstem and then to the facial nerve, which provides motor control of the stapedius muscle. The system acts to control stiffness of the ossicular chain, thereby helping to protect the ear against sustained loud sounds.

The middle-ear system acts as a trans-

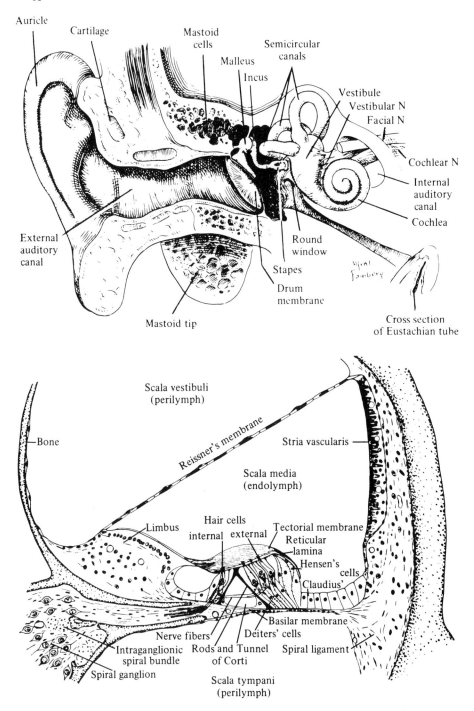

A

Auricle

Cartilage

Mastoid cells

Malleus

Incus

Semicircular canals

Vestibule

Vestibular N

Facial N

Cochlear N

Internal auditory canal

Cochlea

External auditory canal

Round window

Stapes

Drum membrane

Mastoid tip

Cross section of Eustachian tube

Scala vestibuli (perilymph)

Bone

Reissner's membrane

Stria vascularis

Scala media (endolymph)

Limbus

Hair cells

internal external

Tectorial membrane

Reticular lamina

Hensen's cells

Claudius'

Basilar membrane

Nerve fibers

Deiters' cells

Spiral ligament

Intraganglionic spiral bundle

Rods and Tunnel of Corti

Spiral ganglion

Scala tympani (perilymph)

Fig. 6–4. A. Simplified drawing of the peripheral hearing apparatus, showing structures from pinna to VIIIth nerve. (Davis and Silverman, 1970, p. 48.) **B.** Cross section of the cochlear duct, showing structures of the organ of Corti, including the rows of outer and inner hair cells. (From Davis and Silverman, 1970, p. 56.)

former, matching the impedance-to-sound properties of air (outside the tympanic membrane) to those of the fluids within the inner ear. Many mechanical, physiological, and biochemical disruptions may occur within this finely tuned system that can decrease the efficiency of its impedance-matching function and thus interfere with hearing.

The *inner ear* properly includes both auditory and vestibular structures, but we will restrict our discussion to auditory components. From the footplate of the stapes, via the oval window, the auditory functional system continues into the cochlea, a system of three fluid-filled ducts encased within the bony labyrinth of the temporal bone. The floor of the middle cochlear duct is formed by the basilar membrane, on which lies the organ of Corti, the auditory receptor organ (Fig. 6–4B). The organ of Corti contains the auditory hair cells, the primary receptor cells of the auditory system. There are two sets of hair cells in human: one row of inner hair cells and three rows of outer hair cells. Inner hair cells make synaptic connections with dendrites of almost all of the afferent neurons of the auditory nervous system. The cell bodies of these neurons lie in the spiral ganglion, a mass of cell bodies that "spirals" along with the cochlea. Outer hair cells make contact with afferent fibers and also receive efferent input from axons of the olivocochlear bundle. Details of the interaction between outer hair cells and inner hair cells and their central connections are yet to be understood.

The inner ear functions as a transducer; that is, it changes the mechanical energy of sound as transmitted through air and through the outer-ear and middle-ear systems into neural (electrochemical) energy that can be passed into the nervous system. The inner ear functions both as a mechanical system (the basilar membrane *moves* in response to sounds) and as a biochemical system, with essential characteristics including the ionic content of

fluids, structural proteins, and material for synaptic transmission between receptor cells and neurons. Disorders of the inner ear can disrupt either mechanical or sensorineural functioning.

One important mechanical aspect of this system is the construction of the basilar membrane. Portions nearest the stapes footplate (the basal end) react most strongly to high-frequency sounds, whereas portions nearer the apex react to lower-frequency sounds. This is referred to as the tonotopic organization of the cochlea. It is the receptor-surface map of this sensory system, repeated in the topography of neurons from nucleus to nucleus within the auditory nervous system.

The axons of the spiral ganglion cells course centrally as part of the *vestibulocochlear (VIIIth) nerve*, joining the brainstem at the junction level of the medulla and the pons. Axons twist away from the cochlea to form an approximate cochleotopic-tonotopic arrangement within the nerve: neurons from the basal cochlea (high-frequency) to the outside and more apical (lower-frequency) fibers to the inside. Axons within the VIIIth nerve display characteristic responses summarized as tuning curves (see Fig. 6–5A). Such curves illustrate that each neuron responds at the lowest threshold to one frequency (its best or characteristic frequency) and less well (i.e., at higher thresholds) to neighboring frequencies over a limited range. These characteristic frequencies are determined by the site of innervation of the basilar membrane. Thus tone, or pitch, is coded peripherally (and centrally) by labeled lines.

The auditory central nervous system

Once within the brainstem, the VIIIth nerve axons enter the cochlear nuclei and synapse on neurons within subdivisions of that complex. Each fiber divides to send two branches ventrally (one to each of two subdivisions of the *ventral cochlear nu-*

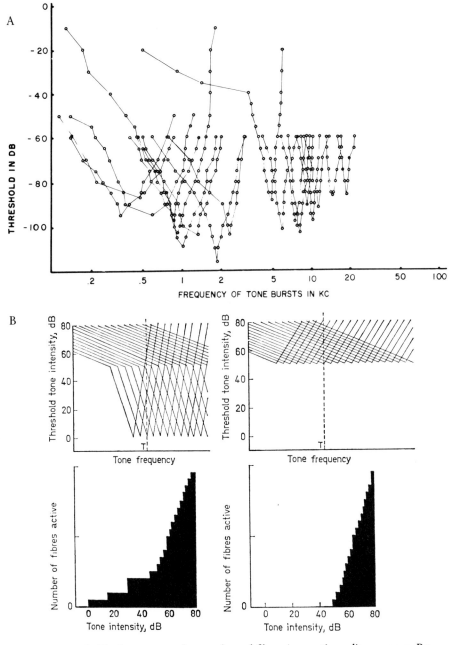

Fig. 6–5. A. Tuning curves of a number of fibers in a cat's auditory nerve. Responses are graphed similarly to thresholds in a behavioral audiogram: The sound intensity at which a fiber shows activity above spontaneous firing rate is plotted as a function of sound frequency. Note that fibers more responsive to higher frequencies are more sharply tuned than those responding best to lower frequencies. (From Kiang, 1965, p. 87.) **B.** Diagrammatic illustration of loudness recruitment. Left: Representation of the normal tuning curves of VIIIth-nerve fibers. As a tone of given frequency (T) is increased in intensity, the number of active fibers, indicated in the lower panel, gradually increases. Right: Pathological situation in which the peaks of the tuning curves are truncated due to sensory or neural damage, resulting in a decreased sensitivity and then a sudden onset in fiber response at a particular intensity of tone T, heard by the patient as an abnormal growth of loudness. (From Evans, 1975, p. 436.)

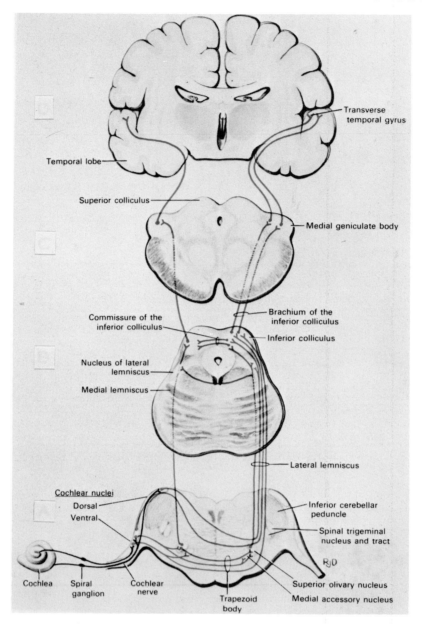

Fig. 6–6. Schematic of the central auditory pathways in humans. Interhemispheric connections between auditory cortical areas via the corpus callosum are not detailed. (From Carpenter, 1972.)

cleus) and a third branch dorsally to synapse on cells in the *dorsal cochlear nucleus* (see Fig. 6–6). There are fine, detailed connections within each of these subdivisions, with structural and functional distinctions. It is sufficient here to note that axons from the basal end of the basilar membrane synapse with cells in the more

dorsal part of each cochlear nucleus, while apical axons connect with more ventral cells within each subdivision. Thus the cochlear nuclei contain several versions of the cochleotopic-tonotopic organization seen in the cross section of the VIIIth nerve. Cells in the ventral cochlear nucleus show responses similar to those of VIIIth nerve axons, with spontaneous activity and tuning curves. In dorsal cochlear nucleus, morphological complexity is reflected in complexity of response, as cells may be excited or inhibited by stimulation and may show different response patterns from cell to cell.

Cell bodies within the cochlear nuclei send axons along one of three paths. Cells in the dorsal cochlear nucleus project ipsilaterally through the pons, via the pathways of the lateral lemniscus, to synapse on cells in the inferior colliculus of the midbrain. Cells in ventral cochlear nucleus subdivisions project to cells in superior olivary complex. These projections may be unilateral or bilateral, ipsilateral or contralateral. However, the majority (>75%) of auditory fibers make contralateral connections. This is the first major crossing of the auditory system, sending left-ear information primarily up the right side of the CNS, with some ipsilateral information also passed on from both dorsal and ventral cochlear nuclei.

The *superior olivary complex,* as its name implies, is composed of a number of subdivisions, each with distinguishing cytoarchitectural characteristics. Tonotopic organization is evident here, as well as an orderly distribution of incoming axons according to contralateral and ipsilateral origin within the cochlear nuclei. Thus, within the different subdivisions of the complex the two principles of auditory organization (cochleotopic-tonotopic and ear of input) are reflected in orderly distributions of axon terminals.

Individual neurons in the superior olivary complex are sensitive to differences in sounds at the two ears: Differences in time of arrival and intensity between left and right ears give rise to selective neuronal responses. Some cells are excited by contralateral stimulation and inhibited by ipsilateral sounds. A number of such combinations, involving excitation-inhibition and ear of input, have been demonstrated, and may be important in the localization of sound in space.

Cells within the complex not only receive afferent input from cochlear nuclei neurons, but some also send axons back toward the periphery, as the *olivocochlear bundle.* These axons bypass the cochlear nuclei, passing directly into the VIIIth nerve and making synaptic connections within the cochlea. The exact function of the olivocochlear bundle is not known, but it has been postulated that these cells provide a feedback mechanism for central control of peripheral response to sensory input.

Axons from cells in the superior olivary complex subdivisions course rostrally on the same side, forming fiber bundles called the *lateral lemniscus.* Axons within these bundles may be either second order (if coming directly from cochlear nuclei neurons) or third order (if coming from superior olivary complex cells). Mixed with the fibers on each side are two *nuclei of the lateral lemniscus.* Axonal distributions to the more dorsal of the two nuclei carry input from both ears, whereas cells synapsing on the more ventral lateral lemniscus nuclei carry only contralateral information. Each nucleus contains a cochleotopic distribution of inputs from lower nuclei, with basal cochlea (high frequencies) ventral, and apical cochlea (low frequencies) dorsal.

All axons of auditory neurons rising through the pons synapse on cells within the *inferior colliculus* of the midbrain. As with other auditory nuclei, a number of cell masses can be differentiated within this structure. Each cell mass can also be further subdivided into groups of cells that differ by structure and connections. In the central nucleus there is a laminar arrangement of cells that seems to correlate with cochleotopic organization, having connections within and across laminae. The pericentral nucleus receives input from lateral leminiscus axons, from auditory cortex and from contralateral inferior colliculus. Cells in the external nucleus receive both auditory and somatosensory inputs. The midbrain is the second level of crossings in the auditory system, as some inferior colliculus axons cross the midline within the midbrain to synapse on contra-lateral inferior colliculus neurons.

Single-cell responses reflect these ana-tomical relations. Some inferior colliculus neurons have narrow tuning curves; oth-ers are more broadly tuned. Cells may se-lectively respond to differences in time of arrival at the two ears on the order of sev-eral microseconds and may show sensitiv-ity to a sound moving in space, toward or away from the midline. Other inferior col-liculus neurons do not respond to a steady-state sound, but will respond if a fre-quency-modulated sound is presented (the responses are independent of the direction and rate of frequency change).

Most axons projecting from the infe-rior colliculus course rostrally to synapse in the ipsilateral *medial geniculate nucleus* of the thalamus. Cytoarchitectural differ-ences distinguish a number of subdivi-sions within the medial geniculate nu-cleus. The ventral division of the nucleus receives most of the input from the infe-rior colliculus. It has tonotopic organiza-tion and projects heavily to primary au-ditory cortex. Neurons of the ventral division show responses that distinguish among sets of speech sounds (see Fig. 6–7A). The physical characteristics of the in-dicated sounds provide an explanation for this distinction, since they differ consid-erably in dominant-frequency region and temporal pattern. Other cells may re-spond only to FM sounds changing at a certain rate, independent of the direction of frequency change.

The dorsal division of the medial ge-niculate nucleus receives few fibers from the inferior colliculus (most come from the midbrain tegmentum), and projects to the nonprimary auditory cortex. Very little cochleotopic organization has been found in dorsal medial geniculate nucleus. Some cells in the medial division of this nucleus receive both auditory and somatosensory input. Cells in this division that respond to auditory stimulation are excited by both monaural and binaural sounds.

In humans, the *primary auditory cor-tex,* called AI in studies on other animals, is represented on the superior plane of the temporal lobe (Brodmann's areas 41 and 42). Both of these areas (the posterior transverse temporal gyrus and the ante-rior transverse temporal gyrus, "Heschl's gyri") have been shown to have the ana-tomical and physiological characteristics of primary auditory cortical areas studied in animals. In this region, cortical cells of layer IV receive input from cells of the thalamic medial geniculate nucleus. These primary auditory cortical cells are there-fore at least fifth-order auditory neurons.

Maps of cell responses to sounds of different frequencies that seem to reflect the tonotopic organization of the cochlea have been demonstrated in the primary auditory cortex of a number of animals. Evidence for a similar organization in hu-mans has been recently reported. Such a frequency organization appears to con-tribute to auditory columns (analogous to those in somatosensory and visual cor-tex), with intersecting dimensions of fre-quency and sound differences at the two ears. Figure 6–8 shows one example of in-tersecting isofrequency and isolaterality bands in a cat's primary auditory cortex.

Another approach to the study of cell responses in auditory cortex is the use of species-specific communication sounds. A number of experimenters have reported results of such testing in squirrel monkeys, with most cells tested responding better to monkey calls than to simple sounds. Often there was no correlation between a cell's response to pure tone stimuli and its re-sponse to calls. Some cells responded to several calls, while others were highly spe-cific to one call type. Still others re-sponded only to portions of a call (see Fig. 6–7B). Some cells had a long latency of response, with sensitivity to temporal ele-ments of a call: If an early segment of the call were omitted, the cell would not re-spond.

Cells in primary auditory cortex have also been shown to be sensitive to behav-

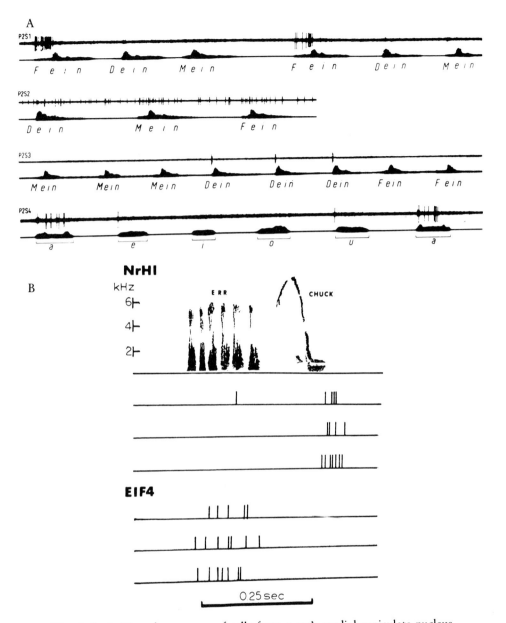

Fig. 6–7. **A.** Neural responses of cells from a cat's medial geniculate nucleus, recorded on presentation of the indicated German monosyllables. Different cells ("P2S1," etc.) seem to respond preferentially to the acoustical patterns of /f/ (versus /d/ and /m/) and /a/ (versus /e/ and /i/). (From Keidel, 1974, p. 223.) **B.** Responses of two single cells (NrH1 and E1F4) in a squirrel monkey's primary auditory cortex showing selective firing to different portions of the temporal sequence of acoustical events comprising a presented species-specific call. (From Funkenstein et al., 1971, p. 311.)

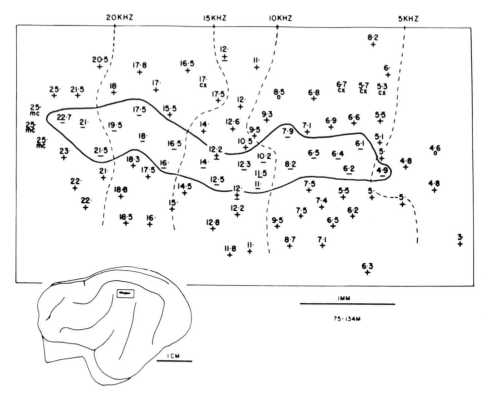

Fig. 6–8. Intersecting isofrequency and isolaterality bands in a cat's primary auditory cortex. Cells responsive to similar frequencies are grouped together in medial-lateral zones by dotted lines. Cells responsive to binaural interaction are indicated when there is summation (+) or suppression (−). The solid line encloses an anterior-posterior band of cells showing binaural suppression. (From Brugge and Imig, 1978, p. 497.)

ioral variables. For example, a cell's response may be determined in part by whether the animal is looking at the source of the sound, is attending to the task, or has been taught to hear the sound as a test stimulus. Also, individual primary auditory cortical cells can be classically conditioned.

Other auditory areas have been found surrounding the primary reception area for medial geniculate nucleus input. These secondary and tertiary fields of association auditory cortex have not been identified physiologically in humans, but they presumably occupy regions of the cortical surface analogous to those defined in other animals. Brodmann's areas 21 and 22

probably contain additional auditory fields. Portions of the cortex beyond this (Brodmann's 39 and 40), which like area 22, have been implicated in the aphasias, are situated in a position suggesting that they receive both subcortical and transcortical input from auditory, visual, and somatosensory systems. This would seem to be an ideal description of a "language area."

Beyond tonotopic mapping, auditory areas surrounding AI have not been studied in nonhuman subjects. However, in humans, it is damage to these areas that leads to the complex of syndromes known as auditory agnosia and sensory aphasia. There have also been a few reports of the impressions of patients who received elec-

Table 6–1. Correlations between positive test results and site of lesion within the auditory system.

	Outer ear	Middle ear	Inner ear	VIII nerve	Lower brainstem	Upper brainstem	Cortex
Behavioral							
Tone audiometry	x	x	x	x	(x)		
Threshold decay				x	x		
Recruitment tests				x	x		
Speech tests:							
normal	(1)	(1)	x	x	x		x
distorted (2 ears)							
fusion				x	x		
separation				(x)	(x)		x
swinging					x		
Tinnitus report		x	x	x	x		
Physiological							
Immittance		x					
Acoustic reflex		x	x	x	x		
Brainstem ERA			x	x	x		
Cortical ERA							x

(1) Speech tests give normal results in presence of outer-ear or middle-ear pathology, given sufficient intensity of presentation. (x) Occasionally lesions at this site will yield positive results on the tests indicated.

trical stimulation to selected auditory regions during surgery. Stimulation on the superior temporal plane (primary auditory cortex) evoked impressions such as tones, buzzes, or knocking sounds, but stimulation in lateral portions of the temporal lobe seemed to arouse memory sequences that had auditory components and sometimes other sensations as well. All sequences had spatial, spectral, and temporal form. One woman heard a tune that after several stimulations to the same point, she was able to sing and identify.

Right and left auditory fields, both in primary cortex and association areas, are connected via the corpus callosum. These are the last major crossings in the auditory system, providing another instance of interaction of information from the two ears. This interaction is probably both supplementary and complementary to that provided at lower levels in inferior colliculus and superior olive.

EVALUATION OF HEARING LOSSES

The possible types of auditory dysfunction can be classified and correlated with the site of auditory-system damage (see Table 6–1). A loss of sensitivity with relatively the same effect at all frequencies is most often due to mechanical disruption at the periphery: blockage of the outer ear canal, puncture of the tympanic membrane, malfunction of the middle-ear ossicular chain. Both mechanical and physiological malfunction within the inner ear can also result in loss of sensitivity, but are more often frequency selective and accompanied by various sound distortions.

Peripheral disorders obviously affect more than merely the patient's ability to detect single sounds. However, damage to more central structures produces even greater losses in speech intelligibility. Though little is known about the influence of brainstem and thalamic injury on speech understanding, it is certain that cortical damage, particularly in relevant regions of the left hemisphere (for most individuals), can disrupt or terminate the ability to communicate verbally, although sensitivity to simple sounds such as pure tones and noises is normal. Thus the hierarchy of malfunction complexity, that is, frequency loss over all pure-tone frequencies to total loss of speech comprehension, matches the hierarchy of anatomical and physiological complexity in the system from the mechanical resonant tube of the outer ear canal to neural excitatory and inhibitory interactions in the cortex. Auditory test design attempts to reflect these two hierarchies by comprising stimulus-response combinations that are evocative of different dysfunction complexities at different levels of the system.

Peripheral signs and symptoms

Many disruptions can occur in the normal sequence of events during development of the pinna and external ear canal. The effect on hearing can range from slight (e.g., a malformed pinna can cause small differences in the filtering effect on sound reaching the eardrum) to significant (e.g., canal atresia can block airborne sound entirely). Outer-ear abnormalities can occur in the presence of normal middle- and inner-ear systems because these structures are derived from different embryological origins.

The outer ear's function may also be disrupted by otitis externa, inflammatory diseases affecting the external ear structures. Infections, impacted cerumen, or foreign matter can lead to blockage of the canal, reflected audiologically by a conductive hearing loss.

To evaluate the effect of such abnormalities and other disruptions in the peripheral auditory system, the threshold of detection for pure tones of different frequencies is plotted on an audiogram (Fig. 6–9A). The zero line is derived from data on thresholds measured in a large population of otologically normal individuals (cf. the threshold curve in Fig. 6–3). This curve is normalized across frequencies to provide a standard of normal threshold (audiometric zero) against which to measure hearing sensitivity. The measure of threshold shown in Figure 6–9A at 500 Hz would be described as 30-dB hearing level, in reference to the audiometric zero.

A tone presented at 40 dB above this threshold for the same subject would be termed 40-dB sensation level, in reference to the individual's threshold.

Sounds delivered by a vibrator applied to the mastoid process can bypass outer- and middle-ear structures. An audiogram can be taken via this route of bone conduction (as opposed to air conduction from earphones or a speaker). A comparison of the two measures, in cases of outer-ear or middle-ear pathology, shows the air-bone gap illustrated in Figure 6–9A: normal hearing (i.e., normal inner-ear function) with bone conduction, but hearing loss with air conduction.

Although pure-tone audiometry is clinically performed with tone generators, an approximation to these more complete results can be obtained at the bedside using tuning forks. A difference between air and bone conduction can be revealed using the Rinne test. A struck tuning fork is held against the patient's mastoid and he reports when the sound goes away. Immediately, the fork is held outside the ipsilateral canal. If the tone is heard again this demonstrates that air conduction is better than bone conduction—the normal expected finding. If the tone is not heard again with air conduction, external or middle-ear abnormality is likely.

Pathologies of the *middle ear* may result from physical causes (e.g., perforation of the tympanic membrane) or disease processes such as otitis media, cholesteatoma, or the bone proliferation of otosclerosis). All disruptions of the middle ear result in a conductive hearing loss that may be slight, moderate, or severe (up to 70-dB loss), with similar effects across frequencies. Small differences between frequencies may be seen in cases involving the tympanic membrane, in which its resonance properties to different frequencies may be differentially affected, or in early stages of otitis media or otosclerosis, in which hearing at lower frequencies is most affected.

Differential diagnosis of middle-ear

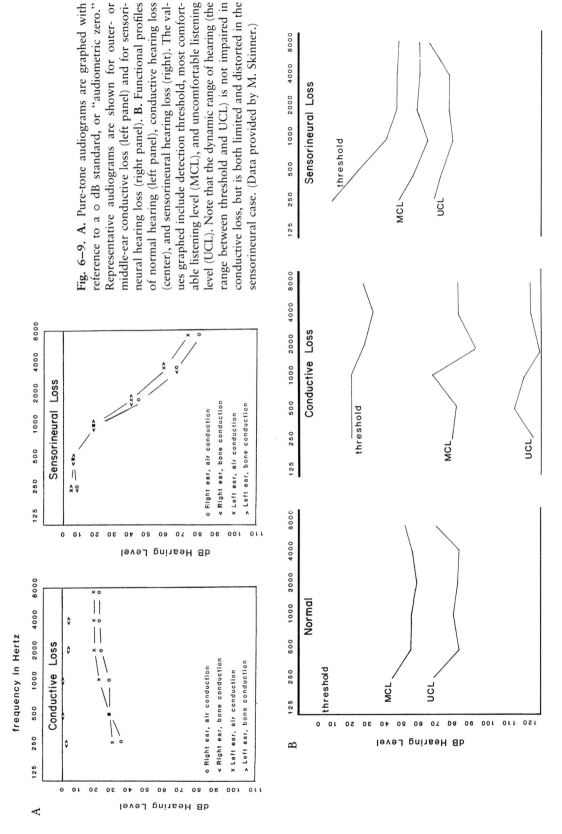

Fig. 6–9. A. Pure-tone audiograms are graphed with reference to a o dB standard, or "audiometric zero." Representative audiograms are shown for outer- or middle-ear conductive loss (left panel) and for sensorineural hearing loss (right panel). **B.** Functional profiles of normal hearing (left panel), conductive hearing loss (center), and sensorineural hearing loss (right). The values graphed include detection threshold, most comfortable listening level (MCL), and uncomfortable listening level (UCL). Note that the dynamic range of hearing (the range between threshold and UCL) is not impaired in conductive loss, but is both limited and distorted in the sensorineural case. (Data provided by M. Skinner.)

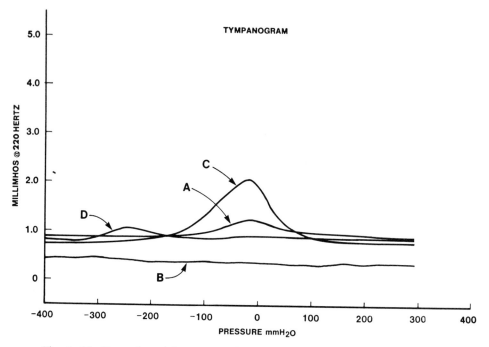

Fig. 6–10. Examples of four types of tympanogram associated with different diagnoses of middle-ear function. **A,** normal function; **B,** a stiffened system, with both tympanic membrane and ossicular chain completely immobilized; **C,** abnormally flexible tympanic membrane or disarticulated ossicular chain (normal pressure in middle ear); **D,** negative pressure in the middle ear, creating partial immobilization of the tympanic membrane and ossicular chain.

disorder depends on otoscopic examination (e.g., a simple case of tympanic membrane perforation is easily distinguished from advanced otitis media), pure-tone testing, and tests to determine the resistance of the middle-ear system to the conduction of sound (immittance tests). A tentative diagnosis of an interrupted or stiffened ossicular chain can be made on the basis of immittance measurements. Tympanograms are types of immittance test results; tympanograms and the correlated pathology are shown in Figure 6–10. The cause of abnormal stiffness (e.g., fluid filling the middle ear or otosclerosis) or laxness (e.g., perforated tympanic membrane or disarticulated ossicles) is determined by tests such as otoscopic examination, biopsy, and exploratory surgery.

In speech testing using lists of mono-

syllables or two-syllable words, the patient is to repeat the word presented. This repetition shows normal speech perception in cases of outer-ear or middle-ear pathology, so long as the speech is presented at high-enough levels to compensate for the conductive loss in sensitivity. Thus hearing aids are of immediate benefit to individuals with such losses.

Peripheral disorders may also involve the *inner ear.* Physical changes in the inner ear, such as the failure in basilar membrane elasticity with age, can result in inner-ear conductive loss. This loss may contribute to problems of hearing in presbyacusis, a condition that also gives signs of both sensory (cochlear hair cells) and neural (spiral ganglion cells) involvement. This is reflected in a sensorineural type audiogram (cf. Fig. 6–9B) indicative of age-related metabolic changes within the inner ear, as well as loss of hair cells and neurons. Traumatic insults such as temporal bone fracture, anoxia, infections such as mumps or measles, and exposure to high levels of noise or to ototoxic drugs can all cause physical and biochemical changes in the delicate inner-ear system. These etiologies can result in damage to and loss of sensory cells within the cochlea and damage to spiral ganglion neurons, leading to hearing loss. Sensorineural hearing loss is characterized by three symptoms: recruitment, selective loss of the higher frequencies, and occasionally tinnitus.

Recruitment is defined subjectively as an abnormal growth in loudness. It is measured by a short increment sensitivity index (SISI) test. A listener with a sensorineural hearing loss has recruitment if he can hear an increment of 1 dB in intensity in a series of tones at 80-dB hearing level. A normal person cannot hear this small change. Current speculation relates recruitment to the shape of neural tuning curves (cf. Fig. 6–5B): In damage to the end organ, the sensitive peaks of the tuning curves are lost, while the broadly tuned bases are spared. Thus, as a test sound is increased in intensity, at some level there is a sudden onset of responses from a number of neurons because the threshold of the bases of many neuronal tuning curves is reached at the same time. This surge in response activity is perceived by the patient as a sudden growth in loudness.

The effect of these two aspects of sensorineural hearing loss (threshold shift at selected frequencies and recruitment) on the *dynamic range* of hearing is indicated in Figure 6–9B, which compares parameters of the hearing range for a normal listener, a listener with conductive hearing loss, and one with sensorineural hearing loss. The range of hearing for the sensorineural case is limited by two factors: a rise in threshold that is uneven across frequencies, and a concomitant lowering of the uncomfortable listening level ceiling. In the presence of physiological changes causing recruitment, sounds sometimes become uncomfortably loud at lower sensation levels than normal. This may be compared with the absence of change in the dynamic range in cases of outer-ear/middle-ear pathology (middle panel of Fig. 6–9B). Because the conductive loss raises both threshold and UCL ceiling and there is no abnormal loudness at higher sound levels, there is no narrowing of the range.

The third common complaint in sensorineural hearing loss is tinnitus, or the perception of sound in the absence of an external stimulus. Tinnitus may be tonal or noisy and may result from abnormal hyperactivity within the cochlea, the VIIIth nerve, or central auditory structures. It can be associated with a number of conditions, from mechanical causes such as impacted cerumen against the eardrum, or otosclerosis, to cochlear pathology such as noise-induced hearing loss or Ménière's disease. Both subjective and objective tinnitus are recognized, though the subjective form is more common. Objective tinnitus refers to spontaneous acoustic emissions that can be recorded in the outer-ear canal. It has been demonstrated that very few instances of subjective tinnitus are accompanied by actual emissions that can be recorded externally.

Ménière's disease (endolymphatic hydrops) presents a striking combination of symptoms. This disorder is apparently associated with changes in the fluids of the inner ear. Endolymph, an inner-ear fluid, is either not absorbed normally or is overproduced. Reissner's membrane is displaced as a result of increased pressure, most dramatically toward the more flexible, apical end. The typical audiogram in Ménière's disease shows a loss predominating at low frequencies (apical cochlea involvement), or a flat loss. Acoustic immittance is normal (indicating a normal middle ear), but speech discrimination scores are poor, often lower than would be predicted from the audiogram. Also, a roaring tinnitus and recruitment may be present, indicating abnormal function of receptor cells and/or spiral ganglion cells, perhaps caused by excessive endolymph pressure affecting the hair cells. Patients with Ménière's also report a sensation of fullness in the ear. The dominant complaint in this disorder is vertigo. The most helpful test for diagnosing the disease and for tracking its progress is electronystagmography, a test in which eye movements are monitored with electrodes during spatial or thermal stimulation of the vestibular system. The glycerin test is also useful. In this test a glycerin solution (given orally) is used to dehydrate the inner ear and will bring about temporary cessation of symptoms if endolymphatic hydrops is the cause. All symptoms typically fluctuate from hour to hour and from day to day.

The VIIIth nerve can be adversely affected by a number of agents, the most common being head trauma, infection, and tumor. Differential diagnosis of VIIIth nerve disorders depends on a test battery that includes pure-tone audiometry (selective loss for frequencies may be seen), speech testing (abnormally low scores are common), loudness-balance tests (usually no recruitment or hyporecruitment), and the short increment sensitivity test. Damage to the nerve also leads to abnormal results on the threshold decay test, with patients reporting that a sustained tone fades after only a short time.

Because damage to the nerve can also result in complaints of vertigo, electronystagmography with caloric stimulation is a useful test to determine whether the vestibular portion of VIII is affected. Tinnitus can also be associated with VIIIth nerve damage. However, unlike the vertigo and tinnitus associated with Ménière's disease, VIIIth nerve problems do not fluctuate with time.

There are similarities between the symptoms of cochlear and VIIIth nerve damage. However, for hearing losses less than 40 dB, it is believed that only outer hair cells are involved, with VIIIth nerve symptoms such as fatigue seldom seen. Hearing loss greater than 40–50 dB may reflect damage to inner hair cells as well (95% of afferent input), resulting in both cochlear and neural symptoms. The distinction between cochlear and "retrocochlear" pathology has been a basic concern in diagnostic audiology and continues to elude satisfactory solution. More sophisticated physiological testing such as electrocochleography (in which a recording electrode is placed within the ear canal or through the tympanic membrane to the inner wall of the middle-ear space), or brainstem evoked-response audiometry (see later discussion) may provide further information about differences in dysfunction between these two sites.

Central signs and symptoms

As we have seen, a fair amount of information is available about the pathological details and etiology of disorders affecting the outer, middle, and inner ear. Much less is known about the effects of damage to auditory structures beyond the VIIIth nerve. This lack of knowledge is due to the factors mentioned earlier: (1) Auditory symptoms for subcortical structures are "hidden" (i.e., patients do not spontaneously notice a decrement in either sensitivity or speech-recognition ability); (2) involvement of neighboring structures in the brainstem often dominates the clinical profile; and (3) behavioral tests have not yet been designed that can provide sophisticated differential diagnosis for the central pathways.

Tumors and vascular lesions are the most common causes of damage within the auditory centers in the *lower brainstem*. Neonatal hyperbilirubinemia (kernicterus), which results from Rh incompatibility, can also affect these centers. Cases of lower brainstem damage studied audiologically are fairly rare because any resultant problems with hearing take second priority to other, more critical symptoms. No tests to date have been designed that can distinguish between lesions separately affecting the cochlear nuclei, superior olivary complex, and their connections. Therefore, central auditory tests for this region are considered diagnostic of nothing more discrete than "lower-brainstem" auditory function. Behavioral tests reveal symptoms very similar to those seen in VIIIth nerve damage, i.e., elevated puretone thresholds, poor scores on speech tests, and abnormal threshold-decay results.

Damage to the lower-brainstem auditory system may also be reflected in brainstem evoked-response audiometry (BERA). Brainstem ERA focuses on the electrical results of averaged, evoked activity in the VIIIth nerve and auditory CNS within 10 msec of stimulus onset. The test is useful for audiological examination of hard-to-test individuals (infants, children, mentally retarded individuals, etc.), and in describing lesions affecting auditory neural pathways. Brainstem ERA is also gaining increasing popularity for a number of diagnostic applications involving the brainstem, e.g., in multiple sclerosis, vascular ischemia, and central pontine myelinolysis, where it can be used to identify dysfunction in acute disease phases as well as to trace recovery of function.

A waveform sequence of seven waves is recorded at the vertex in the first 10 msec post stimulus onset (often called Jewett waves after their discoverer). Wave V is the most prominent and most often used in audiological applications; Figure 6-11 shows the constancy of wave V as an indicator of suprathreshold reception as stimulus intensity is lowered. For audiological uses, the amplitude and latency of individual waves are measured. With appropriate stimulation, this technique can be used to produce an electrophysiological audiogram of responses at several frequencies across the hearing range.

Abnormalities in the waveform caused by lesions include delay in absolute latency of individual waves, interwave latency delay, loss of individual waves, and changes in overall waveform. It has been observed that treatment (e.g., removal of a tumor) can return the waveform to normal. However, because the source of individual waves in the brainstem evoked-response has not been conclusively determined, only the approximate level of a lesion may be inferred from changes in the evoked response.

Individuals with *temporal lobe* damage rarely have lesions restricted to primary auditory cortex. Luria ascribed both auditory agnosia (failure to identify everyday sounds) and problems with phonetic identification of isolated words to damage in primary, as well as secondary, auditory cortex (Brodmann's areas 41, 42, and 22). Some researchers found that electrical stimulation in these areas of cortex caused their patients to hear tones, buzzes, or knocking sounds. Temporal lobe damage seldom affects pure tone thresholds, although there may be peripheral hearing loss unrelated to cortical injury.

Several of the central auditory tests may be abnormal in temporal lobe disorders. Distorted-speech tests show reduced performance in the ear contralateral to a temporal lobe lesion. Tests using two-ear presentation and an auditory fusion task are not dramatically affected by temporal lobe damage. However, all of those tests in which the listener must separate competing signals at the two ears are sensitive to damage in this region, with the greatest decrement in performance found in the ear contralateral to the side of damage. Some patients with damage to the corpus callosum have been found to have poor performance on competing speech tests, presumably due to poor transfer of speech signals to the language-dominant hemisphere.

Lesions have been placed in the primary auditory cortex of animals. The animals were then tested behaviorally to identify subsequent perceptual deficits.

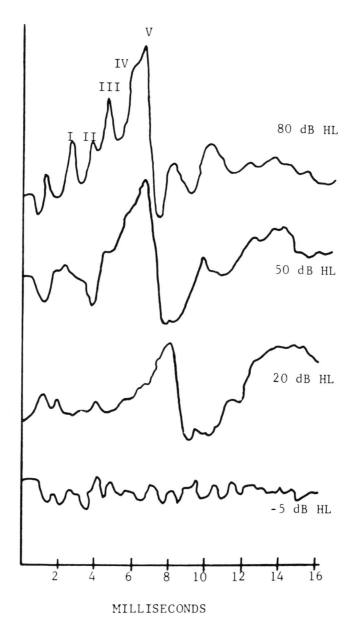

V

IV

III

I II

80 dB HL

50 dB HL

20 dB HL

-5 dB HL

2   4   6   8   10   12   14   16

MILLISECONDS

Fig. 6–11. Waveforms of the brainstem auditory evoked response, evoked at different signal levels. (HL indicates an intensity referred to audiometric zero for the sound, in this case, a broadband click.) Note the prominence of wave V at suprathreshold levels, and the decrease in latency of wave V as the signal level increases. (From Brackmann, et al., 1980, p. 1257.)

These cause a loss of sensitivity to the direction of frequency modulation and problems with temporal discrimination, such as judging the order of three tones of different frequencies. The animals also appear to have difficulty with auditory space in relating body position to side of input. Deficits in frequency and intensity discrimination have also been noted.

Physiological studies on primary auditory cortex suggest that more tests could be designed to analyze primary cortical disorders. Complex sounds, involving both spectral and temporal complexities, could be manipulated to examine an individual's ability to distinguish among such sounds, to identify sounds in isolation, or to make judgments about the location of sounds in space.

Areas surrounding human primary auditory cortex on the temporal lobe have been implicated in the group of aphasic syndromes labeled posterior or fluent (Wernicke's aphasia). Because of the site of lesion, these disorders must be considered, at least in part, auditory disorders. Posterior aphasics have in fact been observed to have difficulty with auditory comprehension. Luria correlates disorders affecting auditory memory, word meaning, and sentence comprehension with damage in such regions (Brodmann's areas 21 and 37). Many reports have noted that aphasics with damage to auditory association areas typically have difficulty comprehending strings of words, although they might be quite accurate in identifying isolated words. Damage to these areas also results in judgment deficits for the temporal order of nonspeech stimuli such as tones or lights.

It is unclear how much specificity is possible in considering the function of any area of cortex. Intrinsic transcortical and subcortical connections complicate the task of inferring function from anatomical relations or site of lesion. More analytical diagnostic tests could surely be designed,

perhaps guided by findings on the physiological organization of auditory association cortex. Functions of auditory cortex that underlie speech comprehension may be most efficiently studied with nonspeech sounds. These sounds may approach speech sounds in complexity, but do not involve "overlearning," familiarity with the language, or semantics. These characteristics of speech stimuli may in fact be a disadvantage in studying the truly auditory aspects of complex auditory perception, including the perception of language.

EXPECTATIONS FOR THE FUTURE

Our understanding of the pathophysiology of outer-ear, middle-ear, and inner-ear disorders will continue to advance, due to developments in both behavioral and physiological techniques that promise to reveal more details about normal and abnormal structural function in each of these peripheral regions of the auditory system. However, the parallel concern in central auditory testing with fixing the site of auditory CNS damage has changed considerably.

Recent advances in the technology of viewing the human CNS, such as evoked responses, computerized axial tomography (CAT), nuclear magnetic resonance (NMR) scanning, and measures of cerebral blood flow and metabolism, such as positron emission tomography (PET), have led a number of authors to suggest that the audiologist of the future will be able to leave the determination of CNS site of lesion to the neurologist. This will then free the audiologist to apply behavioral and physiological testing in analyzing and interpreting the degree of perceptual dysfunction suffered by individuals with damage affecting different levels of the auditory pathways.

This shift in focus should motivate those who deal with such patients to seek guidelines for the design of more sophisticated tests. Data from experiments on auditory electrophysiology and neuro-anatomy using animal subjects, as well as principles of stimulus and response control developed in psychoacoustics, may suggest directions for the design and application of these new tests. Specifically, it is probable that the most useful test design will be one that attempts to correlate behavioral variables such as task and stimulus complexity with the anatomical and physiological hierarchy represented by the auditory nervous system. This attempt would be based on the assumption that lower levels of the nervous system are sufficient to process simple sounds in a simple task (e.g., detection of pure tones in an audiometric exam), whereas increasingly higher levels with more sophisticated processing will be required as the stimulus-task combinations become gradually more complex (e.g., discrimination of tone sequences). Relationships are more subtle than this, of course, since sufficient integrity at lower levels is obviously important for successful function at higher ones.

Ultimately, our understanding of auditory nervous system function in everyday situations will depend on a synthesis of details related to anatomy, physiology, and pathology. Clinical management of patients with damage affecting different levels within the auditory system can possibly be improved both diagnostically and therapeutically by a more sophisticated understanding of the organization of this sensory system. Individualized programs for therapy will depend on coordination between updated behavioral testing and sophisticated neurological evaluation.

GENERAL REFERENCES

Brackmann, D. E., W. A. Selters, and M. Don. Electric response audiometry. In Paparella, M. M., and D. A. Shumrick (eds.) Otolaryngol-

ogy. Philadelphia, W.B. Saunders, 1980, pp. 1250–1242.

Brugge, J. F. Progress in neuroanatomy and neurophysiology of auditory cortex. In The Nervous System. Vol. 3, Human Communication and Its Disorders, D. B. Tower (ed.), New York, Raven Press, 1975, pp. 81–96.

Brugge, J. F., and T. J. Imig. Connections of auditory area AI of cat cerebral cortex. In Naunton, R. F., and C. Fernandez, (eds.) Evoked Electrical Activity in the Auditory Nervous System. New York, Academic Press, 1978, pp. 497–514.

Carpenter, M. B. Core Text of Neuroanatomy. Baltimore, Williams & Wilkins, 1972.

Davis, H., and S. R. Silverman. Hearing and Deafness. New York, CBS College Publishers, 1970.

Evans, E. F. The sharpening of cochlear frequency selectivity in the normal and abnormal cochlea. Audiology 14:419–22, 1975.

Funkenstein, H. H., P. G. Nelson, P. Winter, Z. Wollberg, and J. Newman. Unit responses in auditory cortex of awake squirrel monkeys to vocal stimulation. In Physiology of the Auditory System. Sachs, M. B. (ed.) Baltimore, National Educational Consults, Inc., 1971, pp. 307–316.

Jerger, J., N. J. Wiekers, F. W. Sharbrough III, and S. Jerger. Bilateral lesions of the temporal lobe. Acta Otol. Supp. 258, 1969.

Keidel, W. D. Information processing in the higher part of the auditory pathway. In Facts and Models in Hearing, E. Zwicker and E. Terhardt (eds.) New York, Springer-Verlag, 1974, pp. 216–26.

Keith, R. W. (ed.). Central Auditory Dysfunction. New York, Grune & Stratton, 1977.

Kiang, N. Y. S. Discharge Patterns of Single Fibers in the Cat's Auditory Nerve. Cambridge, MIT Press, 1965.

Newman, J. D., and Z. Wollberg. Multiple coding of species-specific vocalizations in the auditory cortex of squirrel monkeys. Brain Res. 54:287–304, 1973.

Paparella, M. M., and D. A. Shumrick (eds.). Otolaryngology, 2d ed. Philadelphia, Saunders, 1980.

Penfield, W., and L. Roberts. Speech and Brain-Mechanisms. Princeton, N.J., Princeton University Press, 1959.

Stephens, S. D. G. Application of psychoacoustics to central auditory dysfunction. In

Scientific Foundations of Otolaryngology, R. Hinchcliffe and D. Harrison (eds.). Chicago, Heinemann, 1976, pp. 352–61.

Stockard, J. J., and V. S. Rossiter. Clinical and pathologic correlates of brain stem auditory response abnormalities. *Neurology* 27:316–25, 1977.

Suga, N. Feature extraction in the auditory system in bats. In *Basic Mechanisms in Hearing,* A. R. Moller (ed.). New York, Academic Press, 1973, pp. 675–744.

7.

Visual System

ALAN L. PEARLMAN

Humans are highly visual animals. With our visual system we are able to detect light and shadow, form and motion, color and depth. But this list only begins to describe the rudiments of vision and takes no account of such remarkable visual functions as reading or recognizing familiar faces. To carry out this wide range of functions, the pathways and centers within the brain that are involved in vision are extensively interconnected with other systems. The clinical importance of the visual system arises both from these interconnections and from its long traverse through the brain, from the retina to the occipital cortex. Although this long course makes the system susceptible to damage at many different sites, its anatomical features provide important clues to the localization of the disease process. In addition, recent progress in the analysis of the structure and function of the system has proven to be very helpful in understanding some of the symptoms that occur when the system is not functioning normally.

The visual system has also been of considerable importance in advancing our understanding of nervous system func-

tion. It is at present the best understood of the sensory systems, in large measure because the eyes are relatively accessible for experimental manipulation, and each eye provides a separate but highly comparable set of input fibers. The removal of one eye was one of the earliest experiments carried out to trace the course of a degenerating central nervous system pathway. Many recent developments in tract-tracing methodology were tested first by injecting a particular tracer substance into one eye. The visual system has also been extremely important in studies of the development of the central nervous system. These studies have examined the role of early sensory experience in development, the mechanisms involved in establishing the highly ordered connections between afferent axons and their synaptic targets, and the role of competitive interactions among incoming axons for synaptic sites.

This chapter will review the features of the anatomy and physiology of the visual system that have particular clinical relevance, and the ways that altered development and acquired lesions affect visual system function.

RETINA AND OPTIC NERVE

The visual image is focused on the retina by the cornea and lens. Most of the refraction required to form the image occurs at the air–cornea interface; the lens provides the adjustments of focus that occur as we look from distant objects to objects that are nearby. This accommodative ability gradually declines with age as the lens loses its elasticity.

The retina is a part of the central nervous system. It is derived from the optic vesicles that grow out from the brain during early development, and the myelin in its output pathway, the optic nerve, is provided by oligodendroglia. Since the neurons and glia of the retina and its vasculature are subject to many of the diseases that affect other parts of the central nervous system, examination of the retina with an ophthalmoscope is an extremely important part of the neurological evaluation.

The process of transduction from light to chemical and electrical energy takes place in the photoreceptors, the rods and cones. Light must pass through the other retinal elements, which are transparent, to reach the outer segments of the photoreceptors (rods and cones) adjacent to the pigment epithelium. The outer segments of both rods and cones are densely packed with disk-shaped elements that contain the photopigments. Each of the three cone types and the rods contains a different photopigment. Each photopigment is characterized by its absorption spectrum, the curve that indicates that the ability of the photopigment to capture photons differs as a function of the wavelength of the light striking it.

The rod system functions in night vision. It is very sensitive to low light levels, but is color-blind. This inability to distinguish colors is a result of the fact that all of the rods contain the same photopigment, rhodopsin, which undergoes the same conformational change after capture of a photon, no matter what the wavelength of the stimulating light. Since the absorbtion spectrum of rhodopsin peaks in the green region of the spectrum, objects that reflect green will appear brighter than those that reflect red, which is less efficiently absorbed. But the objects will not appear colored when the illumination is dim. It is the event of photon capture that is signaled, not the wavelength, so that the rod system is only able to distinguish brightness differences, not colors.

In order to distinguish colors, at least two photopigments with different spectral sensitivities are required. These photopigments must be contained in separate photoreceptors, and there must be a subsequent neuron that signals the difference in input from the two types of receptor. The cone system, which functions at higher light levels, meets these requirements. Humans have three types of cones, which differ by the absorbtion spectrum of photopigment they contain. The three absorbtion spectra, which are broad and overlapping, are named for their peaks, and the cones are named for the pigments they contain, i.e., red, green, and blue.

Color blindness: About 8% of males have a hereditary defect in their ability to discriminate colors. Although these individuals are commonly called "color-blind," a better term would be color-defective since they are able to make many color discriminations, but their abilities are not the same as those of normal individuals. Protanopia and deuteranopia are two common types of color-vision defect. These are sex-linked heredity conditions, carried on the X chromosome and thus expressed predominantly in males and carried by females. In protanopia the red cone pigment is replaced by one that is identical to the green pigment; in deuteranopia the green pigment is replaced by red. Thus individuals with these two color vision defects have trouble discriminating reds from greens since in effect they have only one photopigment covering that range of the spectrum.

Retinal anatomy and physiology

The retinal photoreceptors are distributed in a characteristic pattern across the retina that gives rise to functional differences in the various retinal areas. The macula, which is very rich in cones, contains a central pit called the fovea (Fig. 7–1A). The foveola, at the very center of the fovea, contains only cones. The other retinal elements have been displaced aside, since although they are transparent, they produce sufficient light scatter to reduce acuity slightly. The cones in the foveola are the smallest and most densely packed in the retina (Fig. 7–1). This combination of small, densely packed photoreceptors and the elimination of light-scattering elements produces the retinal zone of highest acuity. The bipolar cells and ganglion cells subserving central vision are also small and densely packed. The cone concentration peaks sharply in the central 5° of the retina, then falls off abruptly to a low level (4,000–5,000/mm^2) over the rest of the retina (Fig. 7–1B). The rods are completely absent from the foveola. Rod concentration peaks about 20° away from the fovea and then drops off gradually to a concentration of 30,000–40,000/mm^2 over the rest of the retina (Fig. 7–1B). The other neuronal elements are also larger and less densely packed in the areas away from the central retina, and there is more convergence of connections from receptors onto other neurons, resulting in lower acuity, but better sensitivity to low light levels.

The photoreceptors connect to bipolar cells, which in turn connect to the ganglion cells that send their axons into the optic nerve. The photoreceptors are also connected to horizontal cells, which provide extensive lateral interactions in the outer plexiform layer. The bipolar cells also connect to amacrine cells, which carry out lateral interactions in the inner plexiform layer between bipolar cells, ganglion cells, and other amacrine cells. Since the only neuronal elements present in the optic nerve head are the axons of the ganglion cells as they gather to leave the eye, this zone is a blind spot in the visual field.

Each neuron in the retina responds to stimulation in a particular part of the visual field. That part of the visual field is called the *receptive field* of the cell, and the stimulus features that produce a response make up the receptive field properties of the neuron. For example, a retinal ganglion cell with an on-center, off-surround receptive field responds to light in the center of the field with an increase in firing rate (on response, Fig. 7–2A, B), whereas illumination of an area around the central zone inhibits the response elicited by central illumination (Fig. 7–2C). A relative decrease in the illumination of the surround zone increases the cell's firing rate (off response, Fig. 7–2D). The original study of the cat's retina by Kuffler also described neurons with the reverse configuration, that is, off-center, on-surround. Since then, the extensive analysis of retinal ganglion cells that has been carried out in several species has defined many more types of receptive fields. Intracellular injections of various dyes during the course of physiological study have helped to provide correlations between receptive field type and ganglion cell morphology. At present more than 20 types of retinal ganglion cells have been identified in the cat's retina on the basis of their morphology and physiological responses.

Optic nerve

Axons of the retinal ganglion cells come together at the optic nerve head and penetrate the sclera of the eye through the lamina cribrosa to become myelineated just behind the globe (Fig. 7–3). The membranes surrounding the optic nerve are continuous with those that surround the

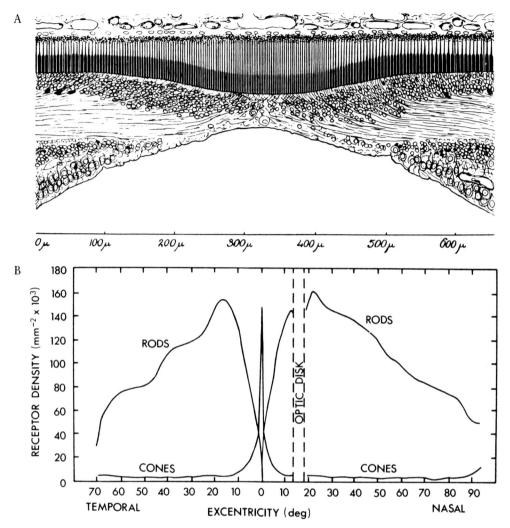

Fig. 7–1. A. Fovea of the human retina. The photoreceptors are shown as dark lines at the top of the figure, their outer ends in contact with the pigment epithelium. The cones are long, thin, and very densely packed in the foveal pit. Cone nuclei are shown as open circles in the outer nuclear layer. Rod nuclei, shown as filled circles, are absent from the foveola in the center of the foveal pit and are present in small numbers at the edges. The other retinal layers are swept aside. (From S. Polyak, *The Vertebrate Visual System.* Chicago, The University of Chicago Press, 1957.) **B.** Density of rods and cones in the human retina. (From M. H. Pirenne, *Vision and the Eye.* London, Chapman and Hall, 1967.)

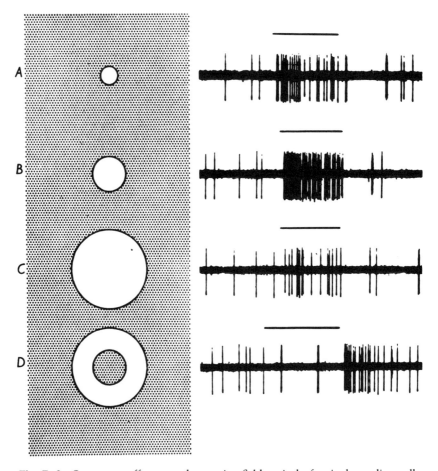

Fig. 7–2. On-center, off-surround receptive field typical of retinal ganglion cells, cells in the lateral geniculate nucleus, and cells in layer IV of monkey cortex. Light stimuli centered on the receptive field are shown at the left on a dark screen; action potentials recorded from a single neuron with an extracellular microelectrode are shown on the right. The bar over each response indicates when the stimulus light is on. A small spot in the receptive field center (**A**) produces an excitatory response when the stimulus is on; a slightly larger spot (**B**) produces more excitation. Illumination of both center and surround (**C**) produces much less response than illumination of the center alone, while stimulation of just the surround with an annulus of light (**D**) inhibits the spontaneous firing of the cell and produces an increase in firing when the annulus is turned off. [From D. H. Hubel and T. N. Wiesel, Integrative activity in the cat's lateral geniculate body. *J. Physiol.* (Lond.) 155:385, 1961.]

brain. The dura of the optic nerve is continuous with those that surround the sclera; the optic nerve is also surrounded by arachnoid and pia and is bathed by cerebral spinal fluid (CSF) in the subarachnoid space (Fig. 7–3). Elevated CSF pressure is thus transmitted to the subarachnoid space around the optic nerve.

Papilledema

Although swelling of the optic nerve head can have many local or systemic causes, the term *papilledema* usually refers to optic disk swelling associated with and caused by increased intracranial pressure.

Several features characterize the early

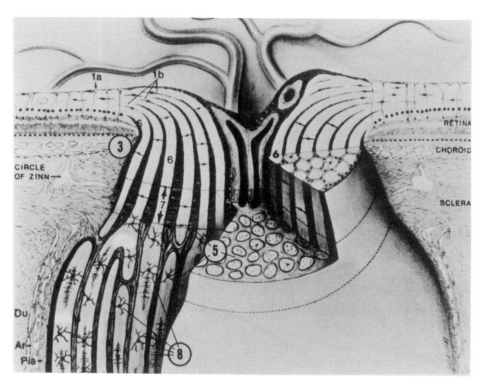

Fig. 7–3. Schematic representation of the optic nerve as it penetrates the sclera to leave the eye. 1a, internal limiting membrane of the retina; 1b, layer of ganglion cell axons; 2, optic cup and central retinal vessels; 3, edge of the optic disk that is visible with an ophthalmoscope; 5, glial and connective tissue columns; 6, fascicles of nerve fibers; 7, lamina cribrosa; 8, oligodendroglia that form the myelin of the optic nerve; Du, dura; Ar, arachnoid. The circle of Zinn is an arterial network with contributions from the posterior ciliary arteries, the pial arteries, and the choroid, that provides blood supply to the optic nerve. (Modified from Glaser, 1978. Original from D. R. Anderson and W. F. Hoyt, Ultrastructure of intraorbital portion of human and monkey optic nerve. *Arch. Ophthalmol.* 82:506, 1969.)

stages of papilledema. These include hyperemia of the optic disk as a result of dilitation of disk capillaries, absence of spontaneous venous pulsations, blurring of the optic disk margins, obliteration of the optic cup by mild swelling of the disk, and small splinter hemorrhages around the disk in the optic fiber layer. As papilledema becomes more fully developed, the disk swelling becomes more pronounced and the retinal veins become engorged. More splinter hemorrhages and small retinal infarcts occur. Subhyloid hemorrhages, which appear between the retina and the vitreous, occur if the increase in cerebral spinal fluid pressure has been rapid. If the papilledema is persistent, damage to the optic nerve fibers occurs with subsequent optic atrophy.

The distinction between papilledema caused by increased intracranial pressure and optic disk swelling caused by lesions in the optic nerve just behind the globe is based in part on examination of the visual fields. Even when papilledema is severe, the visual field defect often consists of nothing more than an enlargement of the blind spot. On the other hand, optic disk swelling produced by inflammatory or vascular lesions at or behind the disk, which cause an ophthalmoscopic picture that is difficult to distinguish from papilledema, produce central scotomas that severely impair vision.

For many years it was thought that elevated CSF pressure caused papilledema by impairing venous return from the optic disk and optic nerve, thereby producing an accumulation of extracellular fluid and swelling of the optic nerve head. More recently it has been demonstrated that the swelling is mainly a result of enlargement of the ganglion cell axons at the nerve head produced by an obstruction to the flow of materials within the axon in the normal process of axoplasmic transport. The obstruction to flow results from increased pressure on the optic nerve as it enters the subarachnoid space just behind the eye. Swelling of the optic nerve head that mimics papilledema can be produced by drugs that block axoplasmic transport in the absence of elevated CSF pressure. Vascular compression must also occur to account for the loss of spontaneous venous pulsations, venous engorgement, capillary dilitation, venous hemorrhages, and infarcts.

OPTIC CHIASM AND TRACT

The fibers of the two optic nerves come together in the optic chiasm; fibers from the nasal half of each retina cross to the opposite side while fibers from the temporal aspect of each retina enter the optic tract on the same side (Fig. 7–4). This crossing brings information from the right visual field into the left side of the brain and vice versa.

The anatomical relationships of the optic chiasm play a critical role in its involvement by disease processes. The chiasm lies above the sella turcica, where it is subject to compression by tumors of the pituitary that grow out of the sella, or by parasellar lesions such as meningiomas of the dorsum sellae. The internal carotid arteries ascend on either side of the chiasm, making it vulnerable to compression by

carotid aneurysms. The optic chiasm forms a part of the anterior-inferior wall of the third ventricle where it is sometimes compressed by tumors of the pituitary stalk or hypothalamus. Lesions compressing the chiasm from above or below characteristically produce damage to the crossing fibers of the chiasm, resulting in loss of the visual field subserved by both nasal retinas, i.e., bitemporal hemianopia (Fig. 7–4; lesion 2). Lesions damaging fibers in the anterolateral aspect of the chiasm produce vision loss in one eye as a result of involvement of the optic nerve and in the contralateral temporal visual field as a result of damage to the crossing fibers in the chiasm (Fig. 7–4; lesion 4).

As the axons of the retinal ganglion cells leave the optic chiasm they form the optic tract, which courses around the cerebral peduncle on its way to the lateral geniculate nucleus in the thalamus and to the several other sites where retinal ganglion cell axons terminate. Lesions that damage the optic tract are relatively rare. When such damage does occur, it produces visual field defects in the contralateral hemifield (Fig. 7–4; lesion 3). Since the axons from the two eyes are not completely intermixed in the optic tract, the resultant visual field defects are usually incongruous, i.e., not involving exactly the same parts of the two hemifields.

Although the majority of optic tract axons end in the lateral geniculate nucleus and in the superior colliculus, they also provide input to several other centers. Fibers from each eye project to both Edinger-Westphal nuclei in the pretectal region of the midbrain, which are the parasympathetic motor nuclei for pupillary constriction. This bilateral innervation results in constriction of both pupils when light is shown on one retina. Damage to one optic nerve will result in a decrease in the pupillary response to light in that eye. This *afferent pupillary defect* is easily demonstrable by the pupillary dilitation that occurs when the light is moved from the

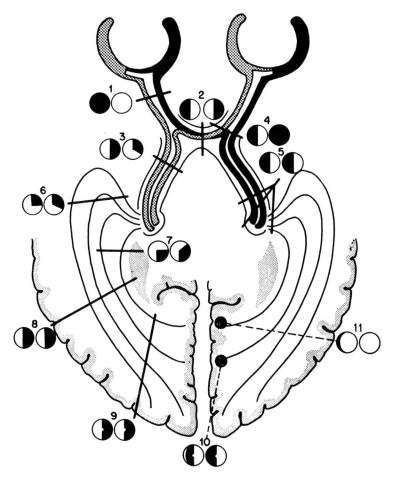

Fig. 7–4. Diagrammatic representation of the visual pathways viewed from the base of the brain and the visual field defects produced by lesions at the sites indicated. Actual visual field defects are seldom as clearly delineated as those shown schematically here. 1. Transection of the left optic nerve, producing total loss of vision in the left eye, sparing the right. 2. Bitemporal hemianopia resulting from a lesion of the crossing fibers in the optic chiasm. 3. Partial lesion of the left optic tract producing an incongruous right hemianopia. 4. Involvement of the anterior aspect of the chiasm at the junction with the optic nerve causing loss of vision in one eye and temporal field loss in the other. 5. Complete lesions in the optic tract, lateral geniculate, or the origin of the optic radiations result in contralateral homonymous hemianopia. 6. A lesion in the anterior aspect of the left temporal lobe produces a right superior quadrantanopia. 7. Interruption of the medial fibers of the left optic radiations causes a right inferior quadrantanopia. 8. Lesion in the left optic radiations producing a right homonymous hemianopia. 9. Lesion of the left visual cortex with right homonymous hemianopia and macular sparing. 10. Lesion involving the posterior aspect of the right visual cortex, producing a left homonymous hemianopia that spares the temporal crescent of the left eye. 11. A small lesion of the anterior aspect of the right visual cortex, causing loss of vision only in the temporal crescent of the left eye. (Adapted from D. O. Harrington, *The Visual Fields: A Textbook and Atlas of Clinical Perimetry,* 4th ed. St. Louis, Mosby, 1976.)

normal eye to the eye with damage to the optic nerve.

Optic tract axons also terminate in the pretectal nuclei and the accessory optic nuclei, which, along with the superior colliculus, are important in the control of eye movements. In addition, optic tract axons terminate in the suprachiasmatic nuclei of the hypothalamus, where they presumably play a role in light-mediated endocrine responses.

ALBINISM AND THE OPTIC CHIASM

The optic chiasm is an extremely important structure in diagnostic neurology. The differences in the field defects that arise with lesions in front of, within, and behind the chiasm provide critical localizing information. For the neurobiologist interested in how the brain develops, the optic chiasm poses questions of a very fundamental nature: What are the factors that guide the ganglion cell axons of the retina toward their several sites of termination in the nervous system? What determines that fibers from a particular part of the retina will head for the left side while others will head for the right? Although the answers to these questions are far from clear, there is a condition that occurs in many mammals, including humans, in which some of the retinal ganglion cell fibers take a wrong turn at the optic chiasm and end up on the incorrect side of the brain. The misdirected fibers arise primarily from a segment of the temporal retina of variable size near the vertical midline. These fibers normally should enter the ipsilateral optic tract; instead they cross in the chiasm and proceed to targets on the contralateral side. Thus an abnormally large extent of the visual field of one eye is represented in the opposite hemisphere. This anomaly was first discovered in Siamese cats, where it was detected because it produced a disruption in the laminar pattern of the lateral geniculate as a consequence of the ab-

normal innervation by fibers from the contralateral temporal retina. Since Siamese cats have a form of albinism, the defect was looked for and found to be present in a wide range of albino mammals. It is now evident that the abnormality in the crossing of retinal ganglion cell axons at the optic chiasm is associated with virtually all forms of albinism that produce an absence of pigment in the retinal pigment epithelium. This is true even though the genetic defects that produce the various forms of albinism are quite different.

A number of studies of albino humans have indicated that the abnormal crossing pattern also occurs in man. Although very few brains from human albinos have been studied, they show a severe disruption of the layering of the lateral geniculate analogous to that seen in the Siamese cat. The visual-evoked response recorded from albino humans is much larger when the eye contralateral to the recording electrode over the occipital pole is stimulated than when the ipsilateral eye is stimulated. Since the visual-evoked responses recorded over one occipital pole in normal humans during monocular stimulation are approximately equal, this observation indicates that albino humans have more input reaching the visual cortex from the contralateral eye than is normally the case, and less from the ipsilateral eye. This abnormality in the connections of the visual system undoubtedly contributes to the visual disabilities that albino humans experience, although the precise extent of this contribution has not been determined. Nor is the presumed relationship between melanin in the retinal pigment epithelium and the course taken by ganglion cell axons understood. But the widespread occurrence of the abnormal crossing pattern at the optic chiasm among so many different mammals with albinism strongly suggests that an understanding of this relationship will provide important clues to the mechanisms by which axons find their targets in the development of the central nervous system.

LATERAL GENICULATE NUCLEUS

The neurons of the lateral geniculate nucleus are segregated into discrete layers. In the human lateral geniculate, there are six layers in the portion of the geniculate that represents central vision. Two of the four dorsal layers receive input from the contralateral eye and two from the ipsilateral eye. Each of the two ventral layers receives input from one eye. Each layer contains a map of the contralateral visual hemifield; the maps are in register so that a microelectrode passing from dorsal to ventral at an appropriate angle will encounter cells in each layer with receptive fields in the same part of the visual field. Complex synaptic interactions occur between the incoming optic tract axons, the principal cells of the lateral geniculate that project via the optic radiations to the visual cortex, and the interneurons of the lateral geniculate. In addition, the lateral geniculate receives a strong projection back from the visual cortex. Studies of the receptive fields of individual lateral geniculate neurons in cats and several subhuman primates have demonstrated a segregation of functionally distinct neurons in the various geniculate laminae. Although the functional significance of this careful anatomical and physiological segregation is not yet understood, the segregation is maintained in subsequent processing; axons from the dorsal and ventral laminae of the geniculate terminate in different layers of the striate cortex.

Identifiable clinical involvement of the lateral geniculate is quite rare, in part because it receives its blood supply from both the internal carotid by way of the anterior choroidal artery and from the posterior cerebral artery by way of the thalamogeniculate branch. Lesions involving the optic radiations are much more common. As the optic radiations leave the lateral geniculate, the fibers run laterally over the temporal horn of the lateral ventricle. The fibers representing the superior aspect of the contralateral hemifield run anterolaterally around the anterior aspect of the temporal horn of the lateral ventricle. Lesions in the anterior aspect of the temporal lobe therefore produce vision loss in the contralateral superior visual field of both eyes, known as a "pie-in-the-sky" defect (Fig. 7–4; lesion 6). The optic radiation fibers then course posteriorly and turn medially to terminate in the striate cortex on the medial aspect of the occipital lobe.

VISUAL CORTEX

The primary visual cortex, also called the *striate cortex* or *calcarine cortex,* extends from the occipital pole anteriorly along the calcarine fissure. Most of the striate cortex is buried in the depths of the calcarine fissure. The superior visual field is represented on the inferior lip of the calcarine fissure while the inferior visual field is represented on the superior lip (Fig. 7–5). The central aspect of the visual field is represented posteriorly; the macular region is represented on the occipital pole. The representation of the peripheral visual field lies anterior in the calcarine cortex (Fig. 7–5). The segment representing the extreme temporal aspect of the contralateral field receives input only from the contralateral nasal retina; there is no matching input from the ipsilateral temporal retina. Thus the extreme temporal aspect of the contralateral visual field is the only portion of the cortical representation of the field that is monocular. Since this region lies so far anteriorly, it is sometimes spared in lesions involving the occipital pole (Fig. 7–4; lesion 10).

The central visual field is disproportionately represented in the visual cortex, just as the thumb and forefinger are disproportionately represented in the sensorymotor cortex (Fig. 7–5). In the monkey, the central 5° of the visual field occupies approximately 30% of the surface of the primary visual cortex. In contrast to the retina, where the receptors and other neural

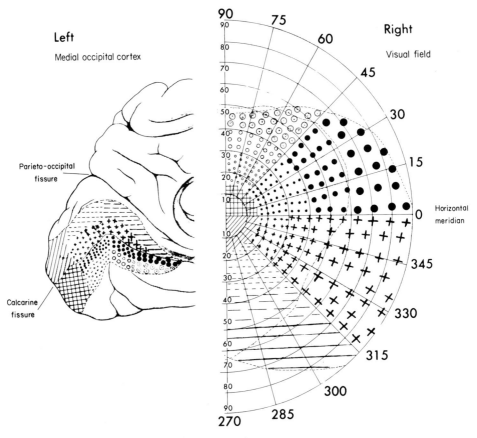

Fig. 7–5. Diagrammatic representation of the right visual field drawn on the striate cortex of the human left hemisphere. The calcarine fissure has been opened to show the cortical surface. The symbols on the cortex indicate the representation of the part of the right visual field that is filled with the same symbols. (From S. Duke-Elder, *System of Ophthalmology*. St. Louis, Mosby, 1961.)

elements are small and densely packed in the fovea to provide the neural apparatus for high acuity, the neural elements in the visual cortex are uniform in size and density. The neural apparatus necessary to process the fine detail of central vision is provided by devoting a much larger area of cortex to each degree of central field than to each degree of peripheral field.

The field defects arising from lesions of the visual cortex are characteristically congruous, since the cortex is the first place where single neurons receive input from both eyes. Lesions of the occipital lobes sometimes produce visual field defects in which the central few degrees of the field are spared (Fig. 7–4; lesion 9). This situation, called *macular sparing*, is sometimes simply an artifact produced by poor fixation during visual field testing. In some instances, macular sparing is a reflection of the large representation of central vision, since a large representation has a better chance of being spared in a destructive process than a small one. The occipital pole, where the central visual field is

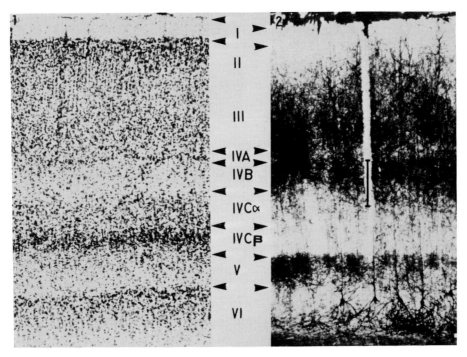

Fig. 7–6. Striate cortex of the monkey, *Macaca mulatta*. The laminar distribution of neuronal cell bodies is evident in the Nissl-stained section on the left, while the extensive processes of cortical neurons are visualized in the section stained with a Golgi method on the right. Roman numerals identify the cortical laminae in both sections. The stria of Gennari is indicated by the vertical bar in the center of the section on the right. Several large pyramidal cells can be seen in layer VI on the right. (From J. S. Lund, Organization of neurons in the visual cortex, area 17, of the monkey. *J. Comp. Neurol.* 147:455–95, 1973.)

represented, receives a variable degree of collateral circulation from the middle cerebral artery in addition to the major contribution from the posterior cerebral artery. Thus a vascular occlusion of the posterior cerebral artery might result in a contralateral visual field loss that does not involve central vision in instances where the collateral circulation is prominent. Finally, there is recent evidence that the dividing line in the retina between retinal ganglion cells that project to the same side and those that cross in the optic chiasm may not be sharp. To the extent that this overlap is greater in the macular region than in other parts of the retina, this bilat-

eral representation might also account for macular sparing.

Neurons of the cerebral cortex are organized in distinct layers separated by zones that are relatively free of neuronal cell bodies (Fig. 7–6). The primary visual cortex has a highly distinctive pattern of lamination that makes it one of the most easily recognized of all of the cortical areas. It contains a dense band of dendrites and axons called the stria of Gennari, which is visible to the unaided eye in both fixed and fresh specimens. It is this stria that gives rise to the name *striate cortex*. The lateral geniculate axons terminate in layer IV (Fig. 7–6) of striate cortex. Although informa-

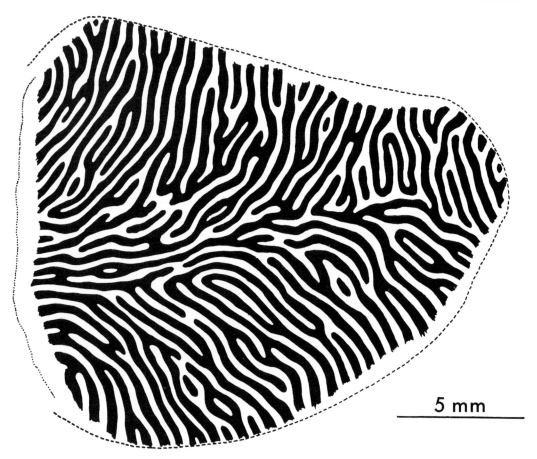

Fig. 7–7. Ocular dominance columns in the striate cortex of the monkey. The view is of a large tangential section of layer IVC viewed from above. Black represents ocular dominance columns of one eye, white the other. (From D. H. Hubel and T. N. Wiesel, 1977.)

tion from the two eyes will eventually come together on neurons above and below layer IV, most neurons in layer IV receive input from only one eye. Afferents representing input from each eye are grouped together in distinct bands with very little overlap. These bands have been demonstrated by several neuroanatomical techniques; they are most clearly evident when the cortex is sectioned tangentially (Fig. 7–7).

Neurons in layer IV of the rhesus monkey's visual cortex have receptive fields with a concentric, center-surround organization that resembles the receptive fields

of lateral geniculate cells (Fig. 7–2). The receptive fields of neurons above and below layer IV are strikingly different. These cells respond best to stimuli of particular orientations (Fig. 7–8). Hubel and Wiesel, who discovered the orientation specificity of neurons in the visual cortex, also discovered that cells responsive to a particular orientation were grouped in columns. A microelectrode passing from the pial surface to the white matter perpendicular to the cortical layers will encounter one neuron after another with the same orientation specificity. A microelectrode

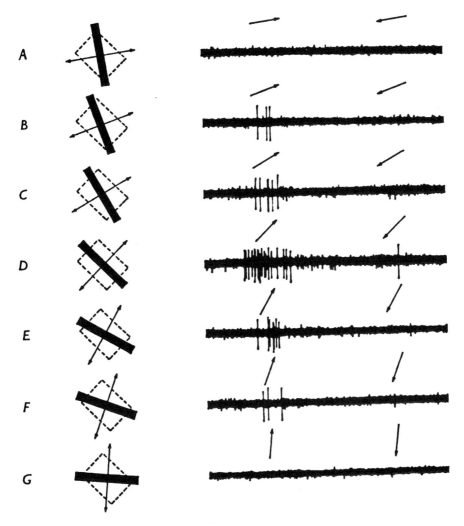

A

B

C

D

E

F

G

Fig. 7–8. Oriented receptive field of a neuron in the striate cortex of the monkey. The receptive field is shown by the dashed outline. In each row the stimulus, indicated by the black bar, is presented in a slightly different orientation, and moved back and forth in the direction of the arrows. The response to each direction is shown in the oscilloscope records on the right, under the corresponding arrow. This cell not only requires a particular orientation (**D**) for the best response, but also responds to only one direction of stimulus movement. (From D. H. Hubel and T. N. Wiesel, Receptive fields and functional architecture of monkey striate cortex. *J. Physiol.* (Lond. 195:215–43, 1968.)

moving downward through the cortex at some angle other than perpendicular to the cortical layers encounters neurons first with one receptive field orientation, and then others with a slightly different orientation (Fig. 7–9). Thus orientation specificity shifts gradually from one orientation column to the next until all orientations have been encountered. The 2-deoxyglucose method, which demonstrates neurons that are responding to a particular stimulus, has been useful in outlining orientation col-

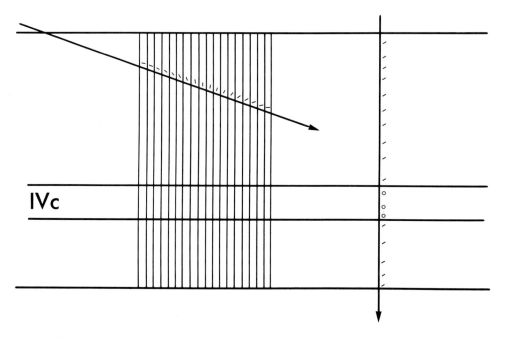

Fig. 7–9. Diagrammatic representation of orientation columns in the striate cortex of the monkey. The arrow on the right indicates a vertical electrode penetration from the pial surface to the white matter. Each neuron encountered has the same receptive field orientation, indicated by the short lines next to the arrow. Receptive fields of neurons in layer IVC (circles) are not oriented. The arrow on the left represents an oblique electrode penetration, which encounters neurons with slightly different receptive field orientations as it moves from one orientation column to the next. (From D. H. Hubel and T. N. Wiesel, 1977.)

umns (Fig. 7–10). As is the case with ocular dominance columns, orientation columns are much more like strips or slabs when viewed in tangential sections of the cortex. However, the term *column* was applied to the original descriptions and has persisted in the literature.

The receptive fields of cortical neurons above and below layer IV have very prominent orientation specificity. They respond best to lines, bars, or edges of a particular orientation and poorly or not at all when the line stimulus is not in that preferred orientation. Neurons in layers above and below layer IV also receive input from both eyes. Neurons in the striate cortex that receive input from both eyes receive that input from corresponding parts of the two retinae. In addition, the input

is organized so that the receptive field properties elicited by stimulation of each eye are exactly the same. Although most cells in the monkey's striate cortex respond to stimulation of both eyes, the response from one eye is often stronger than the response from the other.

Migraine. The visual cortex is frequently involved in the prodromal phase of classic migraine. The attack typically begins with impairment of central vision in one hemifield. The patient then becomes aware of bright, flashing, diagonal lines surrounding the area of decreased vision. The diagonal lines form an arc around the area of blindness *(scotoma);* because of its resemblance to the outer walls of an ancient fortified city, the arc is called a *foritification figure* or *spectrum*. Since the

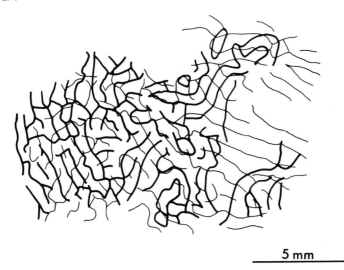

5 mm

Fig. 7–10. Orientation columns and ocular dominance columns in the striate cortex of the monkey. The thick lines show the vertical orientation columns in a tangential section of layer VI demonstrated by stimulating the visual field with vertical stripes while infusing radioactive 2-deoxyglucose. The thin lines indicate the ocular dominance columns in a superimposed tangential section of layer IVC of the same monkey. Thus far no definite relationship between ocular dominance columns and orientation columns has become apparent. (From D. H. Hubel, T. N. Wiesel, and M. P. Stryker, Anatomical demonstration of orientation columns in macaque monkey. *J. Comp. Neurol.* 177:361–80, 1978.)

fortification figure spreads from the center to the periphery of one hemifield in about 20 minutes, and frequently recurs in a similar pattern, several people have been able to draw and write about their own attacks. The neuropsychologist K. S. Lashley provided detailed drawings of his own fortification figures as they enlarged (Fig. 7–11). He noted that the size and shape of the lines that make up the figure did not change as the figure spread across the visual field. Lashley reasoned from this observation and from the constancy of pattern from one attack to the next that "the pattern is a function of the anatomic substratum." It is tempting to speculate, as many authors have, that the "anatomic substratum" may have some relationship to the orientation columns of the visual cortex (Fig. 7–10) that were to be described more than 30 years after Lashley's speculation.

For many years the prodromal phase

of an attack of migraine has been thought to be a manifestation of vasoconstriction. In this formulation, the neurological symptoms, such as the fortification figure and the enlarging scotoma, are the result of cortical ischemia. However, the spread of the disturbance in a manner that takes 10 account of vascular territories, has led many to doubt that cortical ischemia is causal. Recently, cerebral blood flow studies of patients during migraine attacks have shown that although there is a wave of decreased blood flow (oligemia) that begins in the posterior aspect of the hemisphere and spreads forward, the neurological symptoms often precede the oligemia, and the oligemia persists for many minutes after the neurological symptoms have subsided. This evidence supports the hypothesis that the prodromal phase is a manifestation of a phenomenon called *spreading cortical depression*, rather than ischemia. Spreading depression is a brief

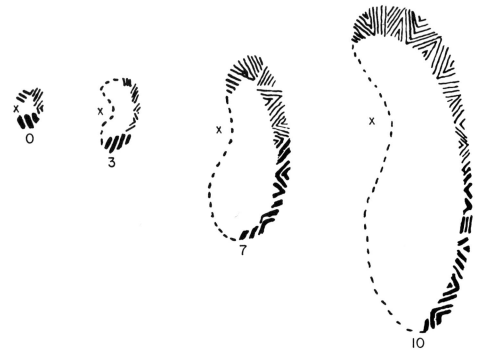

Fig. 7–11. Successive maps of the progression of a scintillating scotoma of classic migraine. The x indicates the fixation point, and the dotted line encompasses the area of decreased or absent vision in the right visual field. The rate of scintillation was about 10 per second. The numbers below each figure indicate minutes from the time when the symptoms started. (From K. S. Lashley, Patterns of cerebral integration indicated by the scotomas of migraine. *Arch. Neurol. Psychiat.* 46:331–9, 1941.)

wave of intense cortical activation that is followed by a marked decrease in neuronal activity and responsiveness that lasts as long as 40–60 minutes. Relative oligemia develops in the depressed region of cortex. The spreading depression hypothesis is supported by the fact that the phenomenon spreads across the cortex at 2–3 mm per minute, the same rate Lashley calculated for the spread of the disturbance across his visual cortex that produced a fortification figure on the edge of an enlarging scotoma. In addition, the oligemia observed in the blood flow studies of patients with migraine spreads from posterior to anterior at the same rate.

Although the spreading depression hypothesis is attractive, it does not account for the headache that usually follows the prodrome, typically on the same side as the involved cortex. In addition, although spreading depression can be elicited in the cortex of experimental animals by intense electrical stimulation, by local increases in extracellular potassium, and by several other rather noxious stimuli, nothing is known about the way it might be produced by humans.

VISUAL DEPRIVATION

Very soon after Hubel and Wiesel began to understand the physiological responses of single cells in the striate cortex, they undertook a series of experiments to determine how these projections might be affected by conditions in which visual input was altered early in the animal's life. These experiments were prompted in part by the clinical observation that children with visual deprivation resulting from lesions like congenital cataracts or corneal scars often have poor vision even after the ocular problem is corrected, and children with congenital strabismus often develop poor vision in one eye. In order to learn something about the pathogenesis of these conditions, as well as to understand more about the role of visual experience in determining the development of the visual cortex, they carried out a series of experiments in which they produced monocular visual deprivation and artificial strabismus in infant kittens and monkeys.

Many of the connections that underlie the function of the striate cortex are established by the time a kitten or monkey is born and thus are not dependent on visual experience. The development of receptive field properties of cortical neurons proceeds normally in the absence of visual experience until the kitten or monkey is three to four weeks old. At that time they enter a period in their development, called the *critical period,* in which further development of the visual system depends in a very important way on the animal's visual experience. In addition, normal visual experience during the critical period, which lasts from 4 weeks to about 12 weeks of age in the cat and about a month longer in the monkey, is essential for the maintenance of the previously established properties of neurons in the striate cortex. *Monocular occlusion* during the critical period, usually accomplished by suturing the eyelid, produces a very dramatic result. Virtually all of the cells in the striate cortex respond only to the eye that remained open and not to the eye that was closed. In addition, the axon terminals of the lateral geniculate cells that receive input from the open eye occupy larger territories in layer IV of the striate cortex than do the terminals of the lateral geniculate

cells that got input from the deprived eye. Thus the ocular dominance columns subserving the normal eye are much larger than those subserving the occluded eye (Fig. 7–12). During normal development, the segregation of lateral geniculate terminals representing each eye appears to take place by a process of competition. The terminals are almost completely overlapping in the early postnatal period. If both eyes are functioning normally or if the animal is reared in total darkness so that neither eye has a competitive advantage, the terminals segregate to form ocular dominance columns. Occlusion of one eye seems to give the other eye a competitive advantage, with the result that the ocular dominance columns representing that eye are much larger and most of the neurons in the cortex respond only to the nondeprived eye.

Not surprisingly, behavioral tests of animals who have had one eye occluded during the critical period demonstrate a severe loss of vision in the eye that was closed. Severity of the vision loss and the severity of the physiological and anatomical changes described earlier depend on when the eye was closed during the critical period and for how long. The changes are reversible to some extent if the eye is reopened during the critical period but not if eye opening occurs later. Eye closure after the critical period does not produce these changes and does not alter the animal's vision.

Experimental strabismus, produced by cutting either the medial or lateral rectus muscle of one eye during the critical period, also induces striking changes. Experimental exotropias (divergent eyes) result in cortical neurons that respond to one eye or the other, but not to both. Vision in each eye remains normal with the exception that stereoscopic depth perception is lost. Experimental esotropias (convergent eyes) produce a more complicated situation. Monkeys reared with this condition have very poor acuity in the in-turning eye

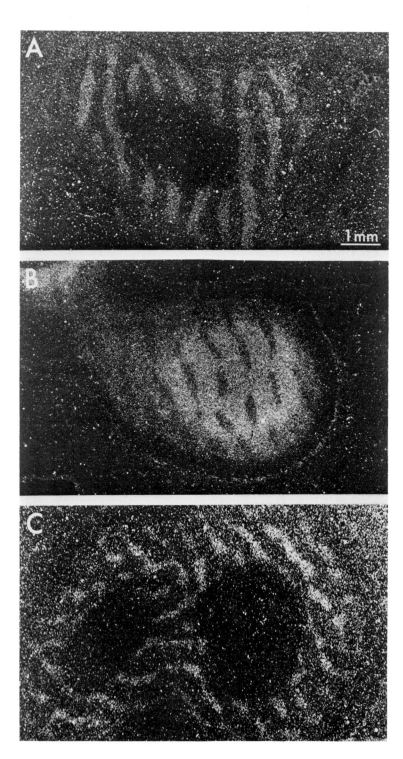

and decreased numbers of cells in the striate cortex that respond to that eye.

In many respects these experimental conditions resemble the phenomenology of human congenital strabismus. Children with exotropias usually alternate fixation. Visual acuity in both eyes is preserved, but stereoscopic depth perception is poor. Children with esotropias often fixate with one eye and lose acuity in the other. The animal experiments have thus far not provided an explanation for this difference between esotropias and exotropias.

Many other alterations in the visual environment have been tried experimentally, and most produce some effect during the critical period. For example, rearing a kitten in a situation where it sees only vertical stripes produces cells in the visual cortex that respond only to stimuli with vertical orientations. This experiment has been likened to the situation in humans in which one or both eyes have severe astigmatism that is not corrected until late in childhood. In the presence of marked astigmatism, lines of a particular orientation are in much worse focus than lines orthogonal to that orientation, in effect producing a kind of deprivation for orientation. When the astigmatism is corrected, these individuals have less ability to detect fine gratings in the orientation that was most severely defocused before correction.

All of these experiments indicate that the striate cortex is extremely sensitive to the effects of visual deprivation during a period early in development. The critical period in humans has not been precisely determined, but monocular deprivation for periods as short as one to four weeks in children under 1 year of age has been shown to produce a significant loss in visual acuity. The critical period for the development of binocularity in humans has been estimated by studying infants who developed convergent strabismus at various ages. Sensitivity to this form of deprivation begins in humans at or soon after birth, peaks between one and three years of age, and probably continues for several more years. Thus, both experimental and clinical observations strongly indicate that strabismus and other conditions that deprive the child of normal visual input should be corrected at the earliest possible time. Once loss of vision occurs, the best hope for recovery is early treatment at a stage when the cortex is still susceptible to alteration.

EXTRASTRIATE VISUAL REGIONS

The traditional view of the organization of the visual regions of the cerebral cortex stems from the cytoarchitectonic observations of Brodmann and others early in this century. This view held that striate

Fig. 7–12. The effect of monocular visual deprivation on the size of ocular dominance columns in the monkey. **A.** Normal ocular dominance columns in a tangential section of layer IV of the striate cortex. The ocular dominance columns have been demonstrated by injecting large amounts of radioactive amino acids into one eye, which are transported up the optic nerve to the lateral geniculate. Some of the radioactive label is taken up by the lateral geniculate cells in the layers innervated by that eye and transported to their cortical terminals. The radioactive label appears as white stripes in these autoradiograms. The large dark areas are zones where the tangential section passes through layers outside layer IV because the cortex is not completely flat. **B.** Ocular dominance columns after monocular eye closure in an infant monkey. In this case the nondeprived eye was injected to demonstrate the wider ocular dominance columns. **C.** Similar to B, but in this case the deprived eye was injected to demonstrate the smaller ocular dominance columns that result. (From D. H. Hubel, T. N. Wiesel, and S. LeVay, *Cold Spring Harbor Symp. Quant. Biol.* 40:581, 1976.)

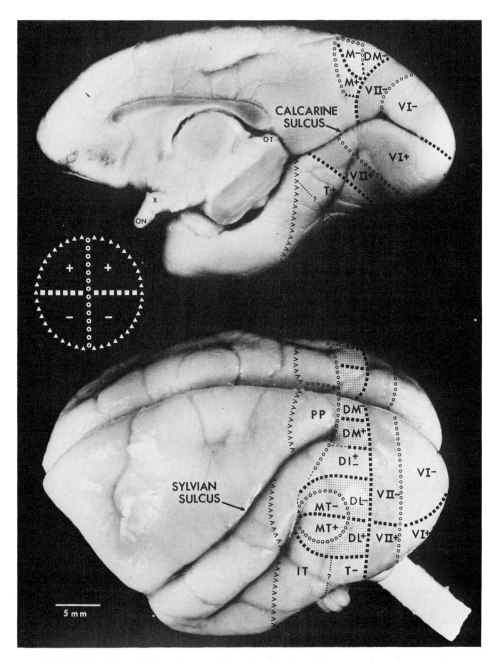

Fig. 7–13. Striate (VI) and extrastriate visual regions demarcated on the smooth cortical surface of the owl monkey. The upper view is of the medial aspect of the right hemisphere. The lower view is of the dorsolateral surface of the brain viewed from the left. The perimeter chart between the two photographs shows the symbols used to indicate the zones of the visual field represented in each cortical map. The outer border of the visual field is represented by triangles, the vertical midline by circles, the horizontal meridian by squares, the upper visual field by plus (+) and the lower field by minus (−). The rows of Vs on the cortical surface represent the limits of visually responsive cortex. VI indicates striate cortex, and VII is the second visual area. The remainder of the abbreviations indicate additional discrete representations of the visual field. (From J. Allman, Evolution of the visual system in the early primates. *Prog. Physiol. Psychol.* 7:1–53, 1977.)

cortex (area 17) is surrounded by two uniform, concentric visual regions, areas 18 and 19. Recent physiological and anatomical observations have led to a major revision of this concept. Instead of two extrastriate visual regions there are a great many, and their arrangement is considerably more complex than the early cytoarchitectonic studies suggested. Each of these several representations contains a partial or complete representation of the contralateral hemifield. These regions have been most extensively studied in the owl monkey, whose cerebral cortex is almost free of the variable and complex cortical convolutions that complicate the analysis of other primates (Fig. 7–13). Areas 18 and 19 and the parietal and temporal cortex adjacent to them contain several visual field representations. The principle of multiple cortical representations of sensory surfaces applies to the auditory and somatosensory systems as well. The extrastriate visual regions receive input from the lateral posterior nucleus and pulvinar of the thalamus, both of which receive visual input from the superior colliculus. The extrastriate visual regions are also extensively interconnected with the striate cortex and with each other.

The anatomical and physiological delineation of the extrastriate visual areas has proceeded further than the understanding of their functional significance. There are indications, however, that some of these regions are specialized for the analysis of particular aspects of vision. For example, an area in the rhesus monkey cortex called the V4 complex contains a high prevalence of cells that respond preferentially to particular colors. These cells are much less prevalent in the other extrastriate visual regions that have been studied. A few patients have been reported with lesions involving the extrastriate visual cortex in the anteromedial aspect of the occipital lobe, at the occipitotemporal junction. These patients have severely impaired ability to discriminate colors even though visual acuity, stereoscopic depth perception, and many other functions are not disturbed. Such patients lend support to the concept that the extrastriate visual regions are specialized for particular visual functions and suggest that a cortical region or regions with functions similar to the V4 complex of rhesus monkey exists in humans.

GENERAL REFERENCES

Boynton, R. M. *Human Color Vision.* New York, Holt, Rinehart and Winston, 1979.

Creel, D., F. E. O'Donnell, Jr., and C. J. Witkop. Visual system anomalies in human ocular albinos. *Science* 201:931–3, 1978.

Daw, N. W. Color vision. In *Adler's Physiology of the Eye*, 7th ed., R. A. Moses (ed.). St. Louis, Mosby, 1980, pp. 545–61.

Gilbert, C. D. Microcircuitry of the visual cortex. *Ann. Rev. Neurosci.* 6:217–47, 1983.

Glaser, J. S. (ed.). *Neuro-opthalmology.* Hagerstown, Md., Harper & Row, 1978.

Guillery, R. W. Visual pathways in albinos. *Scientific American* 230:44–5, 1974.

Hubel, D. H., and T. N. Wiesel. Functional architecture of macaque monkey visual cortex. *Proc. Roy. Soc. London, Ser. B* 198:1–59, 1977.

Miller, N. R. *Walsh and Hoyt's Clinical Neuro-ophthalmology*, 4th ed. Baltimore, Williams & Wilkins, 1982.

Pearlman, A. L. Anatomy and physiology of central visual pathways. In *Adler's Physiology of the Eye*, 7th ed., R. A. Moses (ed.). St. Louis, Mosby, 1980, pp. 427–65.

Pearlman, A. L., J. Birch, and J. C. Meadows. Cerebral color blindness: an acquired defect in hue discrimination. *Ann. Neurol.* 5:253–61, 1979.

Shatz, C. J. Abnormal connections in the visual system of Siamese cats. *Soc. Neurosci. Symp.* 4:121–41, 1979.

Zeki, S. The representation of colours in the cerebral cortex. *Nature* 284:412–18, 1980.

8.

Eye Movements and Vestibular System

RONALD M. BURDE

The primary function of the oculomotor system is to move the eyes so that the image of a particular object falls on the foveas of both retinas simultaneously and stays there. The coordination of both eyes demands continuous neural output to all of the extraocular muscles. Thus, unlike skeletal muscle, there is never total electrical silence in an extraocular muscle even though ocular movements are accomplished according to Sherrington's law of reciprocal innervation, i.e., activation of the agonist is accompanied by inhibition of the antagonist.

NUCLEAR AND INFRANUCLEAR MECHANISMS

The final common pathway for eye movements includes the neurons of the oculomotor, trochlear, and abducens nuclei (cranial nerves III, IV, and VI) in the brainstem and the extraocular muscles that they control.

Extraocular muscles

The extraocular muscles controlling eye movement may be grouped into three antagonist pairs: (1) the superior and infe-

rior rectus muscles, (2) the lateral and medial rectus muscles, and (3) the superior and inferior oblique muscles. Each muscle is active during all extraocular movements, but the action of an individual muscle may be isolated for testing in one particular field of gaze (Fig. 8–1). In that field of gaze an abnormality of its function is determined by the presence of a measurable deviation of the eyes.

The movement of one eye alone is called a *ductional* movement. The medial and lateral rectus muscles primarily act in horizontal movements; the medial rectus muscle moves the eye toward the nose (adduction), and the lateral rectus muscle moves the eye temporally (abduction). Vertical movements are controlled primarily by the vertical recti. The superior rectus muscle is the main elevator in all positions of gaze, and the inferior rectus muscle is the major depressor in all positions of gaze. When the eye is adducted past the primary straightahead position, the oblique muscles play an increasing role in vertical movements with the inferior oblique acting as an elevator and the superior oblique muscle as a depressor. Although the major action of the obliques is

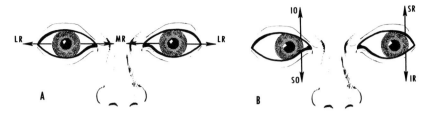

Fig. 8–1. Primary actions of the extraocular muscles. **A.** Horizontal rectus muscles: MR, medial rectus; LR, lateral rectus. **B.** Vertical muscles: SR, superior rectus; IR, inferior rectus; SO, superior oblique; IO, inferior oblique.

torsional, malfunction of these muscles is measured clinically by the presence of a vertical separation of the eyes with the involved eye in adduction (Fig. 8–1).

It is obvious from these statements that the vertical muscles have more than one action, depending on the position of the eye in the orbit. These actions are listed in Table 8–1. The oblique muscles act mainly as torters, rotating the vertical axis of the globe around an imaginary point on the corneoscleral junction near the lateral rectus muscle. The superior oblique muscle intorts, i.e., moves the upper end of the vertical axis toward the nose, while the inferior oblique muscle extorts or moves the upper end of the vertical axis laterally. The vertical rectus muscles act as secondary torters, the superior rectus as an intorter and the inferior rectus as an extorter. The horizontal actions of the vertical muscles, that is, the superior and inferior rectus and oblique muscles, are complex and position dependent and have little clinical importance.

Table 8–1. Actions of extraocular muscles.

	Primary	Secondary
Medial rectus	Adduction	—
Lateral rectus	Abduction	—
Superior rectus	Elevation	Intorsion
Inferior rectus	Depression	Extorsion
Superior oblique	Intorsion	Depression
Inferior oblique	Extorsion	Elevation

Movements of both eyes together are called *conjugate movements* and are activated by input to pairs of homologous muscles. In left lateral gaze, for instance, the left lateral and right medial rectus muscles are stimulated to contract while there is a reciprocal decrease of excitatory input to the left medial and right lateral rectus muscles. These muscle pairs are called *yoke muscles*. The patterns of input they receive follow Hering's law, i.e., appropriate input going to each of the members of the yoke pairs to keep the image of regard on the foveas. Other yoke muscle pairs are the left superior rectus and the right inferior oblique muscles (similarly the right superior rectus and left inferior oblique) and the left inferior rectus and the right superior oblique muscles (similarly the right inferior rectus and the left superior oblique). The eyes also have the ability to tort in a clockwise or counterclockwise direction in order to maintain the objective vertical meridian straight up and down (Fig. 8–2).

Movements of the eyes in opposite directions are called *disjunctive movements*. Typical horizontal disjunctive movements are convergence (bilateral adduction) when the image of regard is closer than 6 m (assumed distance for parallel ocular movements) or divergence (bilateral abduction) as an image of regard recedes to 6 m from the near point of fixation.

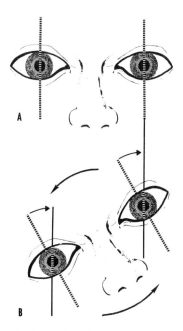

Fig. 8–2. **A.** Dashed line represents the vertical meridian of the retina in the primary position. **B.** With the head tilted toward the right shoulder the right eye must intort and the left eye extort to bring the vertical meridian back to perpendicular. These movements are under the control of the vestibular system.

Cranial nerves III, IV, and VI and their nuclei

As mentioned previously, the nerves supplying the extraocular muscles have their nuclei in the brainstem (Fig. 8–3). The oculomotor nerve (cranial nerve III, Fig. 8–3A) supplies the superior, inferior, and medial rectus muscles as well as the inferior oblique muscle and the levator palpebrae superioris muscle. It also carries the parasympathetic output from the Edinger-Westphal nucleus and the nucleus of Perlia to internal muscles of the eye. The parasympathetic innervation synapses on the cells of the ciliary ganglion, which in turn end on the ciliary muscle (for the control of accommodation) and the sphincter muscle of the iris (which for the most part controls the size of the pupil). The oculomotor fibers arise from a paired group of

motor neurons in the mesencephalon just below the superior colliculus. The fibers course ventrally, passing through the medial longitudinal fasciculus, the red nucleus, and through and medial to the substantia nigra, to form the oculomotor nerve in the interpeduncular fossa. The nerve then travels rostrally in the subarachnoid space, passing ventral to the superior cerebellar artery and dorsal to the posterior cerebral artery. It is in this region that pressure on the nerve causes pupillary dilatation in impending uncal herniation. The nerve then travels through the lateral wall of the cavernous sinus and enters the orbit through the superior orbital fissure, dividing into a superior branch and an inferior branch. The superior branch carries fibers to the superior rectus muscle and levator palpebrae superioris. The inferior branch carries the parasympathetic innervation as well as fibers to the medial and inferior rectus muscles and the inferior oblique muscle. The parasympathetic fibers travel with the fibers to the inferior oblique muscle from which they exit as the motor root to the ciliary ganglion. Here they synapse and enter the globe by way of the short ciliary nerves. The pupillary fibers travel superficially in the superior nasal aspect of the oculomotor nerve. The location of these fibers explains certain clinical observations: (1) the pupil is involved early in compressive lesions such as aneurysms that affect the third nerve, since the fibers are superficial and therefore are most at risk when external pressure is placed on the nerve; and (2) the pupil is spared in vascular lesions of the third nerve associated with diabetes mellitus and hypertension, in which infarction probably occurs as a result of occlusion of one of the small blood vessels supplying the core of the nerve. The superficial layers of the nerve are unaffected, since their blood supply derives from the pial vessels.

The trochlear nerve (cranial nerve IV) (Fig. 8–3B) arises from a paired group of motor neurons just beneath the central gray

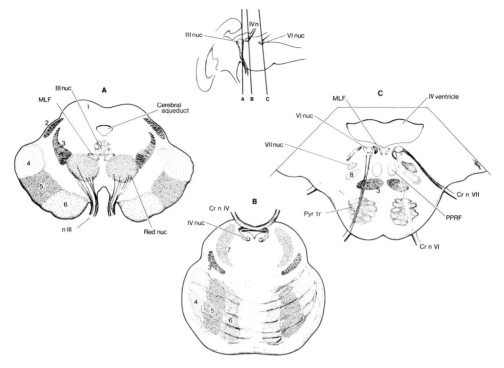

Fig. 8–3. Sections of the brainstem at the levels indicated on the inset to illustrate the three motor nuclei for eye movements and the course of their exiting fibers. Cr n, cranial nerve; nuc, nucleus; MLF, medial longitudinal fasciculus; PPRF, paramedian pontine reticular formation; Pyr tr, pyramidal tract. 1, superior colliculus; 2, brachium of inferior colliculus; 3, medial lemniscus; 4, parietotemperopontine tract; 5, pyramidal tract; 6, frontopontine tract; 7, superior cerebellar peduncle; 8, superior olivary nucleus.

substance under the midportion of the inferior colliculus. The cells are almost continuous with those of the oculomotor nucleus. The fibers course dorsally and cross completely in the superior medullary velum, where they are extremely vulnerable to trauma. Vertex blows, such as often occur in motorcycle accidents, tend to produce bilateral fourth nerve palsies as pressure waves within the fourth ventricle produce a physiologic transsection of this fiber pathway. The trochlear nerve is the only cranial nerve that leaves the brainstem dorsally and then decussates completely. It travels anteriorly and ventrally in the subarachnoid space and enters the lateral wall of the cavernous sinus, just caudal to the posterior clinoid processes.

It lies just below the third nerve and above the first division of the trigeminal nerve in the lateral wall of the cavernous sinus and enters the orbit through the superior orbital fissure to innervate the superior oblique muscle.

The abducens nerve (cranial nerve VI) arises from a paired group of motor cells situated in the floor of the fourth ventricle (Fig. 8–3C). These nuclei are demarcated on the floor of the fourth ventricle by the facial colliculi. The fibers of the abducens nerve course ventrally through the pons to emerge at its base. They travel anteriorly and laterally over the tip of the petrous portions of the temporal bone. The abducens nerve is bound to the tip by the petrosphenoidal ligament. It pierces the dura at the level of the dorsum sellae to enter the cavernous sinus. It is the only cranial nerve to travel within the sinus, where it lies near the carotid artery. It enters the orbit through the superior orbital fissure and supplies the lateral rectus muscle. The sixth nerve has the longest intracranial course through the subarachnoid space and is frequently compromised in conditions that cause raised intracranial pressure, resulting in unilateral or bilateral sixth nerve palsy.

THE PATIENT WITH DIPLOPIA

True diplopia (double vision) is produced when an object at which an individual is looking stimulates the fovea in one eye while simultaneously stimulating extrafoveal retina in the other eye. By definition, true diplopia is a binocular experience: Both eyes must be open, and it disappears when one eye or the other is covered.

Many patients who complain of diplopia are in fact misinterpreting a different sensory experience as diplopia. The most common such experience is "ghosting" produced by aberrations in the ocular media of one or both eyes. Ghosting is a monocular occurrence wherein, with one eye open, the patient perceives the object much like an image on a television set with reception interference, i.e., an overlapping of images. This effect is easy to identify by having the patient cover one eye and then the other. If the diplopia is present when one eye is open, then the sensory experience is that of a monocular or false diplopia and represents a nonneurologic problem isolated to the ocular media.

True diplopia is almost always caused by ocular misalignment. This misalignment may be produced by disturbances of the input to the extraocular muscles or to restrictive changes involving the muscles within the orbit. Disturbances of the efferent supply can occur (1) within the brainstem, affecting the ocular motor fascicles but rarely producing an isolated cranial nerve palsy; (2) in the peripheral nerves; or (3) at the neuromuscular junction (myasthenia gravis).

A paresis of one of the extraocular muscles produces two characteristic findings: (1) the presence of a deviation when the uninvolved eye is used for fixation, the *primary deviation,* which differs from the deviation when the involved eye is used for fixation, the *secondary deviation* (Fig. 8–4); and (2) a change in the measured deviation with a change in gaze position, called incomitance. The secondary deviation is always greater than the primary deviation, and the measured deviation is, of course, greatest in the field of action of the involved muscle. With the passage of time after an acute lesion, if recovery does not occur, this difference in the measured deviation becomes blurred (spread of comitance). Patients with comitant strabismus, i.e., esotropia (crosseyed) or exotropia (walleyed), do not demonstrate such changes in their measured deviations in different positions of gaze.

Total third, fourth, and sixth nerve palsies are not difficult to recognize. The patient with a total sixth nerve palsy will be unable to abduct the involved eye past the midline. Obvious inability to move the involved eye down and in suggests a fourth nerve palsy, and the patient with a complete third nerve palsy will have a drooping lid (ptosis) and the eye will be turned down and out.

Red glass test

If there is no gross deficit of ocular movement, a red filter should then be placed in front of the patient's right eye, and the patient instructed to look at the red image. The red image is the image perceived by the right eye, and therefore the right eye is the fixating eye at that moment. The object used for fixation can be either a penlight or any other convenient target. The patient is asked to demonstrate how far

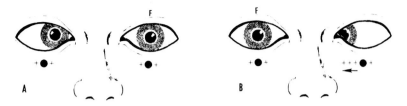

Fig. 8–4. Partial right sixth nerve lesion resulting in a paretic right lateral rectus muscle. **A.** Primary deviation; the left eye is fixating (F) straight ahead. The excitatory output from the motor neurons (indicated by +) to all four horizontal rectus muscles is approximately equal. Since the right lateral rectus muscle does not receive all of its excitatory input, the right eye is deviated medially by the medial rectus. **B.** Secondary deviation; the subject is fixating straightahead with the right eye (F). Since the paretic right lateral rectus will require much more excitatory output from the motor neurons to maintain it in this position, much more excitatory output will also be sent to its yoke muscle, the left medial rectus, resulting in pronounced deviation of the left eye.

apart the images are by using his fingers. The process is then repeated having the patient look at the white image, thus fixating with the left eye. If the image separation is greatest when the patient is looking at the red image, the right eye has the paretic muscle(s) (secondary deviation), and vice versa if the separation is greatest when looking at the white image.

Similar determination of the deviation should be made with the paretic eye fixing in the seven clinically important gaze positions. That gaze position in which the deviation is greatest will identify the paretic muscle if a single muscle is involved (Fig. 8–1), e.g., a sixth or fourth cranial nerve palsy. The third cranial nerve can be compromised in many different ways, ranging from involvement of a single muscle in intrinsic brainstem lesions, to divisional paresis, to partial limitation of all functions. Thus, the diagnosis of an incomplete third nerve palsy is a difficult problem, beyond the scope of this book. Interested readers should consult one of the textbooks of neuro-ophthalmology listed in the references at the end of the chapter.

In the evaluation of a patient with diplopia two other entities must be con-

sidered before proceeding to an extensive evaluation for the presence of intracranial pathology. These disease entities are myasthenia gravis and restrictive orbital disease.

Myasthenia gravis

Of patients with myasthenia gravis, 80% will present with ocular complaints, i.e., ptosis or diplopia. Eventually, 90% of all myasthenic patients will have ocular complaints. Myasthenia gravis can remain isolated to the extraocular muscles. If the disease process does not become more generalized within two years of onset, the patient is likely to remain with only ocular involvement.

The hallmark of myasthenia gravis is fatigue (Chap. 3). The diplopia or ptosis may be absent in the morning and develop later in the afternoon or evening. Due to fatigue, the measurements of the ocular deviation will vary with time. Holding the eyes in upgaze for a prolonged period of time will often induce ptosis of an involved lid that was not present in the primary position.

For the most part, the diagnosis of myasthenia gravis depends on testing with edrophonium hydrochloride (Tensilon). When the ocular signs are being used to judge the response of a patient to the injection of edrophonium, the test must be quantitative; there must be a measurable change in either the ptosis or the ocular deviation for it to be considered positive. Recent evidence has demonstrated that in certain instances the measurable change may be in the wrong direction; the deviation may be increased, but this is still considered to be a positive response.

Restrictive orbital disease

Restrictive orbital disease producing mechanical limitation of extraocular movement can be caused by such diverse entities as a traumatic blowout fracture of the orbital floor with muscle entrapment, or thyroid orbitopathy, which is by far the most common cause of restrictive extraocular muscle disease. The presence of a mechanical limitation is ruled out through the use of the forced duction test, which is performed by applying proparacaine anesthesia and attempting to move the eyes passively with a cotton-tipped applicator or toothed forceps in the direction of gaze limitation. If both the edrophonium test and the forced duction test are negative, the problem is one of neurologic dysfunction. The location and etiologic diagnosis of the particular disease entity will then depend on many other factors.

SUPRANCULEAR MECHANISMS FOR EYE MOVEMENT CONTROL

The control mechanisms for eye movements fit into five functionally distinct groups: (1) the saccadic system, (2) the smooth pursuit system, (3) the vestibular system, (4) the vergence system, and (5) the position maintenance-fixation system. These five systems are defined by the stimuli that evoke their activation and by the response characteristics of the ocular motor movements initiated (Table 8–2). The control mechanisms are represented in supranuclear centers that specify the function of coordinated muscle groups rather than of individual muscles. Therefore, interruption of these centers or their pathways (with the exception of the vergence system) will result in a loss of gaze function, not in diplopia.

The output of these systems is translated into action in one of two modes: rapid eye movements and slow eye movements. Rapid eye movements result from a burst of activity in the motor neurons innervating the eye muscles involved in the movement. Slow eye movements, by contrast, are mediated by a continuous, graded firing pattern in the motor neurons.

Brainstem centers

Pontine Gaze Centers. Lateral gaze movements are coordinated through the pontine centers for horizontal gaze, which are located in the paramedian zone of the pontine reticular formation (PPRF). The PPRF extends from just caudal to the abducens nerve to just short of the trochlear nuclei bilaterally. The portion of the PPRF that is contiguous to the abducens nucleus controls ipsilateral conjugate gaze movements, sending fibers to the ipsilateral abducens nucleus. An interneuron connects the abducens and para-abducens nuclei. Fibers from the para-abducens nucleus travel via the *medial longitudinal fasciculus* to the contralateral oculomotor nucleus, specifically to cells associated with the medial rectus muscle (Fig. 8–5).
oldest myelinated tract, running from the thalamus to the anterior horn cells of the spinal cord. It extends on either side of the midline, forming a V-shaped pattern that is especially well developed between the region of the vestibular and oculomotor nuclei. This tract coordinates the nuclei of the oculomotor, trochlear, and abducens nerves and carries information to and from these nuclei and other brainstem nuclei and centers.

Table 8–2. Control Mechanisms.

	Position maintenance	Pursuit	Saccadic	Vergence	Nonoptic reflex (vestibular)
Function	Maintain eye position with respect to target	Maintain object of regard on fovea; match eye and target	Place object of interest on fovea rapidly	Align visual axes to maintain bifoveal fixation	Maintain eye position with respect to changes in head and body posture
Stimulus	Visual interest and attention(?)	Moving object near fovea	Object of interest in peripheral field	Retinal disparity	Stimulation of semicircular canals, utricle, & saccule
Latency (from stimulus to onset of eye movement)		125 msec	200 msec	160 msec	Very short
Velocity	Both rapid (flicks, microsaccades) & slow (drifts)	To 100°/sec, accurately to 30°/sec	To 600°/sec	Around 20°/sec	To 300°/sec[1]
Feedback		Continuous	Sampled data		
Substrate	Occipitoparietal junction	Occipitoparietal junction	Frontal lobe; occipitoparietal junction; superior colliculus(?)	Unknown	Vestibular apparatus; muscle receptors in neck→cerebellum(?)

[1]Slow phase only. The fast phase, although initiated in the pontine reticular formation, is discharged via the saccadic mechanism.

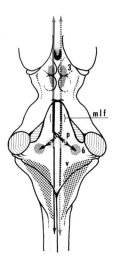

Fig. 8–5. Diagram of the midbrain, pons, and medulla seen from the dorsal surface. Fibers from the pontine gaze center (p) run to the ipsilateral abducens nucleus (6) and para-abducens nucleus, then via the medial longitudinal fasciculus (mlf) to the motor neurons of the medial rectus muscle in the contralateral oculomotor nucleus (3). v, vestibular nucleus.

Lesions of the medial longitudinal fasciculus between the abducens nerve nucleus caudally and the oculomotor nerve nucleus rostrally produce a characteristic movement deficit in horizontal gaze called *internuclear ophthalmoplegia.* Internuclear ophthalmoplegia includes weakness of the ipsilateral medial rectus muscle as demonstrated by a lag in adduction and nystagmus of the abducting eye on conjugate horizontal gaze. Such lesions are often accompanied by an upbeating nystagmus in upgaze. Bilateral lesions of the medial longitudinal fasciculus in a young adult almost always indicate demyelinating disease. Unilateral internuclear ophthalmoplegia in a middle-aged or older patient is usually indicative of small-vessel occlusive disease.

Midbrain Gaze Centers. The PPRF also controls vertical gaze. These pathways are not well worked out, but the following scheme seems reasonable in the face of clinical and experimental data. Fibers arise in the PPRF more rostral to the sixth nerve nucleus than those for lateral gaze, and project rostrally. The fibers end in the rostral interstitial nucleus of the medial longitudinal fasciculus with the fibers for downgaze segregating laterally and those for upgaze segregating medially. The rostral interstitial nucleus of the medial longitudinal fasciculus is located rostral to the third nerve nucleus, medial to the anterior end of the red nucleus, and lateral to the nucleus of Cajal.

This region also contains the intercalated neurons responsible for mediating the pupillary light reflex. The retina projects bilaterally to the pretectal olivary nuclei and sublentiform nuclei, which in turn project bilaterally (via intercalated neurons) to the Edinger-Westphal nucleus. Lesions of any type involving these intercalated neurons produce light-near dissociation, which is characterized by a relatively normal pupillary response to near stimuli in contrast to a relatively poor response to light. The best-known example of this dissociation is the *Argyll Robertson pupils* associated with neurosyphilis (tabes dorsalis). In this syndrome the pupils are miotic, irregular, react poorly to light, react well to near stimuli, and dilate poorly to belladonna alkaloids. The irregularity of the pupils and their poor response to belladonna alkaloids suggest pathology of the pupillary sphincter as well.

Lesions involving the mesencephalon dorsally, either intrinsic or extrinsic, often produce *Parinaud's syndrome,* consisting of: (1) loss of voluntary upgaze movements, which are replaced by convergence-retraction movements that are pathognomonic of a lesion in this area; (2) pupils that are 4–5 mm in diameter but exhibit light-near dissociation; (3) diplopia; and (4) papilledema. These findings are produced by dysfunction of the upgaze center (medial rostral nucleus of the medial longitudinal fasciculus), involvement of the third cranial nerve nuclei, the fourth cranial nerve nuclei or fascicles in the anterior medullary velum, and closure of the aqueduct. Intrinsic brainstem lesions located more rostral and ventral often produce isolated loss of downgaze movements.

Superior Colliculus. Direct projections from the retina to the superior colliculus are well documented. Their role in pattern discrimination is still the subject of disagreement, but recent physiologic evidence suggests that the superior colliculus aids in, but is not necessary for, foveation. That is, the superior colliculus will help initiate a foveation movement to place the image of regard exactly on the fovea, but this can also be accomplished without collicular input.

Cerebellum

The role of the cerebellum in oculomotor function is not yet completely understood. It is likely that it integrates input from the ocular muscle spindles, the vestibular apparatus, the tonic neck receptors, and the gaze centers to control the smoothness of programmed movements initiated in the pontine gaze centers. The central cerebellar structures, which include the vermis, the paravermian structures, and the flocculi, are involved in eye movements. The central structures can be divided in a cephalocaudal direction into an anterior, middle, and posterior portion. The anterior portion does not seem to be concerned with eye movements. The middle portion deals with head motion, upper limbs, and saccadic eye movements. Lesions of this portion cause ataxia of the arms, titubation of the head, and ocular dysmetria and flutter (see below). The posterior portion of the vermis is involved in the visual monitoring of eye movements, including smooth pursuit movements and maintenance of eccentric gaze while viewing an object.

The major oculomotor signs of cerebellar disease are as follows:

Nystagmus is a rhythmic movement of the eyes with an abnormal slow phase drifting away from fixation and a corrective, fast phase, which attemps to foveate the target. Most often the latter is not accomplished. The alternating slow–fast movement is called *jerk nystagmus.* Some patients do not have a fast phase and a slow phase but have pendular oscillations of equal velocity *(pendular nystagmius).*

Cerebellar nystagmus is usually horizontal in nature with its fast component toward the side of the lesion. The oscillations are always greatest when the eyes are deviated toward the side of the lesion. There may be a relative position of rest with the eyes deviated 10–20° to the side opposite the lesion, which may lead to a compensatory head turn.

Dysmetria is the inability of the eyes to stop at the end of a conjugate movement. Dysmetria is most readily elicited when the patient moves the eyes from a lateral to a straightahead position. The eyes will move past the target, move back in the appropriate direction but overshoot, and continue to oscillate around the fixation point in decreasing excursions until fixation is finally established. This movement disorder is similar to limb dysmetria.

Flutter-like oscillations are abrupt breaks in fixation with oscillations around the fixation point. This disorder is seen by observing while the patient tries to hold sustained fixation on an object for a prolonged period. Flutter probably represents a lack in the damping of the microsaccadic system, which subserves fixation maintenance and corrects for normal microdrifts that continually are occurring away from fixation. Microdrifts are thought to be necessary for vision because they prevent the retinal adaptation that causes an image stabilized on the retina to fade.

Opsoclonus is the term used to describe continuous conjugate saccadic eye movements in all directions. These movements probably represent the final breakdown of cerebellar control over the saccadic system in the PPRF. Dysmetria probably represents the earliest sign of cerebellar dysfunction and flutter the intermediate stage. The sudden onset of opsoclonus in an infant requires a thorough search to rule out an occult neuroblastoma that can produce a remote, nonmetastatic effect on the cerebellum. It is most adequately excluded by a CT scan of the retroperitoneal and suprarenal areas.

Microsaccadic following movements occur when smooth pursuit movements are replaced by a series of broken movements (microsaccadic flicks). This type of movement is often termed cogwheeling. Microsaccadic pursuit in itself is nonlocalizing, since it occurs not only with cerebellar disease but also with any disease affecting the pursuit system or its pathways (e.g., Parkinson's disease).

Rebound nystagmus: In patients with lesions of the posterior vermis, if the eyes are held in lateral gaze the cerebellum often attempts to alter the tone of the lateral gaze system in order to obviate gazeholding failure. This alteration of tone may be seen clinically as rebound nystagmus, of which there are two types.

In *type 1*, when the eyes are held in eccentric gaze for a relatively prolonged period of time (often more than one minute), the gazeholding nystagmus will damp and then reverse direction, i.e., the fast phase will be directed medially. This is frequently associated with cerebellar degeneration due to alcoholism.

In *type 2*, when the eyes are held in eccentric gaze for a period of time and then are brought to the midline position, a short burst of jerk nystagmus away from the prior eccentric gaze position can be seen. This type of nystagmus also has been associated with cerebellar disease. It has been suggested that both gazeholding failure and rebound nystagmus involve dysfunction of the dentate nuclei.

Skew deviation is a vertical deviation of the eyes causing vertical diplopia that cannot be attributed to a single muscle or to a group of vertically acting muscles. Its presence is indicative of a lesion in the posterior fossa but has no further localizing value.

Vestibular system

The vestibular system is largely responsible for reflex orientation of the body and head in space and for adaptation to linear and rotatory acceleration. The system includes an anatomically and physiologically balanced pair of labyrinthine end organs located within the inner ear (Fig. 8–6). They are connected to the vestibular nuclear complex at the pontomedullary junction or to the flocculonodular complex of the cerebellum by the statoacoustic division of the eighth cranial nerve (Fig. 8–7). Scarpa's ganglion is the peripheral sensory ganglion of the vestibular system, located in the internal auditory meatus. It contains the cell bodies of the bipolar vestibular neurons that carry information from the hair cell receptors in the ampullary cristae of the semicircular canals and the macula of the utricle.

The flocculonodular complex exerts partial inhibitory feedback control over the four vestibular nuclei on each side of the brainstem. The superior and medial vestibular nuclei project back to the cerebellum. The medial vestibular nucleus also projects to the reticular gray substance of the brainstem, the dorsal efferent nucleus of the vagus nerve, and the spinal cord. The lateral vestibular nucleus primarily projects back to the cerebellum. Projections from the vestibular nuclei also ascend through multisynaptic pathways of uncertain locations to the cerebral cortex.

The vestibular system, through its connections with the brainstem nuclei, the cerebellum, and the spinal cord centers, plays a part in the regulation of muscular tone and the maintenance of postural re-

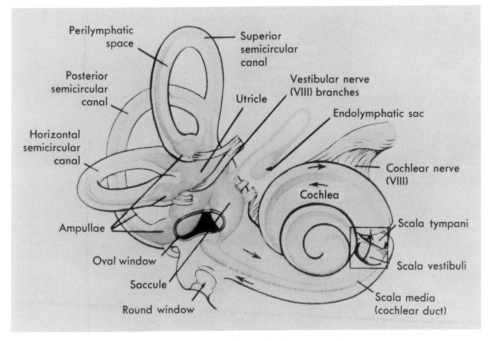

Fig. 8–6. Right labyrinth and cochlea. The three ampullary nerves carry impulses from each of the semicircular canals and from the vestibular segment of cranial nerve VIII. (Drawing by Ernest W. Beck, courtesy of Beltone Electronics Corporation, Chicago.)

flexes. An important function of the vestibular complex, and one that is essential in the clinical testing of the vestibular system, is the reflex coordination of extraocular movements. The vestibular nuclei project to the PPRF as well as directly to the ocular motor nuclei through the reticular substance of the pontine tegmentum and the medial longitudinal fasciculus (Fig. 8–7).

The peripheral receptors subserving vestibular control over the extraocular movements lie in the membranous labyrinth lodged within the petrous portion of the temporal bone. The membranous labyrinth (Fig. 8–6) is divided functionally into three separate entities: (1) the utricle, (2) the saccule, and (3) the semicircular canals. The utricle and saccule are bulbous enlargements of the membranous labyrinth within which are the membranous plaques of hair cells embedded in a gelat-

inous material containing calcium carbonate crystals, the otoliths. These organs are responsible for ophthalmostatic functions. Every position of the head in space has a specified position of the eyes in the orbit with respect to the vertical, and this control is exerted by the otolithic apparatus, which detects the position of the head.

The semicircular canals control ophthalmokinetic functions wherein the eyes respond to angular acceleration of the head. There are three semicircular canals in each side: (1) horizontal, (2) anterior vertical, and (3) posterior vertical, lying at right angles to each other (Fig. 8–6). At one end of each canal is the ampulla, a blister-like enlargement containing sensory hair cells embedded in a gelatinous dome (crista). When the head undergoes angular acceleration, the viscous fluid in the semicircular canals lags behind be-

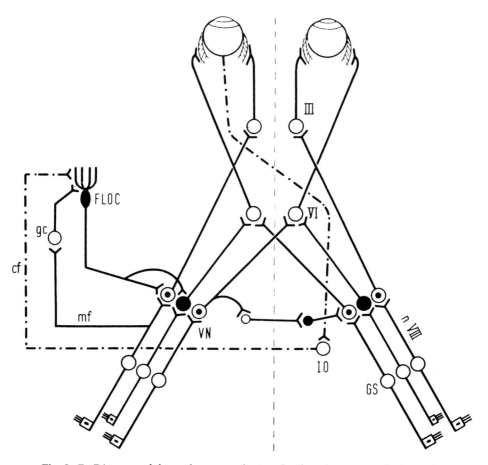

Fig. 8–7. Diagram of the pathways mediating the short latency vestibulo-ocular reflexes and their relationship to the cerebellum. Excitatory neurons are shown as open circles, inhibitory neurons as filled circles. Circles with a dot show second-order excitatory vestibular neurons. The small filled circles are inhibitory neurons mediating inhibition across the midline. The broken line shows the pathway from the retina to the flocculus. cf, climbing fiber; FLOC, flocculus; gc, granule cell; GS, Scarpa's ganglion; IO, inferior olive; mf, mossy fiber; VN, vestibular nucleus; III, motor neurons of the medial rectus; VI, abducens nucleus; n. VIII, nerve fibers in the vestibular portion of cranial nerve VIII from the horizontal canals. (From W. Precht, Cerebellar influences on eye movements. In *Basic Mechanisms of Ocular Motility and their Clinical Implications*, G. Lennerstrand and P. Bach-y-Rita, (eds.). Oxford, Pergamon Press, 1975.)

cause of inertia, causing the cilia on the hair cells in the ampullary cristae to be bent. The hair cells are directional in that they are depolarized by motion of endolymph in one direction and hyperpolarized by motion in the opposite direction. Turning the head to the left causes relative motion of the endolymph in the horizontal canals on both sides, but on the left side the motion is toward the ampulla and produces excitation of the left vestibular nerve fibers, while on the right side the motion is away from the ampulla and decreases the activity of the right vestibular nerve.

In stuporous or comatose patients, passive turning of the head (doll's-head

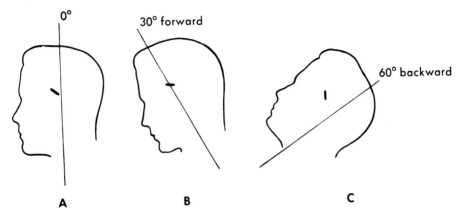

Fig. 8–8. Plane of the horizontal semicircular canal with variations of head position. With the head erect (**A**) the horizontal canal is tilted upward about 30°. The head must be tilted 30° forward (**B**) to put the canal in the horizontal plane for testing in a rotating chair, or 60° back (**C**) for caloric testing when the subject is seated. (From D. G. Cogan, *Neurology of the Ocular Muscles*, 2d ed. Springfield, Ill., Thomas, 1966.)

maneuver) to the left causes the eyes to deviate to the right. This comes about because the combination of increased activity in the left vestibular nerve and decreased activity in the right leads to excitation of the neurons in the vestibular nuclei, which in turn provide excitation to the motor neurons for the right lateral rectus and the left medial rectus. At the same time the motor neurons of the left lateral rectus and the right medial rectus are inhibited (Fig. 8–7).

The anterior vertical semicircular canal of one side forms a unit with the posterior vertical canal at the other side in a manner similar to that described for the horizontal canals. These canals are responsive to anterior-posterior and laterally inclined movements of the head.

The effect of continuous stimulation of the semicircular canals is to produce a jerk nystagmus in the plane of the stimulated canal. This response provides a useful means of testing vestibular function. Since the horizontal canals lie at an angle of 30° to the horizon, the head of the seated patient must be tilted 30° forward to isolate this canal for testing in a rotating chair.

With the head back 60° in the seated patient, or 30° forward in the supine patient, the horizontal canal will be perpendicular to the horizon (Fig. 8–8) and thus in the proper position for caloric testing. Thermal stimulation can then be used to test the vestibular apparatus by injecting either cold or tepid water into the external auditory canal, causing the endolymph in the horizontal canal to move up (tepid) or down (cold). The appropriate response characteristics are most easily remembered by the mnemonic COWS, which indicates the direction of the fast or corrective phase of the nystagmus: Cold, Opposite; Warm, Same. The slow deviation of the eyes is produced by the vestibular apparatus, whereas the fast phase is under the control of the frontal lobe.

Patients being tested with caloric stimulation usually experience *vertigo*, a sensation of spinning or falling, often accompanied by the feeling that the environment is moving (oscillopsia). The patient may also develop nausea and sometimes vomiting. Vertigo is also a major symptom of irritative or ablative lesions in the vestibular system that produce an imbalance of vestibular input from the two sides. Vertigo also results when the vestibular input is not correlated with appropriate proprioceptive and visual input.

The apparent movement of the environment experienced with vertigo is always opposite to the slow phase of the nystagmus. In addition, with the eyes closed the patient will past-point and fall to one side when standing. Past-pointing is consistent pointing to one side of a fixed visual target. The past-point and the fall when standing are always in the direction of the slow phase of the nystagmus. For example, cold-water irrigation of the right external auditory canal, which mimics an ablative lesion of the right vestibular apparatus, will produce left-beating nystagmus with falling to the right and past-pointing to the right. The environment will appear to move to the left.

Lesions of the vestibular apparatus may affect the vestibular end organ, the eighth cranial nerve, or the vestibular nuclei. Labyrinthine disease can be either irritative (rare), mimicked by warm-water caloric stimulation, or as just discussed, ablative, mimicked by cold-water stimulation. Unilateral destructive lesions include Ménière's disease, viral neuronitis, and labyrinthitis. Bilateral destructive lesions may be produced by ototoxic drugs (streptomycin, gentamycin), viral diseases, and infarction. Central vestibular disease can be differentiated from peripheral end-organ disease most readily if there are accompanying signs of brainstem involvement such as oculosympathetic paresis or dysfunction of the fifth or seventh cranial nerves. In addition, pure vertical or rotatory nystagmus, as well as the failure of visual fixation to reduce the degree of nystagmus, is indicative of central involvement.

For the most part, end-organ disease tends to be abrupt in onset, producing severe vertigo with horizontal or mixed horizontal-rotatory nystagmus in one direction that is inhibited by visual fixation.

The symptoms have a finite duration (hours to days) but may be recurrent; they are often associated with tinnitus or deafness. Chronic or slowly developing lesions, such as a cerebellopontine angle tumor, may produce few if any symptoms because functional adjustments are made, probably by the cerebellum, to obviate the imbalance of input. In central vestibular dysfunction, the onset is often not as acute and the vertigo tends to be mild. The nystagmus can be unidirectional or bidirectional and purely horizontal, vertical, or rotatory. Visual fixation has no effect on the vertigo or nystagmus. Auditory dysfunction is usually not associated. Central vestibular disorders are most frequently caused by vascular or demyelinating diseases and tend to be chronic.

Diseases affecting the saccule and utricle (otolithic diseases) are indicated by the presence of positional nystagmus and vertigo. Positional nystagmus is present only with particular head positions. Patients may complain that when they extend the neck to look upward they experience vertigo, or that the room appears to spin when they lie on one side. Thus the history can be helpful in determining which head position the patient should assume during the examination in order to reproduce the problem. Induction of both the vertigo and nystagmus with a given head position is diagnostic.

Four characteristic features of otolithic disease are usually found when a patient is put into a symptomatic position: (1) Nystagmus begins after a *latent period* of 0.5–8 sec; (2) the nystagmus *transiently* increases in rapid crescendo, then abates and disappears; (3) the patient experiences *severe dizziness* (positional vertigo) and wants to change position; (4) finally, with repeated testing, the nystagmus eventually fails to reappear (*fatigability*). The otolith of the ear that is uppermost is stimulated more relative to the other, so that in the case of a destructive lesion, more dizziness will be experienced and greater nystagmus produced with the "bad ear" down. Normal individuals do not experience symptoms or have nystagmus during these maneuvers.

CEREBRAL CENTERS FOR EYE MOVEMENT CONTROL

Horizontal movements

Frontal centers. The frontal center for conjugate horizontal gaze lies in Brodmann's area 8 (Fig. 8–9). It mediates all fast (saccadic) movements to the contralateral side. The fibers to the subcortical centers project through the anterior limb of the internal capsule near the genu and run caudally as part of the frontobulbar projection. The fibers for conjugate lateral gaze decussate in the midbrain before the decussation of the fibers destined for the facial nucleus. They terminate in the PPRF slightly caudal and medial to the abducens nuclei. The fast-phase corrective movements of optokinetic nystagmus and vestibular nystagmus are routed through this frontobulbar center and pathway.

Injury to the frontal center on one side results in a loss of saccadic gaze function to the contralateral side. This loss of function usually slowly improves, i.e., the gaze palsy disappears. It has been suggested that the recovery is due to assumption of function by the opposite intact frontal center. When the lesion is acute and the patient is stuporous or in coma, conjugate deviation of the eyes toward the involved side may be evident. Conversely, during seizure activity in this area, the eyes will be deviated toward the side opposite the seizure focus.

Occipitoparietal Junction. The material upon which the assumptions about the function of these centers are based comes from studies of humans with less than discrete pathology and is thus more speculative than previous discussions in this chapter. This area seems to have some role in three functions: (1) saccadic move-

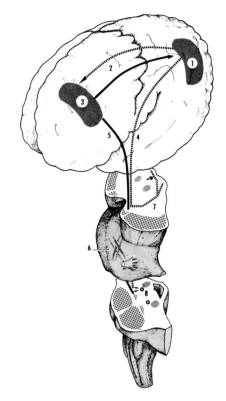

Fig. 8–9. Diagrammatic representation of the postulated gaze centers and their interconnections. 1. Occipitoparietal gaze center for following movements, fixation, and foveation. 2. Interconnecting tracts, ? internal sagittal stratum. 3. Frontal gaze center for saccades-Brodmann's area 8 alpha and gamma. 4. Occipitobulbar tract. 5. Frontobulbar tract. 6. Decussation of corticobulbar tracts dealing with eye movements. 7. Occipitotectal projection. 8. Pontine gaze center.

ments that produce foveation of visual stimuli, (2) smooth pursuit or following movements, and (3) maintenance of fixation. It is unlikely that these functions are subserved by precisely the same anatomical substrate. These centers appear to be located in and around the angular gyrus and Brodmann's area 19 (Fig. 8–9). The projection pathways from this area are less certainly known than the frontobulbar pathways. At this time, the best evidence suggests that the occipitobulbar tract courses medially along with the visual radiations, then caudally through the posterior limb of the internal capsule. The sites for synaptic termination of this pathway are somewhere in the thalamus, superior colliculus, or pons. Evidence from patients with lesions in this area indicates that smooth pursuit movements toward the right are lost with a lesion on the right side. It has therefore been suggested that the pathway from the occipitoparietal center to the brainstem undergoes a double decussation, although there is no anatomical evidence to support this suggestion. Whether the pathway for saccadic foveation is ipsilateral or contralateral is not known. The pathway from the occipitoparietal center to the brainstem eventually terminates in the pontine reticular formation, with the fibers subserving smooth pursuit apparently ending just rostral to the sixth nerve nucleus, contiguous but rostral to those dealing with the production of saccades.

In addition, three tracts connect the occipital cortex and the frontal lobe centers for conjugate gaze. It is believed that these pathways are necessary for the initiation of microsaccades in fixation and the corrective fast phase of optokinetic nystagmus.

Lesions involving the occipitoparietal gaze center produce two clinical signs: (1) contralateral deviation of the eyes with forced lid closure (Cogan's sign), and (2) jerky microsaccadic movements rather than smooth following movements ipsilateral to the lesion. These signs are explained on the basis of a loss of function; that is, when the eyes are closed and ocular fixation is broken there is tone only from the normal center, which leads to a deviation of the eyes away from the damaged occipitoparietal center. Similarly, imprecise following movements are made to the ipsilateral side as the only functioning mechanism is saccadic in nature.

Vertical movements

Purely vertical movements require bilateral supranuclear input. Vertical conjugate gaze movements are represented in the cerebral cortex as part of the frontal gaze center. The projection of the pathways subserving vertical movements to the PPRF is assumed to accompany the projections for horizontal saccadic movement. As was previously described, there are supranuclear brainstem centers for vertical movements in the mesencephalon that receive input from that part of the PPRF rostral to the sixth nerve nuclei. At this time the vertical gaze centers in the mesencephalon are considered to be the rostral interstitial nuclei of the medial longitudinal fasciculus.

Dysjunctive movements

Convergence. Convergence is the act of foveating both eyes on the object of regard at some relatively near point. The supranuclear centers for convergence are not known, but these movements can be seen when both frontal and occipital gaze centers are stimulated bilaterally. The final common excitatory pathway is funneled through the oculomotor nerve (medial rectus subnucleus), and inhibitory impulses are sent to the abducens nuclei simultaneously. Paresis of convergence is seen with midbrain disease and is most often accompanied by accommodative and pupillary paresis. Rarely, lesions of the midbrain can produce convergence spasm or convergence-retraction nystagmus.

Divergence. The centers for divergence are much more obscure than those of convergence. Recent evidence has demonstrated that divergence is an active process, but its substrate remains unknown. Divergence paresis is generally a benign syndrome with the pathologic lesion assumed to be in the region of the sixth nerve nuclei.

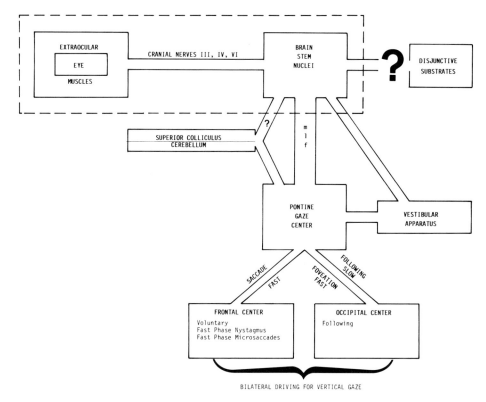

Fig. 8–10. Block diagram summarizing eye movement control centers. mlf, medial longitudinal fasciculus.

Torsional conjugate movements. These movements are unique in that they are not subject to voluntary control. They are stimulated by input from the membranous labyrinth through the vestibular nuclei with some minor input from the proprioceptive mechanisms in the neck.

SUMMARY

Figure 8–10 provides a diagrammatic summary of the centers and pathways controlling eye movements. Lesions within the dotted line produce nuclear and infranuclear diplopia. Lesions outside the dotted line produce loss of one or more supranuclear control functions, depending on the site of the lesion.

GENERAL REFERENCES

Bach-y-Rita, P., Collins, C. Hyde, J. E. (eds.). *The Control of Eye Movements.* New York, Academic Press, 1971.

Burde, R. M., and J. S. Karp. Clinical approach to disorders of the third, fourth, and sixth cranial nerves. In *Neuro-opthalmology.* Symposium of the University of Miami and the Bascom Palmer Institute, vol. VIII, J. S. Glaser and J. L. Smith (eds.). St. Louis, Mosby, 1975, pp. 191–215.

Cogan, G. D. *Neurology of the Ocular Muscles,* 2d ed. Springfield, Ill., Thomas, 1956.

Cohen, B. (ed.). Vestibular and Oculomotor Physiology. *Ann. N. Y. Acad. Sci.,* 374, 1981.

Glaser, J. S. (ed.). *Neuro-ophthalmology.* Hagerstown, Md., Harper & Row, 1978.

Lennerstrand, G., and P. Bach-y-Rita (eds.).

Basic Mechanisms of Ocular Motility and Their Clinical Implications. Proceedings of the International Symposium, Wenner-Gren Center, Stockholm, June 4–6, 1974. Oxford, Pergamon Press, 1975.

Moses, R. A. (ed.). *Adler's Physiology of the Eye*, 7th ed., St. Louis, Mosby, 1981.

Walsh, F. B., and W. F. Hoyt. *Clinical Neuro-opthalmology*, 3rd ed. Baltimore, Williams & Wilkins, 1969.

9.

Motor System

W. THOMAS THACH, Jr. and ERWIN B. MONTGOMERY, Jr.

Many different brain diseases can give rise to defects of movement. Nevertheless, a patient with movement defects may suffer in only two ways: He may have a *negative* defect (loss of ability to perform particular movements), and/or a *positive* defect (presence of involuntary movement or stiffness).

Since a large portion of the brain's structure is concerned with the control of movement, movement defects can be caused by virtually any disease that damages the brain: infections, environmental poisons and drugs of abuse, aging, hereditary disorders, a diet lacking protein and vitamins, trauma, cancer, stroke, and specific brain diseases such as multiple sclerosis and parkinsonism. Because so many different diseases can cause movement disorders, millions of patients are afflicted by them.

It is our purpose here to describe the abnormal postures and movements that result from damage to the motor system, in terms both of the normal functions of its various parts, and of the aberrant physiological mechanisms that cause the abnormal behaviors.

COMPONENTS OF THE MOTOR SYSTEM

The movement control system contains five major subdivisions: cerebral cortex, basal ganglia, cerebellum, portions of the brainstem, and the spinal cord.

Figures 9–1 to 9–3, 9–5, 9–7, and 9–8 show simple schematic diagrams of the motor systems. Essentially, it consists of a *hierarchical* arrangement of interconnected groups of nerve cells, each higher group controlling a lower group. These neuronal groups range from areas of cerebral cortex concerned with mental functions down to the spinal cord, which controls the muscles of the body. From the figures one can see that there are *parallel* paths in the system, which may be important in recovery of function after damage to a particular part, as will be pointed out. For example, the cerebral cortex has direct connections to spinal cord and thence to muscle, plus indirect connections to the spinal cord via the cerebellum and the brainstem.

Studies of behavior after ablation of the various parts of the motor system support the idea that the system functions in a hi-

151

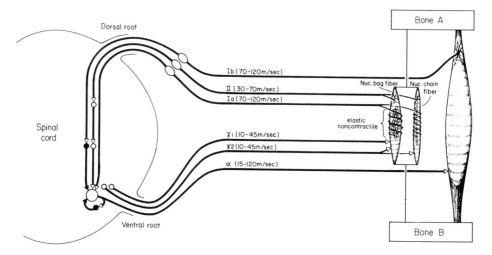

Fig. 9–1. Diagram of muscles and muscle spindles and their motor and sensory innervation. The Ib endings (Golgi tendon organs) sense force that is actively generated by the muscle contraction and they fire proportionately, returning to the spinal cord to inhibit the alpha motor neuron via inhibitory interneurons. By contrast, the Ia (primary annulospiral receptors) and II (secondary flower spray receptors) of the muscle spindles sense length of the muscle and fire proportionately when it is stretched or shortened, returning to the spinal cord to excite the alpha motor neuron. In most kinds of movement, alpha and gamma motor neurons fire together (coactivation). The gamma motor neurons excite the spindle fibers and thereby the Ia and II endings, so as to maintain spindle sensitivity to length despite muscle shortening. The tendon and spindle reflexes act as servomechanisms for force and length, respectively, of muscle contraction. Thus, if the muscle fatigues and produces less force, the Ib ending will be activated less and will cause less inhibitory drive (via the interneuron) to the alpha motor neuron, which will allow it then to increase its firing to drive the fatigued muscle to greater contraction. And, if the fatigued muscle fails to shorten as much as it otherwise would, that extra amount of length will add to the gamma motor neuronal drive of the Ia and II endings, which will then excite the alpha motor neuron more to make up the deficit in length.

erarchical manner. The spinal cord contains nearly all the neural circuitry that is needed for many fundamental motor functions. These functions include the two mechanisms whereby the alpha motor neurons cause muscle to contract and generate force: *recruitment* and *rate coding*. In the process of recruitment, motor units are activated one by one until they add up to the critical number required to generate the desired amount of force. In general, the smallest motor units (generating the least amount of force) are recruited before the larger. This apparently fixed recruit-

ment order is referred to as the *size principle*. Rate coding indicates that each motor unit can be made to fire at higher frequencies to generate more force, at the same time that more motor units are being added by the process of recruitment.

Neural circuits in the spinal cord provide for the reciprocal innervation of agonist and antagonist muscles, the linkage of groups of muscles to a peripheral receptor that forms the segmental and propriospinal reflexes, and finally, for more complicated activities like locomotion (quadripedal gait, swimming). Vestibular

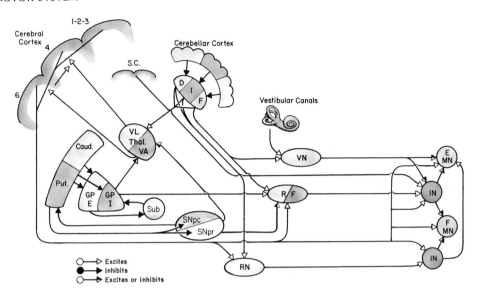

Fig. 9–2. Descending pathways to the spinal cord, and their origins in brainstem, cerebellum, and cerebrum. Caud., caudate; Put., putamen; GP_E, globus pallidus, external segment; GP_I, globus pallidus, internal segment; Thal., thalamus; VA, ventroanterior nucleus; CL, corpus luysi(subthalamic nucleus); SN, substantia nigra; SC, superior colliculus; O, dentate nucleus; I, interpositus nucleus; F, fastigial nucleus; RN, red nucleus; RF, reticular formation (reticular nuclei in pons and medulla); VN, vestibular nuclei; IN, interneuron; E MN, excitatory motor neuron; F MN, inhibitory motor neuron.

and reticular nuclei and the colliculi are superimposed on spinal cord mechanisms to control movements that are guided by vestibular, somatosensory, visual, and auditory input. The basal ganglia and thalamus allow the further elaboration and refinement of motor responses so as to produce effective antigravity stance (including bipedal stance in humans), skin-contact-induced foot placing, body righting, stretch-induced stepping, tonic neck (muscle stretch) reflexes acting on the body, and visually targeted, coordinated eye/limb/body responses. The cerebral cortex adds the ability to vary movement of a single limb, especially its digits, over a wide range, independent of the relatively few and stereotyped whole-body synergies. This is known as *fractionation* of individuated movements of separate members; the same principle presumably also applies to the various muscles of speech, leading to the

wide range of special synergies needed for the sounds of speech, independent of the more automatic uses of eating and breathing. The cerebellum contributes a "fine control" of all these activities, since its ablation impairs all—but is essential to none—of these various movement patterns. Any one act is likely to involve many brain parts acting together, in parallel. For example, visual and vestibular components each add their own unique controlling input to the movement of one body part. Parallel processing thus occurs at the same time as hierarchical processing.

PRINCIPLES OF MOTOR PATHOPHYSIOLOGY: NEGATIVE AND POSITIVE DEFECTS

Before beginning a discussion of the effects of lesions of the different neural parts, and the motor abnormalities that are produced, one must appreciate the meaning of the terms *negative* and *positive* defects of movement, and how they have been used as tools to study both normal and abnormal movement and posture. Essentially, a negative defect refers to the movement that one would like to do that one can no longer do, and a positive defect is that which one involuntarily does that one does not want to do. Paralysis is a negative defect; grand mal seizures, tremor, and the hemiplegic posture are positive defects.

Positive defects are of three kinds. One kind is caused by the overactivity of a neural part because of its being stimulated abnormally, as occurs with electrical stimulation or epilepsy. A second kind is due to a release of the activity of one neural part from the inhibitory control of another neural part. For example, after cerebellar cortex ablation, cerebellar nuclear cells are "released" from the tonic firing of inhibitory Purkinje cells, and do what they normally do, but in augmented degree and all the time. A third kind of positive defect occurs some time after neurons are deprived of excitatory inputs. This type is illustrated by what happens in muscle after a lesion of the motor nerve to it. Immediately after the lesion of the nerve, no nerve impulses can get to the muscle, and it is paralyzed and inactive (a negative defect). However, with the passage of time, the membrane of the muscle becomes more sensitive to circulating cholinergic substances, and begins to fire autonomously, independent of any neural input. Since single muscle fibers discharge and contract without spread to neighboring fibers, these are called *fibrillations;* they can be seen through the thin covering of the tongue and observed with electromyography in any other denervated muscle. The excitability of the muscle, once strictly controlled by the nerve, now occurs spontaneously, independent of the nerve. The muscle's activity can be thought of as being released from the control of the nerve.

The analysis of negative and positive defects after ablation has been used as a tool in animals and humans to infer the normal function of parts of the motor system. Thus, damage to motor cortex permanently disables individuated movements of digits of the hand and foot and of the muscles of the mouth, pharynx, and larynx. The damage may excite the motor cortex in an epileptic seizure to cause individuated movements of these same parts, and it may release the activity of lower structures that then take over the control of these and other muscles for a smaller range of purposes, such as postural support. These defects of posture and movement that result from damage to neural structures have been very influential as clues to what the structures normally do. In addition to the use of ablation and stimulation there is another research strategy for studying how the motor system works. This is recording of the activity of single nerve cells one after another in the various motor system nuclei as an awake animal makes normal movements, to try to see what particular movements a neuron is coupled to and may be causing. Together, these strategies allow one to test a hypothesis about the putative role of the brain part in causing a movement in three different ways: (1) Does the movement disappear with the ablation of the part? (2) Is the movement produced by stimulation of the part? (3) Are neurons in the part active in relation to the normal movement? No one of these strategies is adequate to pinpoint the function of a group of neurons; each plays a unique role. The observations provided by these three strategies will be considered as we explore the physiology and pathophysiology of the motor system's components.

SPINAL CORD

In animal experiments, the isolated spinal cord has been shown to subserve a number of motor functions beyond simply carrying information to motor neurons. These include: (1) *Force of muscle contraction:* two interdependent mechanisms, i.e., recruitment (number of motor units active) and rate coding (frequency of motor unit firing), comprise the manner in which muscles are caused to contract to generate graduated forces. (2) *Reciprocal innervation:* inhibitory connections to the motor neurons of antagonist muscles guarantee that when an agonist contracts, the antagonist automatically relaxes proportionately. (3) *Reflexes:* various sensory motor reflex arcs serve to orient cord motor mechanisms toward environmental events, and control activity of one body part contingent on the movement of another. Because spinal reflexes are so often altered by diseases that affect the motor system, they will be dealt with in some detail.

Stretch of a muscle and of the muscle spindle within it automatically causes the muscle to contract, as if to provide a mechanism for holding constant length (Figs. 9–1, 9–3). The sequences of events is that the lengthening of the muscle also lengthens the muscle spindles that lie parallel within the muscle fibers, exciting the spindle afferent terminals to fire trains or bursts of impulse activity. The impulses travel over the spindle afferent nerve into the spinal cord, where some of the many nerve branches synapse directly onto alpha motor neurons. These synapses are excitatory, and the combined activity at many such synapses drives the motor neuron to fire a train of action potentials out of the spinal cord to the terminals on the muscle fibers that comprise its motor unit. Each spike in the axon causes a contraction in each contacted fiber, and a twitch of all of the fibers in the motor unit. Since the twitches result from nerve impulses and the impulses are in trains, the twitches also are in trains and they fuse together to make the muscle contract and generate force. This sequence of events occurs when a clinician stretches a muscle by tapping its tendon with a reflex hammer; the contraction that occurs is called a stretch reflex or deep tendon reflex.

The *Golgi tendon organ* is most sensitive not to lengthening, but instead to force generated by active contraction of the muscle, and presumably confers the ability of the motor system to monitor the force it itself generates as the muscle contracts (Fig. 9–1, 9–3). Length feedback provided by the muscle spindles and force feedback provided by the Golgi tendon organs could give the motor system accurate information as to whether the motor neurons and muscles had indeed properly carried out the CNS motor commands. Such a feedback system could be used to regulate the constancy of muscle contraction. For example, as muscle fatigues and generates less force and shortening, spindle excitation of the alpha motor neuron would be increased and Golgi tendon organ inhibition decreased, and there would be a tendency for the feedback to increase the activity of the motor neuron and therefore the muscle. This could be used to keep length constant despite load, which would help, for example, in carrying such things as cafeteria trays and coffee cups automatically and with precision.

Two other features of spindle afferents are of note. The first is that the afferents enter the cord and travel to a number of synergistic alpha motor neurons above and below the motor neurons that innervate the muscle of origin, as if to coordinate activity of many muscles in relation to the one. Second, the spindle stretch reflex has a tendency to oscillate in cycles of stretch → contraction → relaxation → stretch → contraction → relaxation, which may produce tremor. This tendency to oscillate becomes more severe in several neurological diseases, which in turn implies that one function of the motor system may be to hold this tendency in check.

Skin contact reflexes activate groups of alpha motor neurons and inhibit others so as to cause the limb to be pulled away from the stimulus (Fig. 9–3). In the leg, this may be accompanied by the extension of the opposite leg, as if to support the body as the stimulated foot and leg flexes up from the stimulus. Stimulation of the skin may also evoke *autonomic reflexes* within the

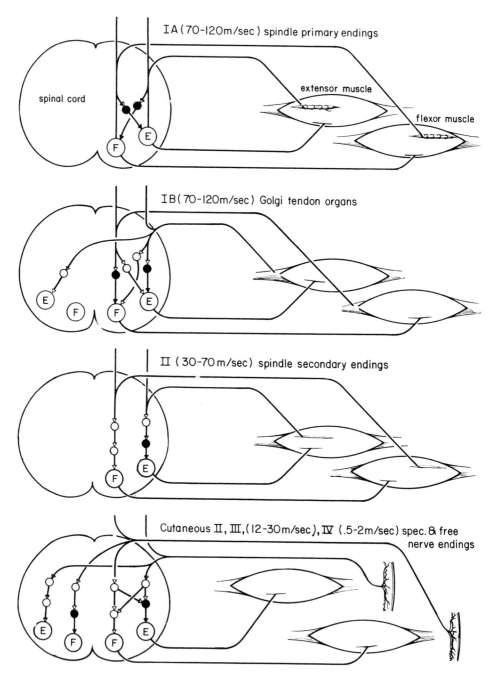

Fig. 9–3. Circuitry for segmental spinal reflexes. Ia spindle reflexes are activated by stretch of the muscle and cause excitation of that muscle and its sy-
nergists and reciprocal inhibition of its antagonists. Ib tendon reflexes are activated by force produced by muscle contraction and inhibit that muscle and
reciprocally excite the antagonist. II. spindle reflexes may excite and inhibit the
agonist and antagonist muscle through several interneurons. Skin reflexes (activated by a noxious stimulus) may cause withdrawal of limb away from the
stimulus and a supporting reaction in the opposite limb.

isolated spinal cord, which may cause changes in blood pressure, sweating, piloerection, and penile erection.

Finally, in many animals, the cord contains enough of the machinery essential for the production of locomotion that it can do so when cerebral hemispheres and brainstem are removed. Thus, fish, frog, turtle, snake, bird, and cat, and even primates, may make more or less effective movements of swimming, jumping, walking, wriggling, flying, or running after transection of the upper spinal cord. This may be more easily produced or maintained if trains of high-frequency pulsatile electric current are applied to the ends of severed descending brainstem paths and to the dorsal roots, and if the feet are passively moved posteriorly by a treadbelt. But the current and treadbelt motion are maintained and steady, whereas the oscillatory activity is generated entirely by neuronal circuits within the spinal cord.

In humans, however, the nervous system has evolved so as to place more of the "spinal" motor control apparatus in the brain, and it is unclear how much of the motor machinery still exists within the spinal cord. One might think that the motor cortex, with its descending corticospinal pathways, would be absolutely essential for movement, but this is not so. In newborn infants, the cortical neurons lack much of their dendritic development and may not even fire at all, and even if they did, the corticospinal tracts have not yet become myelinated and therefore could not conduct the impulses in anything like the normal manner. Yet infants make rhythmic stepping movements when they are held upright with the feet against the floor and are moved forward or sideways. Furthermore, the motor behavior of anencephalic infants who lack any brain rostral to the midbrain is remarkably like that of normal infants for several weeks after birth.

Immediately following brainstem lesions or transection of the human cervical spinal cord, no patterns of movement are produced that resemble locomotion. Initially there is a period (usually lasting one to six weeks) of *spinal shock,* in which the muscles are flaccid and may be refractory to contraction by any reflex pathway. This shows the great extent to which humans rely on the descending controls to operate cord machinery: Presumably, simply the tonic activity in the descending excitatory inputs is necessary to maintain a baseline level of excitation for the interneurons and motor neurons to be effectively excited by the peripheral nerve inputs to the somatomotor reflexes that remain. In this period, the autonomic reflexes are also deprived of descending excitatory control from hypothalamus; they are depressed, and the blood pressure may fall dangerously low, requiring the use of sympathomimetic pressor drugs to maintain it. Nevertheless, in time, the cord reflexes become active—indeed, much more active than in the intact individual. Stretch reflexes are exaggerated. Painful or even innocuous stimulation of the skin may trigger reflex withdrawal of a limb, and sometimes a semblance of "spinal" walking may be seen in chronic cord transections. Superficial or deep stimuli (distension of the bladder) may cause transient elevations of the blood pressure to dangerously high levels, accompanied by sweating and piloerection. Such autonomic hyperreflexia frequently occurs in complete spinal cord lesions above the thoracic level.

Segmental spindle stretch reflexes and spasticity

The term *spasticity* is used vaguely in the literature, but usually includes, as it should, increased stretch reflexes. It also includes a pattern of muscular resistance to continuous slow passive stretch. A more variable feature is that the resistance to lengthening may increase up to the point of a sudden give-away decrease in resistance, the so-alled claspknife reaction. An important generalization is that spasticity has the property of increased muscle *reactivity* to stretch; in contrast to rigid and dystonic states, the spastic muscle *at rest* is flaccid and electrically silent.

Muscle spindle stretch reflexes are both poly- and monosynaptic. Normal motor neurons can be brought to the reflex firing level only by highly synchronized volleys in many afferent fibers, as in the temporal summation of impulses produced by a sudden pull on the tendon that occurs when a reflex hammer is used to elicit a tendon jerk. Slower passive stretch produces asynchronous spindle afferent activity, which causes no consistent EMG activity or tension in the normal muscle. Thus, the earliest evidence of stretch reflex hyperreactivity is the increased amplitude of the tendon jerk. Spasticity seldom appears suddenly, but usually evolves from the state of increased tendon jerk stretch reflexes through to the claspknife reaction, which is a mounting resistance to slow stretch, with or without a distinct give-way phase of decreased resistance, like opening a pocketknife. The release phase of the claspknife reaction probably represents several factors, among which are (1) decrease of excitatory input to the motor neuron from the spindle sense organs due to their unloading by the contraction of the muscle; (2) inhibition from the Golgi tendon organs, which are excited by the contraction of the muscle; and (3) inhibition from the small, secondary spindle stretch receptors (see Fig. 9–3).

The simplest explanation for spasticity is that it represents a lower threshold for synaptic excitation at the level of the alpha motor neuron. There is an increased (population) response of motor neurons to a sudden syncrhonized excitation and a lack of the normal adaptation to a less intense, gradual, tonic excitation. The most direct proof of this in humans is the observation that the maximal response to direct electrical stimulation of the spindle afferent fibers (the H reflex) is increased on the involved side in hemiplegia. Long-term changes have been attributed to sprouting of additional primary afferent neuron collaterals to form new synaptic endings on anterior horn cells, and to postsynaptic sensitization. Theoretically, long-term changes could also be based on changes in the presynaptic terminal, the transmitter agent, or the postsynaptic membrane, including both excitatory and inhibitory mechanisms.

Is the *fusimotor system* involved in spasticity? This system is made up of the small gamma motor neurons of the ventral horn that send their axons directly to the muscle spindles, causing them to contract. Normally, a fraction of these specialized small motor neurons are tonically active at rest, causing contraction of the intrafusal (spindle) muscle fibers and keeping the stretch receptors taut and sensitive to stretch. Since the small axons of gamma motor neurons are more sensitive to local anesthetic agents, it is possible to block them in the normal human subject and thus to desensitize the stretch receptors and grossly depress the stretch reflexes. This does not affect muscle strength. Similarly, a diffuse anesthesia produced by spinal or eipidural block that spares the large axons of alpha motor neurons produces remarkably little motor disability, only a peculiar feeling of looseness similar to what may be noted after sitting in one position a long time. Similar treatment of spastic patients will abolish spasticity along with the hyperactive tendon jerks, but the impaired motor performance (the negative symptom) does not improve; it may be worse. This proves that sensitive muscle spindles are necessary for spasticity to occur. It is not true, however, that spasticity is entirely or even largely due to increased fusimotor tone; both tonic gamma firing and maintained alpha hyperexcitability operate together to cause (1) the increased segmental reflex to a quick "jerk" stretch, and (2) the claspknife reaction to a slow stretch.

Clonus may occur in patients with damage to corticospinal pathways, after the stretch reflexes have increased. It consists of a tremor that oscillates at about 5 beats per second that is elicited by a suddenly applied, maintained ("step") stretch of muscle. This maneuver produces a series of rhythmic, phasic stretch reflex contractions, interrupted by silent periods. The first sudden passive stretch to the tested muscle produces a reflex contraction of the muscle that unloads the spindles that are in parallel with the muscle fibers. The resulting transient loss of excitatory input to the spinal cord lowers the alpha motor neuron excitability and is the major cause of the silent period. Additional factors in the silent period are (1) the inhibition of alpha motor neurons directly by the Renshaw interneurons that are activated by the previous alpha volley, (2) disynaptic inhibition of the alpha motor neuron by the Golgi tendon organs that are activated by the previous muscular contraction, and (3) the relative refractory period of the alpha motor neuron membrane to excitation. The silent period in the alpha motor neurons allows the muscle to relax; the maintained stretching force applied by the examiner suddenly encounters no resistance and again stretches the muscle, setting up another stretch reflex contraction. The cycle can often continue indefinitely. The patient may inadvertently start clonus by such maneuvers as stepping on the gas pedal of his car.

It is important to emphasize that, for the patient, spasticity is not the most troublesome symptom. Indeed, it may be a functional asset. For example, the hemiparetic patient whose knee tends to buckle finds that the spasticity provides a useful bracing action. In this situation, the release of the reflex by the lesion in the corticospinal tract may indeed implement its putative automatic function of maintaining the body upright against gravity. To be sure, clonus can be annoying, and adductor spasticity in young patients may lead to a scissor gait, but, for most patients, release of stretch reflexes is of no symptomatic significance. This conclusion is based on simple clinical observation and is confirmed by the experiments cited earlier, where abolition of spasticity by fusimotor blockade did not improve motor function.

Skin and other flexor reflexes

Applying a sharp, moving stimulus to the lateral aspect of the plantar surface of the foot in normal humans causes the big toe to plantar flex. In humans with lesions of the corticospinal pathways the entire leg may undergo reflex withdrawal, and the dorsiflexion of the big toe to plantar stimulation is the earliest manifestation of this response. This first sign of the *released flexor reflex* is called the *Babinski response*. It is an involuntary reflex dorsiflexion of the big toe, sometimes with lateral spreading ("fanning") of the remaining toes, caused by slowly stroking the lateral edge of the sole or side of the foot from heel to toe. Babinski's sign (the extensor plantar reflex) is one of the most subtle and reliable signs of impairment of the upper motor neuron system. The normal plantar flexion and the abnormal dorsiflexion of the big toe elicited in this reflex share the following features: Specific activation is by pain endings, the minimal threshold is in the S_1 dermatome, and there are both temporal and spatial summation. The central latencies of the normal and abnormal reflexes are identical and indicate a polysynaptic segmental linkage. The motor locus of contraction is in the short flexor muscles of the hallux, with associated flexion at ankle, knee, and hip. But after corticospinal lesions, the neurons supplying the extensor hallucis longus (a dorsiflexor of the big toe) become hyperexcitable, so that the same stimulus causes the normal response to reverse. Peroneal nerve block of the hallux extensor does not abolish the reflex but permits the flexors to dominate. In both the normal and abnormal response, there is an actual mechanical competition between the hallux flexors and the extensor hallucis longus. The abnormal extensor reflex is thus not a *different* reaction from the flexor, but rather an addition to it in which the extensor of the great toe is included, almost by accident, in the radiation of normal reflex activity.

In chronic spinal cord damage, stimulation of skin and deeper structures may cause the limbs to flex at all joints so forcibly that, if sufficient ascending pain paths remain to convey the message to the brain, the patient feels intense pain. Less commonly, extensor spasms of all limbs may also be observed. The extent to which these opposite limb reactions use the same circuitry that underlies normal human walking is not known; suffice it to say that rhythmic alternation between the two in a periodicity resembling normal gait is only rarely observed.

Three other superficial, polysynaptic reflexes that also depend on slow, small-diameter afferent fibers and nociception behave quite differently. The abdominal, corneal, and cremasteric reflexes are all segmental reflexes. Yet these reflexes are depressed, not enhanced, by upper motor neuron lesions. This suggests that there is a normal dependence upon tonic excitation from above for the response by the reflex pathway to a transient stimulus input. In sum, these three reflexes contrast with the plantar response: The latter is present and changes character with corticospinal disease (the toe goes up instead of down), whereas the former disappear.

CONTROLS DESCENDING FROM THE BRAIN TO THE SPINAL CORD

All too commonly, strokes, tumors, multiple sclerosis, and other human diseases interrupt the pathways that descend from the brain to control the spinal cord machinery. The pathways can be grouped into two categories that are spatially and functionally different. These categories have been termed the medial and the lateral spinal systems by Kuypers, and the relative effects of damage to one or the other have been most clearly demonstrated by Lawrence and Kuypers in monkeys.

The *lateral system* consists of the corticospinal and rubrospinal paths that run together in the medullary pyramid and the lateral funiculus of the spinal cord. In monkeys, interruption caused a transient, complete paralysis of the body, with a remarkable degree of recovery. Within weeks, the damaged monkeys could stand, walk, run, and climb with little indication of neurologic impairment. The only movements found to be severely and permanently impaired were individuated movements of the digits, manifested in these studies as difficulty picking small bits of food out of deep, narrow food wells with the fingers. If only the corticospinal or the rubrospinal path were lesioned, survival of the other allowed even greater recovery of function, including some control of the individual digits. These studies, more than any other, suggest that an important function of these paths and the parts of the brain from which they arise is the movement of an individual digit independent of others, such as the precision grip of the thumb and forefinger.

Movements of the digits are also severely affected by lesions of the corticospinal pathway in humans. The delicacy and finesse ("dexterity") of these movements will usually be affected before there is measurable loss of strength or increase in muscle stretch or skin-withdrawal reflexes. *Fine finger movements* are commonly tested by such tasks as turning a coin over and over with the fingers in one direction and then in the reverse, buttoning and unbottoning, turning a screw in a nut, opening and closing safety pins, opposing the thumb to the tip of each of the fingers in rapid succession, and tapping the forefinger quickly, accurately, and rhythmically on the crease of the distal joint of the thumb.

A patient suffering complete destruction of the corticospinal fibers within the internal capsule or at the medullary pyramid may have an initial flaccid hemiplegia, yet within a year may recover almost full function of the extremities except for the digits. The capacity for recovery is most dramatic in younger individuals. This sort of recovery, or plasticity, does not necessarily imply redundancy within the organization of the motor system, but rather suggests that few individuals use the capacities they are born with to the full extent. A pianist, typist, or tailor suffering such a lesion might be expected to appreciate a greater and longer-lasting impairment than someone who does not depend so heavily on fine manual skills.

The same argument cannot be used to say that the lateral system controls *only* individuated movements of the fingers. For within the acute phase of the lesion, the hemiplegia may be profound, involving not only fine movements, but all movements of the fingers, and not only the distal muscles, but the proximal muscles as well. After recovery, are the surviving movements of digits and trunk more than normally subject to reflex and postural control? Are the proximal and trunk muscles, like the distal muscles, impaired for fractionated and individuated movements? Can exercise of the remaining control systems be used in physiotherapy to promote functional recovery? These questions may hold clues to improved understanding and treatment, but at this stage they have not been satisfactorily answered.

As the second component of the descending motor pathways, Lawrence and Kuypers defined a *medial system* that originates from the vestibular nuclei, the pontine and medullary reticular nuclei, the interstitial nucleus, and the optic tectum (superior colliculi). In monkeys, these can be selectively damaged by lesions at the site of origin, and by medial lesions at the pontomedullary junction and in the ventral funiculus of the cord. Monkeys thus impaired initially could not right themselves from a lying position, sit, walk, climb, place limbs upon skin contact, or orient body posture to visual stimuli. Movements most affected were those of the trunk and proximal limb musculature used to support or move against gravity or to orient toward visual or tactile stimuli. Movements least affected were those of the distal digits in exploratory, palpatory activities. In time, these animals recovered much of their capacity for the whole-body postures and movements. Presumably, some of the compensation was carried out by the corticospinal-rubrospinal lateral system: Animals in which these structures were previously damaged failed to recover.

In human disease, one rarely sees lesions of the medial system that neatly spare the lateral system. There are situations, however, in which acute disease processes (anoxia/ischemia from vascular occlusion or the pressure from hemorrhage or tumor) irritate the components of the medial system in the pons and midbrain and may give rise to movements of the trunk and limbs that in some ways resemble normal postural reactions. One of these reactions is the so-called *decerebrate response,* which, in the brainstem lesions noted above, occurs either spontaneously or in response to noxious stimulation of the upper part of the body. The response consists of lowering the shoulder, extension at the elbow, and intorsion of the humerus, with flail fingers; the legs extend at the hip and knee, and the foot plantar flexes and turns in (Fig. 9–4). This pattern of extensor movement of the four limbs has been likened to what one sees if one "decerebrates" a cat either by transecting the midbrain at the level of the red nucleus or by tying off both carotids and the basilar artery (which accomplishes the same effect and ablates the cortex of the anterior lobe of the cerebellum as well). It has been

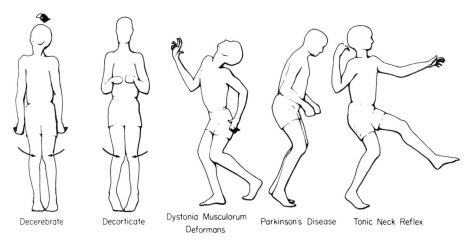

| Decerebrate | Decorticate | Dystonia Musculorum Deformans | Parkinson's Disease | Tonic Neck Reflex |

Fig. 9–4. Patterns of rigidity: increased muscular activity at rest.

suggested that decerebration in the cat re-leases the basic neural mechanism that normally generates four-legged stance in the normal behavior of the cat, and that in human the circuitry is vestigially pre-sent, though less often used, because sub-sequent phylogenetic development has re-sulted in a "higher" mechanism that dominates the lower one to produce two-legged stance. Others have pointed out that the decerebrate response is usually a tran-sient affair, both in cat and in humans, that occurs acutely, and it is therefore more likely to reflect irritation of the parts in question rather than a true release of a posture-generating mechanism. Which-ever view one takes, the clinical picture of the transient extension of both arm and leg in a comatose patient should be inter-preted as a brainstem in dire jeopardy (Chap. 10).

It has been suggested that the two-legged stance depends on neural genera-tors located just above the midbrain, since removal of the cerebral cortex in monkeys results in an obligatory two-legged stance, with arms flexed and legs extended. Pa-tients with destruction of the internal cap-sule, which cuts off input to structures in the midbrain and below, develop the same postural reaction ("hemiplegic posture")

with the passage of time. The arm is flexed at the elbow, wrist, and fingers; the leg is extended at the hip and knee, with plantar flexion in equinovarus of the ankle and foot. This posture is often not interrupti-ble by willed attempts at movement, yet may change during other involuntary ac-tivities like coughing, sneezing, and laugh-ing: The arm may rise at the shoulder or straighten at the elbow, presumably under some other controlling mechanism. As in the monkey, the mechanism is to some ex-tent under vestibular control, since when the patient is turned upside down, the head and neck extend (head-righting vestibu-lar/optical reflex), and then (because of both the labyrinthine and the tonic neck reflexes) the arms extend and the legs flex, as if the arms were to be used to support the body against gravity.

The hemiplegic posture is similar in appearance to the tonic neck reflexes, which also appear after lesions of the in-ternal capsule or upper midbrain. In these reflexes, when the head is actively or pas-sively turned to one side, the arm and leg that the face is turned toward extend and the opposite limbs flex (Fig. 9–4). These tonic neck reflexes are also seen in normal newborn infants and are interpreted as being the activity of brainstem nuclei that have not as yet come under corticobulbar control because of immaturity. The circuitry that causes these reflex whole-body synergies has not as yet been delineated more precisely. Stimulation of the interstitial nucleus in the midbrain may cause a similar turn of the head away, truncal incurvation, and the opposite limbs to extend. A lesion in this nucleus may cause the reverse pattern, presumably due to the release from competition of the activity of the intact nucleus on the opposite side. Patients with an inherited disease called dystonia musculorum deformans frequently have forced postures of head and neck that resemble the normal patterns of tonic neck reflexes and that may represent overactivity at these midbrain structures.

Role of cerebral motor cortex

The postulated role of the cerebral motor cortex in contributing to individuated, precise movements of small parts of the body is supported by various studies of animals. Electrical stimulation of the cortex can cause movement of an individual digit, the eyelid, or corner of the mouth, and even of one muscle. Neurons in the motor cortex are arranged in radial columns in which the cells appear to be directly and indirectly connected through to the muscles that act mainly at one joint. The same cortical cells receive somatosensory feedback from the skin, muscles, and joints of the same limb they cause to move. This feedback may be used in palpatory, exploratory movements and may contribute to the accuracy of movements of precise distances and forces. Speed of movement is provided both by the direct connection of about 20% of corticospinal neurons to alpha motor neurons of the distal muscles and by the ability to "preset" motor cortex for complex movements (organized by other parts of the brain), which may be triggered by sensory stimuli delivered to the part that is to be moved. The "programs" for complex

movements are thought to be delivered to motor cortex from the supplementary motor, premotor, prefrontal, and parietal cortical areas, both directly and possibly by way of the basal ganglia and cerebellum.

The motor cortex has been studied extensively by Evarts, who recorded neuronal discharge in trained monkeys as they performed movements with the upper limb; the results support the conclusions of the ablation and stimulation studies. Thus, many of the neurons in motor cortex discharge before the movement and relate to specific sets of muscles (e.g., extensors), and to the force generated by those muscles. Small cortical neurons reach peak activity during tiny, precise movements of small force and are sensitive to feedback from the limb; large cortical neurons discharge only in relation to large, fast movements of greater force. These properties are rather like those of the spinal alpha motor neurons, which also have a recruitment order from small to large neurons (size principle) as force requirements are increased. Moreover, the motor cortex neurons (especially the smaller ones) have a fast afferent pathway to them from muscle spindles and skin receptors, which enables them to function in *long looped* reflexes in a manner very similar to that of the alpha motor neurons in the segmental stretch reflex. Thus, a neuron in the motor cortex that appears to be coupled to a flexor muscle will be activated when that muscle is stretched and will generate an output that can help cause the muscle to contract. This might seem redundant, and merely additive to the segmental reflex, but Evarts and Brooks have evidence to suggest that the long looped reflex may be used to initiate useful movement, whereas the segmental stretch reflex is not. These properties of corticospinal neurons in the motor cortex thus appear so similar to those of alpha motor neurons as to justify the clinician's term *upper motor neurons.* Evarts has taken the view that their function is indeed as though they were upstream representatives of alpha motor neurons, their main role being to serve as nodal points for the various, more complex motor programs from other parts of the brain to gain access to the lower motor neuron.

These programs are viewed as coming from the basal ganglia and the cerebellum (both via the ventral thalamus) and from other parts of cerebral cortex. Indeed, neurons have been found in the supplementary motor cortex (a somatotopically organized region just anterior to the motor cortex on the medial surface of the hemisphere) that fire during motor performance as if they were supplying a gating signal to motor cortex neurons to either respond, or not respond, to sensory inputs. Thus, depending on what the subject wishes to do, he can either make or not make a quick (60-msec) response to a perturbation of the hand in the *transcortical reflex*. The movement is like a reflex in that it has a short reaction time, but it is like a voluntary movement in that it is subject to the will or intent.

It is not clear yet how these capacities of motor cortex and its input structures are normally used in human behavior, nor how they are impaired by diseases that affect the motor cortex. The fact that motor cortex is wired for speedy, sensory-initiated or sensory-guided movement may explain why palpatory and exploratory low-force, fast, accurate fine finger movements are so badly impaired by motor cortex lesions.

Premotor lesions of cerebral cortex can result in a forced grasp of the patient's hand on any object that touches the palm. It is possible that the grasp reflex may be produced by a "released" transcortical reflex. The grasp reflex may be graded in degrees, from something the patient may overcome when attention is directed to it, to a response that he cannot overcome, or even to one that is generated by a visual stimulus. Some have interpreted this as a release of the parietal lobe's normal activity

of exploring and manipulating the environment. Single unit recordings in the awake monkey's parietal lobe by Mountcastle and others have discovered single neurons that discharge preferentially in relation to a limb movement but only when it reaches toward an "object of interest." *Gegenhalten* ("hold against") is the curious behavior of a demented individual who "perversely" resists virtually any passive displacement of the limb. This also could be due to a parietal position-holding mechanism that is released from control of the frontal lobe.

Role of basal ganglia

The basal ganglia—masses of neurons at the base of the cerebrum—are well developed in vertebrates that have little cerebral cortex (fish, amphibia, reptiles, birds). They have therefore been viewed as phylogenetically "old" parts of the motor system that regulate brainstem and spinal reflexes, and they add motor programs of their own. The consequences of lesions of these structures are compatible with this view: The deficits caused by damage are mainly (if not exclusively) motor and consist of too little (negative defect) or too much (released or irritative function, positive defect) movement. Indeed, the lack of movement after lesions of the basal ganglia may be so severe *(akinesia)* as to support the idea that the basal ganglia are indeed fundamental to motor control.

The components and circuitry of the basal ganglia are diagramed in Figures 9–2 and 9–5. The inputs to the basal ganglia come from the entire cerebral cortex and parts of the thalamus and are received by the *striatum,* which consists of the *caudate nucleus* and the *putamen.* The striatum provides an inhibitory projection to the *globus pallidus* and also projects to the *substantia nigra.* The globus pallidus and substantia nigra, pars reticulata together constitute the major source of outputs from the basal ganglia to the thalamus and

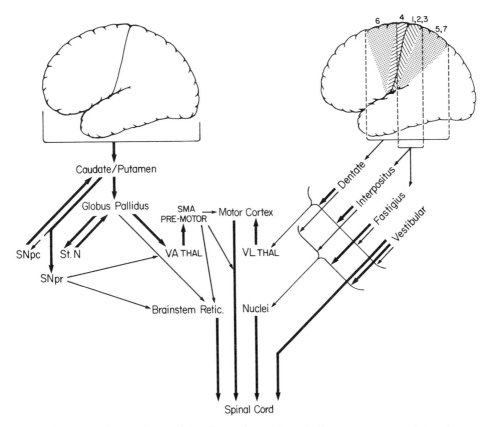

Fig. 9–5. Connections of basal ganglia and cerebellum: extrapyramidal and prepyramidal. SMA, supplementary motor area of cerebral cortex; PM, premotor area of cerebral cortex; VA Thal., ventral anterior nuclei of thalamus; VL Thal., Ventral lateral nuclei of thalamus; St. N., Subthalamic nucleus; SNpc, substantia nigra pars compacta; SNpr, substantia nigra pars reticulata. The basal ganglia receive from the entire cerebral cortex and project to brainstem nuclei and VA thalamus, which in turn projects indirectly to motor cortex and to brainstem nuclei. The cerebellum receives from sensorimotor cortex (and the immediately adjacent regions) and projects directly to spinal cord, brainstem nuclei, and (via VL thalamus) motor cortex.

brainstem. From the thalamus (ventroanterior and ventrolateral nuclei) fibers project onto the premotor and supplementary motor cortex. Other structures important in the physiology of the basal ganglia include the *substantia nigra, pars compacta* the *subthalamic nucleus.* The substantia nigra, pars compacta is the major source of inhibitory dopaminergic input onto the striatum. The subthalamic nucleus receives input from the external segment of the globus pallidus and sends inhibitory outputs to the internal segment of the globus pallidus.

Historically, differing views of the function of the basal ganglia have been based on the output projections. Neurologists at the turn of the century (e.g., Wilson) believed that the output was mainly to the recticular nuclei of the brainstem, which in turn gave rise to reticulospinal pathways. Since these motor pathways were in parallel with the corticospinal (pyramidal) tracts, they were termed *ex-*

trapyramidal. Recent anatomical studies in cat and monkey suggest that the pallidothalamic projection ends upon thalamic neurons that project to premotor cortex and the supplementary motor area. To the extent that these cortical areas in turn project to motor cortex, this basal ganglia → thalamic → cortical circuit could be viewed as *prepyramidal*. In sum, both the appellations—extrapyramidal and prepyramidal—are correct but are oversimplifications, and the future view should incorporate *both* pathways as expressing the output of the basal ganglia.

Much of our understanding of the pathophysiology of basal ganglionic disease comes from observations of patients and experimentally lesioned animals. Large bilateral lesions of the globus pallidus in monkeys produce profound akinesia, an inability to generate volitional movement. This is usually combined with an involuntary rigid posture (dystonia) of flexion of the neck, trunk, and all joints of the limbs. The rigidity has a characteristic "plastic" quality, similar to the resistance one experiences when bending a lead pipe. There is a yielding that is independent of the velocity of the displacement, and the limb keeps the position to which it is displaced. This is distinctly different from the spring-like, velocity-dependent resistance of the claspknife reaction that characterizes the spasticity of corticospinal lesions.

By contrast, small, one-sided lesions of the subthalamic nucleus usually produce a very striking abnormality of the contralateral limbs called *hemiballismus*. The contralateral arm and/or leg are involved in constant, wild, flinging movements, chiefly at the shoulder and hip. This occurs within days after the lesion and may persist. Small lesions of the putamen and caudate can give rise to involuntary movements of the contralateral limbs called *chorea*, from the Greek word meaning "dance." Chorea is a rapid movement spanning several muscles and joints so as to give the appearance of a normal "coordinated" movement.

While choreic movements are often mistakenly called "jerky" because of their speed, which may be of the order of two to three excursions per second, they are usually sufficiently coordinated across muscles and joints that they appear sinuous or writhing. These movements may involve face, arm, leg, neck, trunk, but when least severe they most commonly involve distal musculature (face, hand, foot). The tempo of the movement may also be much slower, with "worm-like" writhing that lasts many seconds or even many minutes. These slower movements are called *athetosis* (changing posture). The movements may also occur at differing tempos in the same individual; they are then called *choreoathetosis*. Chorea occurs most dramatically in Huntington's disease and after streptococcal infections (Sydenham's chorea). In the latter situation there is evidence for an antibody against a streptococcal antigen that cross-reacts with a membrane protein in the striatum. The slower, athetoid movements occur after anoxic birth injury to the basal ganglia and in the inherited disease, dystonia musculorum deformans.

Akinesia, the profound decrease of spontaneous movement that is characteristic of Parkinson's syndrome, is thought to be the result of decreased output of the globus pallidus. As indicated earlier, lesions of the globus pallidus result in akinesia in experimental monkeys. Cooling of the globus pallidus by a probe placed in the brain interrupts the monkey's ability to make alternating movements, with recovery when the globus pallidus is allowed to return to normal temperature. In humans, the syndrome of multiple small (lacunar) infarcts in the globus pallidus is associated with akinesia and bradykinesia. Carbon monoxide poisoning produces marked necrosis of the globus pallidus bilaterally and parkinsonian akinesia. However, since akinesia is also associated with lesions in other parts of the motor system, the pathophysiologic mechanism is not straightforward. A decrease in the activity of the globus pallidus may occur in idiopathic Parkinson's disease, even though there is degeneration of the substantia nigra, pars compacta and not of the globus pallidus (Chap. 19). Lesions of the substantia nigra, pars compacta result in decreased inhibition of the striatum. Some evidence suggests that this disinhibition results in increased striatal activity, increasing inhibition of the globus pallidus and therefore decreasing its output. Drugs acting like dopamine, such as L-dopa (converted to dopamine), bromocriptine, and apomorphine, are thought to improve parkinsonian symptoms by reestablishing inhibition onto the striatum, thereby disinhibiting the globus pallidus. The clinical and pharmacological aspects of Parkinson's syndrome are covered in more detail in Chapter 19.

Conversely, involuntary movements such as chorea, athetosis, and hemiballismus may be associated with excessive abnormal output of the globus pallidus due to loss of inhibitory input. The subthalamic nucleus is inhibitory on the globus pallidus, and lesions of the subthalamus are associated with hemiballismus. Similarly, a lesion of the striatum, which also inhibits the globus pallidus, can produce chorea and athetosis. In Huntington's chorea there is marked neuronal degeneration in the striatum. Other types of lesions in the human striatum, including cysts and infarcts, have been associated with chorea and athetosis. Clinical manifestations of disordered globus pallidus output are probably mediated via the VA and VL thalamus and their projections to the premotor, supplementary motor, and motor cortex. However, the mechanisms involved are controversial. Current hypotheses part company over the nature of the pallidothalamic projection. One model holds that this projection is inhibitory. There is evidence, however that the pallidothalamic projection is excitatory or at least both excitatory and inhibitory (Fig.

9–2). In the model advanced in this chapter, the symptoms of Parkinson's disease might result from the loss of the capacity to send motor programs from the globus pallidus to the thalamus and thence to the cortex, resulting in the inability to initiate voluntary movements (akinesia). If the pallidal-thalamic pathway proves to be inhibitory, the absence of pallidal input may cause thalamic overactivity, driving motor cortex to produce rigidity and tremor. However this would not explain bradykinesia or akinesia. If the pallidal-thalamic pathway proves to be excitatory, then decreased drive to the thalamus and motor cortex would explain akinesia and bradykinesia, but would not readily explain rigidity or tremor.

ROLE OF THE CEREBELLUM

The cerebellum occupies about a quarter of the cranial cavity and is exclusively concerned with the control of movement. Yet its total removal does not abolish movement and rarely even causes muscular weakness. Instead, ablation causes a unique kind of incoordination of the contractions of all the muscles used in any one act, which is called *ataxia* (loss of order). Lesions also produce a 3–5- second side-to-side tremor of the moving part (Fig. 9–9). That so much tissue should be devoted to so subtle a function is reason enough for the cerebellum to have been regarded as rather mysterious. Yet its vulnerability to most of the nonspecific disease processes that attack the CNS, and to several diseases unique to the cerebellum, is reason enough to know something of its functions.

Most of the abnormalities resulting from cerebellar damage may be seen in the contraction of a single muscle. Occasionally there is reduced resistance of the muscles to passive lengthening *(hypotonia)*, and more rarely a slight weakness *(asthenia)* of voluntary contraction. Some have argued that these abnormalities are basic to

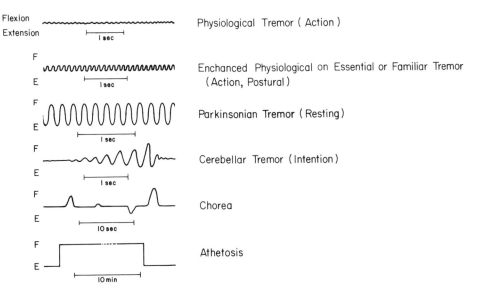

Fig. 9–6. Patterns of involuntary movements showing frequency, relative amplitude, and regularity.

all of the others that are always present and are more severe. For example, lesions of the cerebellum produce an inability to hold a muscle at a given fixed length when unexpected perturbations lengthen or shorten it. When tapped, the outstretched arm or leg is displaced farther than normal, and on the return swing, it overshoots the previous position and then continues to oscillate around that position, much like a weight on the end of a spring. Another example of this is the pendular knee jerk. When the quadriceps is stretched by a tap of the patellar tendon, the leg rises, then falls, and swings to and fro around its initial position for several excursions of underdamped oscillation. In volitional movements, there is a slight delay (100–200 msec, Fig. 9–9) in the start and stop of the movement, and often great irregularity of the shortening of the active muscles so as to cause errors in velocity and trajectory. In the finger-to-nose and heel-to-knee-to-shin movements, there are large errors in the direction of movement as the target is approached (Figs. 9–6, 9–9). In rapid alternating movements (slapping the palm and then the dorsum of one hand against the other, pronation-suppination of the wrist, tapping the forefinger against the thumb), there is gross inability to maintain regularity of amplitude and tempo. In tandem gait (heel-to-toe walking a straight line), there are frequent teeterings of the trunk and arms, and side steps of the feet, to prevent a fall. So great may the abnormalities be in these and other clinical tests, in the complete absence of hypotonia or weakness, that it is difficult to view the disorder as other than a fundamental impairment of coordination.

Microanatomy: fundamental cerebellar circuit: The histological architecture of the cerebellum appears rather simple, and this has led to many speculations concerning its function (Fig. 9–7). The cerebellum receives only two types of afferent fibers, the *mossy fibers* (mf) and the *climbing fibers* (cf). These arise from different sources and project upon the cerebellum in quite different ways. Mossy fibers have many different origins; each fiber projects upon the cerebellar cortex, where it divides to send branches to reach several adjacent folia, terminating in excitatory synapses on up to 50 granule cells (gr). Each granule cell sends its axon upward to the most superficial layer of the cerebellar cortex, where it branches dichotomously in the coronal plane to form parallel fibers. Each parallel fiber synapses on up to 500 Purkinje cells along its coronal trajectory, and each Purkinje cell receives the convergent projections of more than 200,000 parallel fibers. This excitatory input to the Purkinje cell causes action potentials of a simple form, called the *simple spike* (Fig. 9–7). Purkinje cells discharge simple spikes at a maintained frequency of 50–100 per second. The parallel fibers also converge upon the inhibitory neurons of the cerebellar cortex, the stellate, basket, and Golgi cells. The stellate and basket cells terminate in inhibitory synapses on Purkinje cell dendrites and somata, respectively, thus producing a form of feedforward inhibition.

The termination of the climbing fiber differs strikingly from that of the mossy fiber: It enters the cortex to end in excitatory synapses on one or a very few Purkinje cells; each Purkinje cell receives only one climbing fiber. The climbing fiber terminates in massive synaptic contacts upon the soma and proximal dendrites of the Purkinje cell, which differs from the single synapse of a parallel fiber on a single dendritic spine of a Purkinje cell. An action potential in a climbing fiber evokes a multispiked action potential in the Purkinje cell, called the *complex spike* (Fig. 9–7), which occurs sporadically at an average rate of about one per second. The climbing fiber also synapses on all of the inhibitory neurons of the cerebellar cortex. The cerebellar cortex possesses a single output channel, the projection of the Purkinje cell axons upon the cells of the deep cerebellar and vestibular nuclei; this output has been shown by Ito to be inhibitory. The cerebellar output that is excitatory is then generated by the deep cerebellar and ves-

tibular nuclei. The neurons of the cerebellar nuclei also receive an excitatory input from collaterals of the mossy fibers and to a much lesser extent from those of the climbing fibers. There may be some mossy fibers that only project to cells of the deep nuclei.

In summary, four features of cerebellar circuitry figure prominently in physiological theory: (1) All nuclear output is excitatory, whatever its destination; (2) the cortical circuitry is much the same in all parts of the cortex, and all cortical output is inhibitory whether it is destined for the deep cerebellar nuclei or the vestibular nuclei; (3) all input to the cerebellum, both that to the cortex and to the deep nuclei, is excitatory; and (4) the Purkinje cell receives two excitatory inputs that differ markedly in terminal synaptic distribution and action upon the Purkinje cell. The circuit has been caricatured as an inhibitory "side loop" superimposed on an excitatory "main line"; though oversimplified, this concept is useful in thinking about cerebellar function.

The three cerebellar zones and their ablation syndromes

While the basic circuitry is the same throughout the cerebellum, there are regional differences defined by where the input mossy fibers come from, what kind of information they carry, and where the output from the different deep nuclei goes (Fig. 9–8). By convention, there are three major subdivisions according to the input–output connections; each of these has developed to different degrees in different animal phyla, and each has its own unique ablation syndrome in humans. Fish have a well-developed cerebellum, receiving mossy fiber input chiefly from vestibular nerve and nuclei; the output from cerebellar cortex is sent back to the vestibular nuclei. In humans, this portion remains as the *vestibulocerebellum*: the *flocculus, nodulus,* and *parafloccular lobes.* Carnivores have, in

A

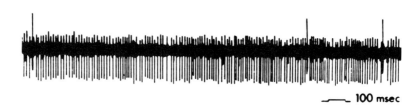

B

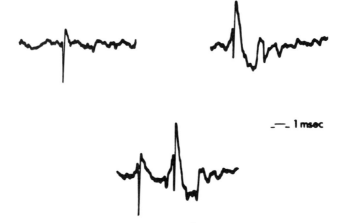

100 msec

1 msec

Fig. 9–7. **A.** Simplified diagram of cerebellar circuitry. mf, mossy fiber; cf, climbing fiber, gr, granule cell; Go, Golgi cell; b, basket cell; s, stellate cell; P, Purkinje cell; n, nuclear cell. White cells are excitatory, black are inhibitory. Diagram shows only what types of cell one type contacts and whether contact is excitatory or inhibitory. The recently discovered nucleocortical fibers are not included. **B.** Maintained discharge of a Purkinje cell, recorded extracellularly, showing its two spike potentials; the simple (left) and the complex (right). The slow trace (top) shows their different patterns of discharge, and the fast traces (bottom three) their different shapes. Positivity is up.

addition, a portion of the cerebellum with especially well developed mossy fiber systems from the spinal cord, the rapidly conducting spinocerebellar pathways. The output from the cerebellar cortex and the fastigial and interposed nuclei in turn goes to systems that project back again to the spinal cord: the lateral vestibular nucleus, the brainstem reticular formation, and the red nucleus. In humans, this portion is called the *spinocerebellum,* and it consists of the entire vermal and paravermal portions rostral to the vestibulocerebellum: the *anterior lobe, folium, declive, tuber, pyramis,* and *paramedian lobules.* Primates have particularly well developed lateral hemispheres of the cerebellum, which receive mossy fiber input from the pontine-cerebellar nuclei that in turn carry information from the cerebral cortex. The output is carried from the lateral (dentate) nucleus mainly to the ventral "motor" thalamus, which then projects back to cerebral (motor) cortex. This is called the *neocerebellum,* or *cerebrocerebellum,* because of its presumed unique relationship to cerebral neocortex. However, it has just been discovered that in primates there is rerouting of much of the output from the vestibulocerebellum (vestibular nuclei) and the spinocerebellum (fastigial and interposed = globose and emboliform nuclei) to the ventral thalamus, where it interdigitates with cerebrocerebellar output (dentate nucleus) to project ultimately back to motor cortex (Figs. 9–5, 9–8a). Thus, primates have not only added a new cerebellar region to process cerebral information in the control of movement, but have

also directed it along with much of the vestibulocerebellar and spinocerebellar information to a phylogenetically "new" nodal point "higher" than the brainstem: the motor cortex.

Vestibulocerebellum. The vestibulocerebellum functions to coordinate the movements of the eyes and the body with respect to gravity (utricle) and the turning of the head in space (semicircular canals) (Chap. 8). Damage to it results in ataxic stance and gait, such that the patient reels and staggers drunkenly, makes many surprisingly agile "saves" from falling, but falls frequently. Vestibular control of limbs and body against gravity is specifically lacking; when gravity is eliminated and the patient is lying in bed, the movements are completely normal. This discrepancy is frequently so striking as to give the incorrect impression that the patient is consciously or subconsciously feigning illness. Since a tumor in this area of the cerebellum may produce its next symptoms by compressing the brainstem, interfering with such vital functions as respiration, it is important to think of this diagnosis before dismissing a bizarre gait as due to hysteria or malingering. The symptoms of vestibulocerebellar damage constitute a negative defect, where muscles are controlled fully normally *except* when they are required to compensate for gravity (standing and walking erect) and to keep the eyes fixed on a distant target despite the constant turnings of the head (the vestibulo-ocular reflex).

A number of other oculomotor abnor-

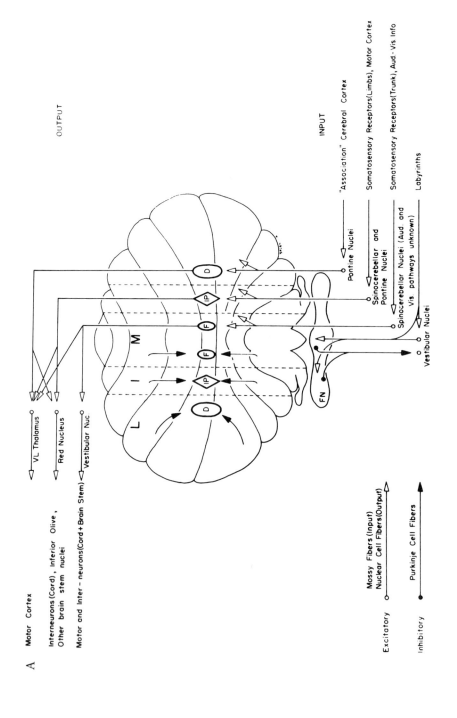

A   Motor Cortex

OUTPUT

VL Thalamus

Interneurons(Cord), Inferior Olive,
Other brain stem nuclei

Red Nucleus

Motor and Inter-neurons(Cord+Brain Stem)   Vestibular Nuc.

L   I   M

D   P   F   F   P   D

FN

Pontine Nuclei

Spinocerebellar and
Pontine Nuclei

Spinocerebellar Nuclei (Aud. and
Vis. pathways unknown)

Vestibular Nuclei

INPUT

"Association" Cerebral Cortex

Somatosensory Receptors(Limbs), Motor Cortex

Somatosensory Receptors(Trunk), Aud.-Vis Info

Labyrinths

Excitatory   o———   Mossy Fibers (Input)
             ▷———   Nuclear Cell Fibers(Output)

Inhibitory   •———   Purkinje Cell Fibers

B

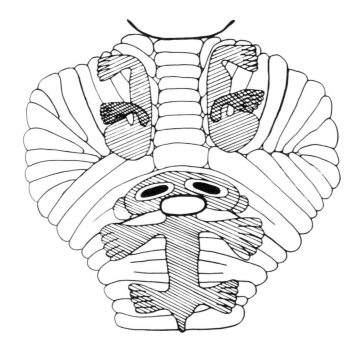

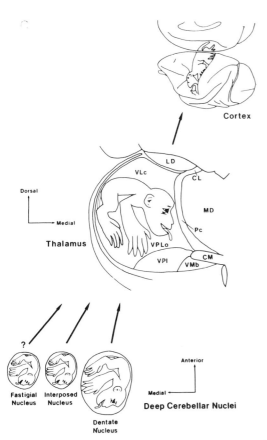

Fig. 9–8. A. Diagram of overall cerebellar organization. Transverse cortical folds comprise folia, lobules, and lobes. The longitudinal pattern of projection of cortical Purkinje cells onto deep nuclei and their targets is indicated. Mossy fiber inputs often branch to reach both nuclei and cortex. Also shown is the origin of mossy fibers supplying different subdivisions and modalities of information they are likely to carry. Pontine and medullary tegmental reticular nuclei supply all of cerebellum with mossy fibers (not shown). VL, ventrolateral (nucleus of thalamus); lateral (L), intermediate (I), medial (M) cerebellar cortex; D, dentate nucleus; IP, interposed nucleus; F, fastigial nucleus. B. Tactile receiving areas of cerebellum. Pattern of tactile representation in cerebellum of macaque. Representation is ipsilateral in anterior lobe and bilateral in paramedian lobules. C. Somatotopy in the cerebellothalamocortical pathway. Each deep cerebellar nucleus contains a complete representation of the body and projects in overlapping fashion onto the VL nuclei of the thalamus. CL, central lateral nucleus; CM, centre median nucleus; LD, lateral dorsal nucleus; Pc, paracentral nucleus; VLc, ventral lateral nucleus, caudal division; VMb, basal ventromedial nucleus; VPI ventral posterior nucleus, inferior division; VPLo, ventral posterior nucleus, oral division.

malities have been described with lesions of the vestibulocerebellum. One is a tendency for the gaze to come to rest slightly deviated from the midline, away from the side of the lesion. This is due to the removal of the tonic inhibitory discharge of the vestibulocerebellar Purkinje cells onto the ipsilateral medial vestibular nucleus. When excited by electrical stimulation (and by a turn of the head), the medial vestibular nucleus acts to drive the eyes away from the stimulated side; removal of tonic Purkinje cell inhibition is the equivalent of nuclear excitation, and the resting discharge of the uninhibited medial vestibular nucleus cells jumps to a higher level. The same mechanism explains nystagmus: When gaze is attempted *toward* the side of the cerebellar lesion, there is a tendency for the eyes to drift back to midline, corrected by a jerk back in the direction of the attempted gaze. The gaze mechanisms have difficulty in overcoming the uninhibited vestibular nuclear drive on that side and must keep correcting with a saccadic jerk. In vestibulocerebellar lesions, there may also be a tilt of the head, with the occiput lower and toward the side of the lesion and the face away. This may also be a vestibular drive, released from the tonic Purkinje cell inhibition, which turns not only the eyes but also the head and neck away from the overactive side. True *vertigo* (spinning or falling sensations) and the nausea and vomiting that often accompany it result only from disease of the labyrinth, the vestibular nerve, and the vestibular nuclei; it is absent in pure cerebellar lesions. When vertigo and vomiting are present, they are due to pressure on the vestibular nuclei, nerves, and brainstem.

Another oculomotor deficit of considerable interest is the loss of the adjustability of the vestibulo-ocular reflex (VOR). This reflex usually remains precisely adjusted throughout life, apparently as a result of supplying the correct amount of Purkinje cell inhibition onto the vestib-

ular nuclei (Fig. 9–7). Indeed, the *gain* (head movement) of the reflex can be altered drastically simply by wearing magnifying, reducing, or reversing goggles. The work of Ito and colleagues suggests that the gain of the reflex is caused by changing the amount of Purkinje cell response (and thus the inhibition onto the medial vestibular nucleus) to the head rotation. The proposed mechanism is as follows: When the head is turned one way, the semicircular canals are activated, and they excite the mossy fibers projecting both to the vestibular nuclei and to the cerebellar cortex (Fig. 9–7). When excited, the vestibular nuclear cells activate oculomotor neurons to medial (ipsilateral eye) and lateral (contralateral eye) rectus muscles and cause the eyes to move in the direction *opposite* the head turn. The Purkinje cells are activated by the head turn at the same time as the vestibular nuclear cells, and inhibit the nuclear cells, thus preventing the eye from turning too much. If the eye turn *is* too much, the world will slip past the retina in one direction; if not enough, the world will slip past in the other direction. It has been proposed that when there is retinal slip during head turning, the cerebellum "learns" to correct it: The inferior olive, which receives the visual error signal, causes (via the climbing fiber) the strength of the granule cell synapses that carry the head-turn information onto the Purkinje cell to change, so that the Purkinje cell becomes appropriately more (or less) active, giving more or less inhibition to the medial vestibular nucleus cells and the eye movement.

Quite surprisingly, several studies appear to support this imaginative theory. Damage to Purkinje cells prevents the adjustment, but not the VOR itself; stimulation of the climbing fibers together with stimulation of the mossy fibers appears to change the Purkinje cells' sensitivity to that mossy fiber–parallel fiber input. In a single unit recording experiment, when monkeys learned to adjust limb movements,

Purkinje cells behaved in response to climbing fiber and parallel fiber inputs in the way the theory predicts.

If these ideas and interpretations are correct, then the "mainline" would be a hardwired mechanism more or less essential to some sort of motor performance, and the inhibitory side loop through cerebellar cortex would provide for its adjustment. If this operation is essentially correct for the vestibulocerebellar control of the horizontal vestibulo-ocular reflex, how might it apply for the rest of the cerebellum, and the rest of the body? The fundamental role of the VOR is to accurately, rapidly, and automatically move one body part (eyes) contingent on movement of another body part (head) so that the gaze (eye and head) stays fixed in space. A moving limb, with its many joints, faces the same problem in trying to keep the finger on a fixed target or a straight-line trajectory through space. The same mechanism could apply to the limb joints as applies to the head and eye: Movement at one joint would be made to covary with movement at another joint—and indeed all the joints—so as to keep the tip of the finger on the target in space. Indeed, the skeleton with its many joints, the muscles with their mass elasticity and many imperfections as motors, and the neural control loops with their long conduction delays would certainly require some control mechanism at least this sophisticated in order to work at all!

Spinocerebellum. The spinocerebellum has both a tonic drive and a modulatory effect during movement that influence independently both alpha and gamma motor neurons, interneurons, and higher nodal points as well. It has been proposed that it collects information via the very rapidly conducting spinocerebellar pathways on the ongoing movement and that it informs and updates the movement while it is in progress. The spinocerebellum does not play a role in the initiation of voluntary movement since its change of neural activity is at or after the onset of movement. The analogy to the VOR mechanism is one suggestion as to what it might do and how it might work. In addition, it seems to be especially concerned with the inherent problem of tremor as well.

Ablation of the human spinocerebellum is most commonly seen in the atrophy of the anterior lobe due to alcoholism and thiamine deficiency. Usually, the initial damage is to the anterior portion of the anterior lobe cortex; this area is known to receive information from and to send it to the legs (Fig. 9–8A). Ablation results in the following behavioral defect: The subject behaves as if he had some ability to stand and walk against gravity, but cannot control his muscles properly to do so. Thus, the trunk and legs tend to set up a violent anterior-posterior tremor of one part of the spine on another at the rate of three to five per second *(titubation)*. The steps are hesitant, small, shuffling, and tentative; the legs are held stiff at knee and hip, and spread wide apart. The wide base of the gait is a volitional correction in an attempt to achieve some stability; whether the stiffness at hip and knee is also purely volitional or instead is due to release of antigravity postures because of abolished Purkinje cell inhibition is debated. Nevertheless, it is clear that the difficulty applies to muscles and their neural control generally, and not just to their use against gravity, since the subject has both ataxia and tremor of the legs when lying in bed and performing any type of movement that is attempted (heel-to-knee-shin test, heel tapping, drawing a square with the toe, etc.) (Fig. 9–9).

As previously stated, oscillation is an inherent problem in the design of the neuromuscular skeletal system: The skeleton has many joints, the muscles are elastic, the body parts have mass, the segmental and transcortical neural loops have long conduction delays, and there is normally a tendency for oscillation at each of the

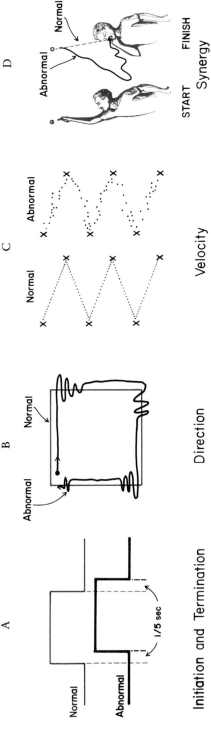

Initiation and Termination Direction Velocity

Fig. 9–9. Patterns of abnormal movement seen in cerebellar ataxia. **A.** Initiation and termination. There may be a delay of 1/10–1/5 second of start and stop of movement. **B.** Direction. In attempting to trace a square with the extended arm and finger, the oscillations are extreme on change of direction. **C.** Velocity. When attempting to touch targets in sequence, the velocity is extremely irregular (time exposure photograph with flashing light attached to finger, spacing of "flashes" is irregular). **D.** Synergy. On attempting to touch the nose with the tip of the finger, shoulder and elbow do not coordinate so as to produce a straight-line trajectory.

many joints. The segmental reflexes tend to amplify the oscillation: Stretch of a muscle causes it to contract, which stretches the antagonist, causing it to contract. The agonist muscle then becomes silent and relaxes just as the antagonist contracts to again stretch the agonist, and the process may continue indefinitely. In its least degree, this tendency is present in all people as physiological (or enhanced physiological) tremor (Fig. 9–6) and in its worst, as clonus and cerebellar tremor. It has been suggested that the cerebellum has damping action on the tendency to oscillate by its action both on the afferent-efferent long loop through motor cortex and also on the segmental loop. The nuclei of the spinocerebellum (interpositus) are known to receive signals, probably from muscle spindle afferents, that very sensitively monitor all perturbations of the limb including the tremor—possibly in order to damp the tremor. These nuclei also generate tonic levels of activity in relation to tonic forces and different postures, and thus seem most likely to control tremor and other properties of the neuromuscular apparatus both for posture as well as movement. Loss of their tonic excitatory drive due to nuclear lesions may also explain the hypotonia sometimes seen with cerebellar lesions, and also the impaired responses to muscle stretch, as demonstrated by the pendular reflexes, the rebound phenomenon, and the oscillation of outstretched arms when they are tapped by the examiner.

Cerebrocerebellum. Because of its connections to the cerebral cortex the neo- or cerebrocerebellum has long been thought to play a special role in volitional, learned, skilled movements. In monkeys performing trained reaction time movements, the dentate nucleus becomes active as much as 100 msec prior to the movement, some 40 msec or so earlier than does motor cortex, to which it projects. Moreover, damage to the dentate delays the onset of activity in motor cortex, and this probably explains the delay in initiating voluntary movements. Unlike spinocerebellum, the cerebrocerebellum does not receive feedback from the moving limb. Furthermore, it discharges in relation to the direction of movement, regardless of what pattern of muscle activity is used to cause the movement. These timing and coding properties, plus the observation that ablation may affect only skilled movements, are (aside from the connections to cerebrum) the main proofs that cerebrocerebellum is exclusive in its role in controlling volitional learned movements.

Clinically, damage of the cerebrocerebellum often does not produce any behavioral defect that is apparent to either the patient or the physician. It is sometimes possible, however, to show severe impairment of highly trained movements, such as playing a musical instrument, when all other movements are normal in clinical tests. Whether lesions in the lateral hemisphere would cause more obvious difficulty in individuals who depend more on learned, skilled movements than those who do not is not known.

Part of the problem is in knowing what it is in the learned movement that the cerebellum controls. As originally stated in the cerebellar learning theories, the cerebellum "learned" and stored the entire program for a complex sequence of movements; the movement was "triggered" from the cerebellum by a brief simple instruction from cerebrum and thereafter maintained by the cerebellum alone, one movement component triggered by the occurrence of the context of the previous movement component. This does not seem likely to be the case, since *any* movement or series of movements—even a musical composition—can be performed without the cerebellum, albeit slowly and imperfectly. The evidence is more in favor of the lateral cerebellum, to use the phrase of Gordon Holmes, "'keeping the motor apparatus "tuned up" so that it may be used for accurate rapid "automatic" movements, rather than providing the strategy and the programs for the steps in the movement itself. Yet it is still possible that the "timing" itself is highly controlled and adjustable.

SUMMARY

The motor system works as an integrated unit, with many parts and many processes functioning simultaneously at any one time, but it is built along modular lines. Focal disease in humans—more than any experimental strategy—reveals a hierarchical plan of function. The alpha motor neurons cause the muscles to contract, and interneurons and afferent nerves within the spinal cord and brainstem control the muscles with regard to the generation of force, agonist-antagonist cooperation, and simple patterns of stance and progression. The brainstem adds antigravity strategy, head-neck-body synergies, and visual orienting. The basal ganglia presumably elaborate on these mechanisms and may provide more complex motor programs as well. Motor cortex collects information from the entire motor apparatus and uses it to fractionate the mass synergies of body parts into larger varieties of independent movements of body parts, especially the digits and the oral-vocal apparatus. The cerebellum is essential for no one movement, but modulates and refines the performance of all.

GENERAL REFERENCES

Creed, R. S., D. E. Denny-Brown, J. C. Eccles, E. G. T. Liddell, and C. S. Sherrington. *Reflex Activity of the Spinal Cord.* Oxford, Clarendon Press, 1932.

Denny-Brown, D. *The Basal Ganglia and their Relation to Disorders of Movement.* London, Oxford University Press, 1962.

Dow, R. S., and G. Moruzzi. *The Physiology and Pathology of the Cerebellum.* Minneapolis, University of Minnesota Press, 1958.

Evarts, E. V. Representation of movement and muscles by pyramidal tract neurons of the precentral motor cortex. In *Neurophysiological Basis of Normal and Abnormal Motor Activities,* M. D. Yahr and D. P. Purpura (eds.). Hewlett, N.Y., Raven Press, 1967, pp. 215–53.

Brookhart, J. M., V. B. Mountcastle, V. B. Brooks, and S. R. Geiger. *Handbook of Physiology,* sec. I, vol. II, parts 1 and 2. Bethesda, Md., American Physiological Society, 1981.

Holmes, G. The cerebellum of man (The Hughlings Jackson Lecture). *Brain* 62:1–30, 1939.

Landau, W. M. Spasticity and Rigidity. In *Recent Advances in Neurology,* F. Plum (ed.). Philadelphia, Davis, 1969, pp. 1–32.

Lawrence, D. G., and H. G. J. M. Kuypers. The functional organization of the motor system in the monkey. I. The effects of bilateral pyramidal lesions. *Brain* 91:1–14, 1968a.

Lawrence, D. G., and H. G. J. M. Kuypers. The functional organization of the motor system in the monkey. II. The effects of lesions of the descending brainstem pathways. *Brain* 91:15–36, 1968b.

Parkinson, J. *An essay on the shaking palsy.* London, Whittington and Rowland, 1817.

10.

Hypothalamus and Brainstem

CLIFFORD B. SAPER

One of the most important functions of the brain is to integrate a variety of autonomic, endocrine, and behavioral responses to insure the maintenance and preservation of the individual and the propagation of the species. The coordination of these responses in such basic functions as fluid and electrolyte balance, energy metabolism, thermoregulation, reproduction, and emergency responses to physical threat requires the critical participation of neural mechanisms in the brainstem and the hypothalamus.

DISORDERS OF INTEGRATIVE FUNCTIONS OF THE HYPOTHALAMUS

The hypothalamus is a remarkably small area at the base of the brain, surrounding the third ventricle, occupying just 4 gm of the normal 1,400-gm adult brain weight. It contains a large number of closely packed but often ill-defined cell groups interwoven with a bewildering variety of fiber systems. With the introduction of modern neuroanatomical tracer methods and single unit recordings, there has been remarkable progress in the last decade in disentangling this web. While most of the experimental data have been obtained in other species, there appears to be little difference in the organization of these very basic mechanisms throughout the mammalian line, up to and probably including humans.

Hypothalamic anatomy

For descriptive purposes the hypothalamus may be divided into three parts medial to laterally and rostrocaudally (see Figs. 10–1–10–4). The most medial part of the hypothalamus, adjacent to the third ventricle, is the periventricular zone. This region contains the neurons that secrete releasing hormones important for anterior pituitary regulation. The next most lateral part, the medial zone, contains both the oxytocin- and vasopressin-secreting neurons of the paraventricular and supraoptic nuclei, and a number of nuclei with integrative functions, including the medial preoptic nucleus, the dorsomedial, the ventromedial, and the premamillary hypothalamic nuclei and the anterior and posterior hypothalamic areas. The lateral zone is traversed by the longitudinally directed medial forebrain bundle, which

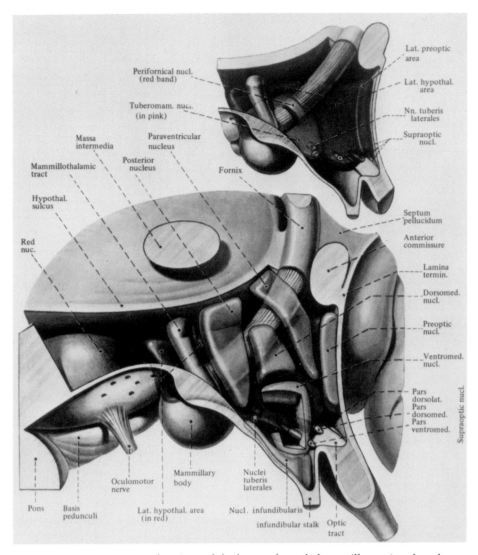

Fig. 10–1. Cut-away drawings of the human hypothalamus illustrating the relative locations of hypothalamic nuclei and areas. In both drawings, the view is from the medial surface. In the upper figure, the periventricular and medial groups of nuclei have been removed to show the relationship of the lateral hypothalamic area to the column of the fornix. In the bottom figure, the medial nuclei are shown projected against the lateral hypothalamic area. (From *The Hypothalamus,* W. J. H. Nauta, W. Haymaker, and E. Anderson (eds.). Charles C. Thomas, Springfield, Ill., 1969, by permission of the publisher.)

conveys axons connecting the various hypothalamic cell groups with areas of the brainstem caudally and the forebrain rostrally. Scattered among the fibers of the medial forebrain bundle are the neurons of the lateral hypothalamic and lateral preoptic areas.

The anterior third of the hypothalamus, roughly from the anterior commissure to the caudal edge of the optic chiasm contains the anterior hypothalamic and preoptic areas (Fig. 10–2). These areas appear to participate in the integration of fluid-electrolyte, thermoregulatory, and reproductive responses. The middle third, because it forms a bulge at the base of the

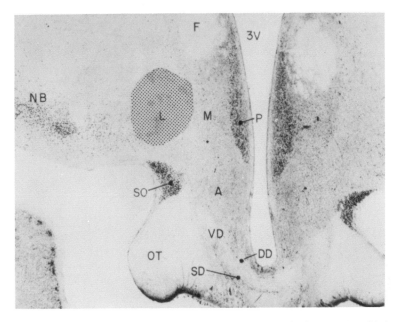

Fig. 10–2. Photomicrograph of a coronal section through the anterior third of the human hypothalamus at a level just caudal to the optic chiasm. The supraoptic (SO) and paraventricular nuclei (P) are prominent, but the anterior hypothalamic area (A), medial preoptic area (M), and lateral preoptic area (L) are more poorly differentiated. The stippled area indicates a cross section of the medial forebrain bundle. F, fornix; NB, nucleus basalis; 3V, third ventricle; DD, dorsal supraoptic commissure; VD, ventral supraoptic commissure; SD, nucleus of the supraoptic decussation. (From *The Hypothalamus*, W. J. H. Nauta, W. Haymaker, and E. Anderson (eds.). Charles C. Thomas, Springfield, Ill., 1969, by permission of the publisher.)

brain extending from the optic chiasm to the mamillary body (Fig. 10–3), is often called the tuberal region (from the older Latin name for this region, *tuber cinereum*, literally "gray swelling"). The tuberal region contains most of the endocrine regulatory mechanisms of the hypothalamus and is important in the integration of energy metabolic and reproductive responses. In the midline, the floor of the tuberal part of the third ventricle forms a highly specialized structure, the median eminence, from which emerges the pituitary stalk, or infundibulum. The posterior third of the hypothalamus contains the enigmatic mamillary body (Fig. 10–4), whose limbic connections are among the most well defined in the hypothalamus, but whose function remains un-

known. Adjacent to the mamillary body are the posterior and lateral hypothalamic areas and premamillary nuclei, which seem to be important integrative areas for a variety of thermoregulatory and emergency responses.

Hypothalamic physiology: basic mechanisms

The hypothalamus is important in regulating autonomic response in at least three ways (Fig. 10–5). (i) It contains a system of neurons that project directly to parasympathetic and sympathetic preganglionic nuclei of the medulla and spinal cord. Many of these neurons are located in the paraventricular nucleus, and some contain oxytocin or vasopressin, but they

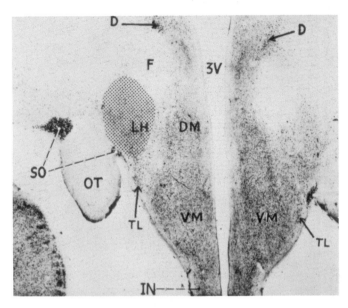

Fig. 10–3. Photomicrograph of a coronal section through the tuberal third of the human hypothalamus. The ventromedial nucleus (VM) and dorsomedial nucleus (DM) are dorsal to the arcuate or infundibular nucleus (IN), which extends down to the pituitary stalk (off picture at bottom). Along the floor of the lateral hypothalamic area (LH) are several clusters of large-celled lateral tuberal nuclei (TL). Portions of the supraoptic nucleus (SO) are located both medial and lateral to the optic tract (OT). The stippled area indicates the median forebrain bundle. D, dorsal hypothalamus; F, fornix; 3V, third ventricle. (From *The Hypothalamus*, W. J. H. Nauta, W. Haymaker, and E. Anderson (eds.). Charles C. Thomas, Springfield, Ill., 1969, by permission of the publisher.)

do not project to the pituitary gland. Other hypothalamic autonomic neurons are found in the dorsomedial nucleus and the lateral hypothalamic area. (ii) Hypothalamic neurons receive projections from and project to other cell groups involved in autonomic control. An entire system of central autonomic control nuclei, with representations at every level of the neuraxis from the cerebral cortex to the medulla, has been identified. Virtually all of these nuclei are reciprocally connected with the hypothalamus, particularly the hypothalamic autonomic neurons and an autonomic integrative area in the posterior lateral hypothalamus. (iii) The lateral hypothalamus is traversed by a number of fiber pathways from higher centers (e.g., amygdala, septum, cerebral cortex), which

innervate central autonomic nuclei of the brainstem.

There are two main endocrine systems in the hypothalamus. The *magnocellular system* consists of large neurons in the supraoptic and paraventricular nuclei whose axons traverse the median eminence and infundibulum. These fibers enter the posterior lobe of the pituitary gland, where they secrete oxytocin and vasopressin (antidiuretic hormone, or ADH). Each hormone is secreted by a separate population of neurons in each nucleus. The *parvocellular system* comprises smaller neurons in the periventricular zone, including the arcuate nucleus, at the base of the third ventricle, which secrete releasing and release-inhibiting hormones. Releasing hormones for thyrotropin (TRH), corticotropin

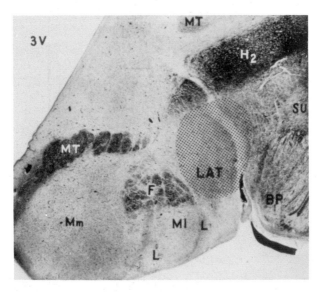

Fig. 10–4. Photomicrograph of a coronal section through the human hypothalamus at the level of the mamillary body. The relationships of the fornix (F) and mamillothalamic tract (MT) to the mamillary nuclei are apparent. The medial mamillary nucleus is divided into medial (Mm) and lateral (Ml) portions, the latter of which is surrounded on its ventral and lateral aspects by the lateral mamillary nucleus (L). Stippling indicates the course of the medial forebrain bundle. LAT, lateral hypothalamic area; BP, basis pedunculi (cerebral peduncle); H_2, field H_2 of Forel; SU, subthalamic nucleus; 3V, third ventricle. (From *The Hypothalamus*, W. J. H. Nauta, W. Haymaker, and E. Anderson (eds.). Charles C. Thomas, Springfield, Ill., by permission of the publisher.)

(CRF), growth hormone (GHRH), and gonadotropins (GnRH) and release-inhibiting hormones for growth hormone (somatostatin) and prolactin (dopamine) have been identified. All are secreted by axon terminals of parvocellular neurons into the hypothalamic-hypophysial portal vessels in the median eminence. The portal veins run from the median eminence longitudinally along the pituitary stalk, conveying the releasing hormones to the capillary bed in the anterior lobe of the pituitary gland. The secretion of each of the above-mentioned anterior pituitary hormones is therefore brought under neural control.

A third type of hypothalamic endocrine control is mediated by the autonomic nervous system, which innervates most glandular tissue. Secretions of renin by the kidney and of insulin and glucagon by the pancreas, for example, are strongly influenced by the autonomic innervation of these organs.

The influence of hypothalamic mechanisms on behavior is controversial. On the one hand, it is clear that certain stereotyped behavior patterns such as the arched back, hissing, and clawing during "sham rage" in decorticate cats, are dependent on the activity of hypothalamic neurons. Various lesion studies also indicate a hypothalamic contribution to drinking, feeding, thermoregulatory, and reproductive behaviors. On the other hand, there has been a tendency to assume that these more complex behaviors are primarily organized at a hypothalamic level, and recent evidence indicates that this supposition may not be correct. For example, a popular theory of feeding behavior sug-

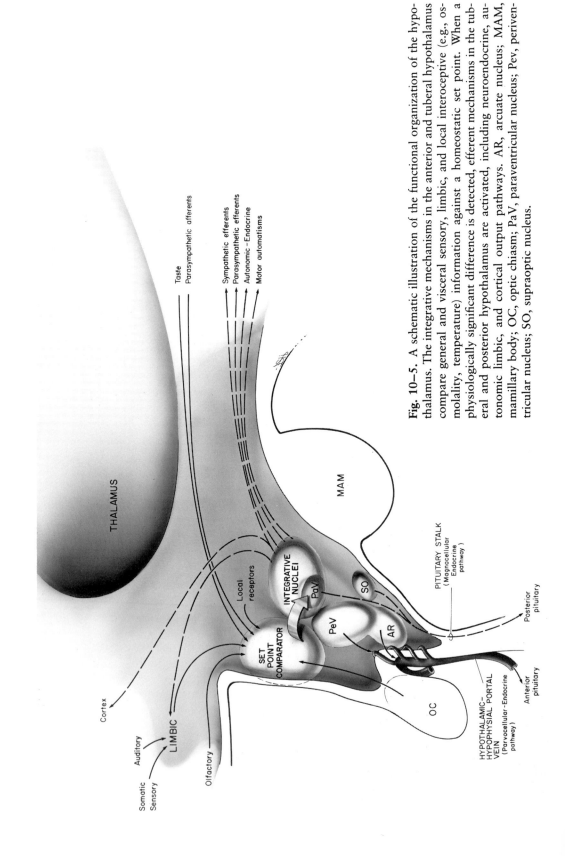

Fig. 10–5. A schematic illustration of the functional organization of the hypothalamus. The integrative mechanisms in the anterior and tuberal hypothalamus compare general and visceral sensory, limbic, and local interoceptive (e.g., osmolality, temperature) information against a homeostatic set point. When a physiologically significant difference is detected, efferent mechanisms in the tuberal and posterior hypothalamus are activated, including neuroendocrine, autonomic limbic, and cortical output pathways. AR, arcuate nucleus; MAM, mamillary body; OC, optic chiasm; PaV, paraventricular nucleus; Pev, periventricular nucleus; SO, supraoptic nucleus.

gests a tonically active lateral hypothalamic "feeding center" that, in times of high blood levels of energy substrates, is inhibited by a ventromedial "satiety center." This view is largely based on the results of lesions of the lateral hypothalamus, which produce aphagia, and lesions to the ventromedial nucleus, which produce hyperphagia. However, recent data suggest that much of the aphagia following lateral hypothalamic lesions may be due to injury to dopaminergic and other fibers of passage in the medial forebrain bundle, which results in a diffuse slowing and suppression of all behaviors. The overeating and obesity seen in animals with ventromedial hypothalamic lesions are mainly due to disordered autonomic control of the pancreas and gut and are abolished by transection of the abdominal vagus nerve. These experiments demonstrate that the behavioral effect of a lesion may not be due to damage to a "center" that organizes the behavior, but rather to disruption of neuronal cell bodies and axons whose function it is to maintain an appropriate physiological setting in which the behavior may be expressed. This view that the hypothalamus plays a permissive role, allowing the timely unfolding of complex behaviors, is probably more consistent with available data.

Hypothalamic physiology: integrative responses

Broadly stated, the main role of the hypothalamus is the integration of autonomic, endocrine, and behavioral responses necessary to maintain and preserve the individual. The organization of this function can be viewed as encompassing three mechanisms: detection, integration, and output (see Fig. 10–5).

The hypothalamus detects relevant stimuli both by exteroceptive and interoceptive means. Exteroceptive olfactory and visual inputs enter the hypothalamus directly; the access to auditory, vestibular, and somatosensory inputs proceeds via relays in the brainstem reticular formation. Exteroceptive information also converges, at a cortical level, in the cingulate and hippocampal cortical areas, both of which innervate the hypothalamus. Interoceptive pathways include the visceral afferent information from the cranial nerves (VII, IX, and X) that reaches the nucleus of the solitary tract and is directly and polysynaptically relayed to the hypothalamus. Other interoceptive cues derive from direct receptors (e.g., osmoreceptors, glucoreceptors) on hypothalamic neurons.

In each regulatory system, integrated sensory information appears to be compared to a set point in evaluating the necessity for initiation of responses. For each integrative response, the hypothalamus regulates the internal milieu around the set point to maintain homeostasis.

Finally, the hypothalamic output involves control of a variety of autonomic, endocrine, and behavioral responses. These will be discussed with respect to the individual integrative responses described later.

In general, disorders of hypothalamic detection mechanisms are characterized by apparent resetting of regulatory set points with integrative and output mechanisms allowing appropriate regulation around a new, albeit abnormal, homeostatic level. Disorders of body temperature and serum osmolality are two examples that are discussed. Hypothalamic lesions that involve integrative mechanisms may result in the loss of ability to coordinate multiple output mechanisms around the established setpoint. Output mechanism disorders may be defined as autonomous lack of activity or hyperactivity, usually of a single output mechanism, whereas the remaining outputs are appropriately regulated. Diabetes insipidus is an example of this type of disorder.

Hypothalamic pathophysiology

While disorders may occur at any of the regulatory steps, focal isolated deficits of hypothalamic function are rather unusual.

The hypothalamus is subject to the same disease processes as the rest of the brain but is peculiarly resistant to trauma and vascular disease. Lying at the base of the brain, it is protected from trauma by the base of the skull below and by the entire thickness of the cerebral hemispheres above. Furthermore, it is literally surrounded by the circle of Willis and receives its vascular supply directly from perforating branches of the arteries that make up the circle (see Fig. 10–6). Finally, each hypothalamic nucleus is present bilaterally so that only an extensive lesion of this area is symptomatic.

Thus, the diagnosis of a structural lesion in the hypothalamic area often depends on the presence of signs pointing to concomitant involvement of neighboring structures. Dysfunction of the optic nerves, chiasm, or tracts is quite common and often pinpoints the area of damage. Less often, dysfunction of one or more of the cranial nerves that traverse the cavernous sinus (oculomotor, trochlear, abducens, ophthalmic branch of the trigeminal nerve) will indicate a lesion in the area of the sella turcica. A large tumor in this area may even extend laterally to involve the medial temporal lobe, with subsequent partial complex seizures.

Primary hypothalamic signs and symptoms occasionally occur. These are usually due to chronic meingitis or another granulomatous process (sarcoid, eosinophilic granuloma) with a predilection for the base of the brain, or to tumors of the suprasellar area (particularly pituitary adenomas and craniopharyngiomas). Symptomatic hypothalamic plaques have been reported in multiple sclerosis, but they are rare.

Fluid and electrolyte balance

The hypothalamus receives peripheral interoceptive inputs concerned with intravascular volume from arterial, venous, pulmonary circulation and cardiac atrial and ventricular distension receptors. Intrinsic hypothalamic osmoreceptor information is combined with volume inputs and compared to volume, osmolality, and electrolyte set points. An example of pathological involvement of this system is seen in certain cases of the syndrome of inappropriate secretion of ADH (SIADH) due to pulmonary disease. Often such patients develop metabolic encephalopathy or seizures and are found to have serum sodium levels below 120 mEq per liter. In these cases, disordering of inputs from intrathoracic volume receptors occurs, with the result that the volume/osmolar set point is effectively lowered. These patients conserve urinary volume at the expense of solute (sodium) until a new, lower osmolar set point is reached. They then regulate around the lower set point until the pulmonary disease resolves or the vagus nerve is cut.

The integrative mechanisms for fluid-electrolyte balance are located in the preoptic-anterior hypothalamic region. Restricted lesions in this area are rare, but localized granulomas have been reported to disrupt mechanisms of regulation of body water and salt in an unusual way. In response to a low vascular volume patients reduce urine output appropriately, but do not drink or reduce perspiration. As a result they are often admitted to hospitals for dehydration.

The autonomic output of the hypothalamus in maintaining fluid and electrolyte balance includes both venous and arterial vasoconstriction. Reduced parasympathetic and increased sympathetic tone in the heart cause a chronotropic and inotropic response, increasing cardiac output. Endocrine adjustments include control of secretion of ADH, with direct volume conserving and weaker vasopressor properties, and of ACTH, which regulates secretion of cortisol, which has a weak mineralocorticoid effect. In addition, increased renal nerve sympathetic activity arguments release of renin, which

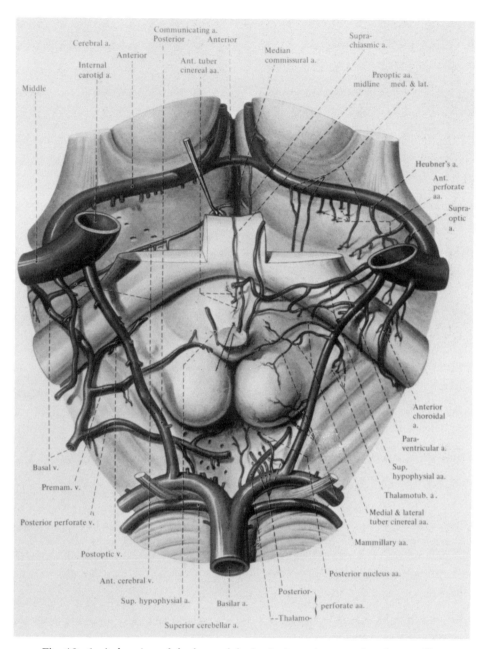

Fig. 10–6. A drawing of the base of the brain from the ventral surface to illustrate the blood supply of the hypothalamus. Notice that the circle of Willis literally surrounds the floor of the hypothalamus. For this reason, discrete hypothalamic vascular infarcts are rare. (From *The Hypothalamus*, W. J. H. Nauta, W. Haymaker, and E. Anderson (eds.). Charles C. Thomas, Springfield, Ill., 1969, by permission of the publisher.)

increases angiotensin II levels. Angiotensin II not only causes vasoconstriction directly, but also increases secretion of the potent mineralocorticoid, aldosterone. Angiotensin II also leaks across the blood-brain barrier at the subfornical organ and the area postrema, where it stimulates neurons important in drinking behavior. This latter response is the only natural way to replete volume. Another hypothalamic influence on drinking behavior is autonomically induced dry mouth, which may then serve as a further exteroceptive cue to higher centers for the need for fluid intake.

An example of a disorder of the hypothalamic output in fluid and electrolyte regulation is diabetes insipidus. The pituitary stalk is vulnerable to a variety of insults, from trauma to tumor and meningitis. When the paraventricular and supraoptic axons to the posterior lobe of the pituitary gland are injured, loss of ADH secretion occurs, with consequent inability to regulate renal water loss. Patients have marked polyuria with secondary polydipsia. Fortunately, exogenous ADH may be administered while the paraventricular and supraoptic axons regenerate over a period of several weeks.

Energy metabolism

The detection of depletion of substrate for energy metabolism involves peripheral interoceptive inputs signaling such information as gut distension and the presence of nutrients in the hepatic portal blood (e.g., by hepatic glucoreceptors). Central receptors for glucose have been claimed to exist in both the ventromedial nucleus and the adjacent lateral hypothalamic area. The existence of liporeceptors, as well as a mechanism for monitoring body weight, has also been proposed. Although traditional models of "lateral hypothalamic phagic center" and "ventromedial satiety center" may be too simplistic, there is lit-

tle doubt that neural mechanisms involved in regulating blood glucose around a set point are located in this area. A body weight set point, particularly necessary for reproductive function (discussed later), may also be maintained. Bilateral lesions in the area of the ventromedial nucleus result in food intake's being regulated around a much higher set point. Patients are markedly obese. This apparently occurs by disordering autonomic and endocrine control of the digestive system, thereby altering the meaning of critical inputs to the hypothalamus concerning substrate availability.

The integration of responses to substrate depletion also appears to take place in the region of the ventromedial nucleus and adjacent lateral hypothalamic area. Congenital tumors involving this area in infants produce severe wasting called the diencephalic syndrome of infancy. Curiously this occurs in the setting of a good appetite, normal linear growth, and a euphoric affect. These children are unable to regulate food intake and energy metabolism about appropriate nutritional set points and are markedly thin.

The autonomic outputs in response to substrate depletion include increased lipolysis and myolysis to provide substrate for hepatic β-oxidation of lipids and gluconeogenesis. Increased gastric motility and acid secretion provide additional interoceptive cues, which may be interpreted by higher centers as hunger. Endocrine regulation includes decreased secretion of anterior pituitary hormones and of pancreatic hormones, e.g., insulin and glucagon. The behavioral responses to substrate depletion include lethargy (to conserve energy) and repletion of substrate, i.e., eating if food is available. Bilateral lesions of the lateral hypothalamic area are rare in humans, but have been reported in patients with multiple sclerosis. They suffer aphagia and inanition similar to experimental animals with lateral hypothalamic lesions. This phenomenon appears to be due largely to disruption of ascending dopaminergic and arousal pathways in the medial forebrain bundle in the lateral hypothalamic area, and as such represents a generalized disorder of behavioral output. Anorexia nervosa is a syndrome occurring predominately in adolescent females and is characterized by near starvation of presumed psychogenic origin. It is not associated with any structural hypothalamic lesion. Changes in autonomic and endocrine regulation seem appropriate for a starvation state. Thus the amenorrhea seen in anorexia nervosa appears to be due to the body weight's dropping below a minimum set point necessary for reproduction.

Thermoregulation

Detection of body temperature occurs at multiple levels of the central nervous system, but the most important control mechanism seems to be a thermoreceptor area in the anterior hypothalamus and adjacent preoptic area. Insertion of heating or cooling probes into this area induces consequent adjustments of body temperature. Fever is a pathological alteration of this mechanism. Endogenous pyrogen, secreted by leukocytes in the inflammatory response, causes neurons in the anterior hypothalamic-preoptic region to interpret body temperature as being too low, thereby functionally resetting the thermostat upward. Lesions of the anterior hypothalamic-preoptic area result in loss of the febrile response as well as reduction in the usual accuracy of thermoregulation. Tumor or congenital defects (e.g., agenesis of the corpus callosum) in this region may induce either periodic or chronic hyperthermia or hypothermia in which there is thermoregulation around a new higher or lower set point.

The integrative mechanisms for thermoregulation in the preoptic thermoreceptive region appear to depend on connections with the more caudal tuberal hypothalamus. Although thermal probes in this latter region in animals do not affect thermoregulation, lesions of this area in humans cause loss of normal thermoregulation, resulting in poikilothermia—the state in which body temperature drifts toward the ambient temperature. These patients not only fail to thermoregulate but also do not appreciate extremes of body temperature that normally cause discomfort.

The autonomic outputs involved in thermoregulation involve both heat dissipation and conservation and calorigenic mechanisms. In response to cold temperatures, heat is conserved by redirecting blood flow from peripheral vascular beds in the extremities and near the body surface to deeper vascular beds. The reverse occurs during warming, and heat dissipation is augmented by the evaporation of increased perspiration. Calorigenesis is facilitated by increased lipolysis and gluconeogenesis, making additional substrate available. The main calorigenic regulation, however, is by means of control of output of thyroid hormone, which promotes increased utilization of ATP by Na-K ATPase in many organs. The Na-K ATPase reaction is believed to use a large proportion of the body's energy output and to be a main source of heat production. Behavioral adjustments to temperature change involve decreased somatomotor activity (lethargy) during heating and increased activity, both voluntary and involuntary (shivering), during cooling. More complex behavioral responses include attempts to manipulate the environmental temperature or to move to a different environment. Patients with low cervical spinal cord transection are unable to utilize the hypothalamic autonomic sympathetic outflow to thermoregulate. Despite normal endocrine function and some motor control of the upper extremities, the absence of autonomic response results in wide swings in body temperature.

Reproduction

The detection of appropriate conditions for reproduction involves both exteroceptive (olfactory, auditory, visual, and somatosensory) and interoceptive inputs. The latter involve both peripheral receptors (awareness of autonomic adjustments in the presence of a possible mate) and a continuing effect of sex steroids on the central nervous system's development and function. Neurons in the medial preoptic and anterior hypothalamic areas and the ventromedial and arcuate nuclei are known to bind sex steroids. Anatomical differences are found between the sexes in the structure of these regions, and the development of the male conformation is dependent on the presence of testosterone during early life. A clinical disorder of this sytem may occur in genetic males with the testicular feminization syndrome due to nonfunctioning testosterone receptors. These individuals develop both morphologically and psychologically as females, with normal female sexual behavior. None of the brains of these patients has yet been examined for pathological verification, but based on the study of testosterone-deprived male animals, a normal female hypothalamic morphology would be expected. Whether a similar pathology may underlie other gender identification or preference syndromes remains to be studied.

The integration of sexual responses probably occurs in the region of the ventromedial nucleus of the hypothalamus. Lesions in this region in animals and in humans cause loss of genital maturation in children and disruption of sexual behavior and endocrine function (e.g., amenorrhea) in adults. More subtle alterations in the function of these integrative mechanisms may underlie amenorrhea at times of stress and perhaps in some cases of delayed puberty.

The autonomic outputs of the hypothalamus in reproduction involve general responses (e.g., cardiovascular adjustments in anticipation of copulation) and specific sexual responses (e.g., erection and ejaculation in males; secretion of lubrication by females). Endocrine adjustments include the regulation of menstrual cycles by LH and FSH in women and possible changes in testosterone secretion in anticipation of sexual activity in men. Furthermore, there is evidence that sex steroid feedback on the brain may increase the likelihood of sexual behavior. In female rats, for example, the lordosis response appears to be under the critical control of appropriate levels of sex steroids. Human behavior is more complex, but one study found that the incidence of female-initiated sexual contacts increased during the preovulatory phase of the menstrual cycles. An example of a clinical disorder due to malfunction of hypothalamic reproductive output is the occasional case of precocious puberty caused by hypersecretion of gonadotropin-releasing hormone due to a functioning hypothalamic harmartoma.

Emergency response

The detection of a threatening situation may involve a variety of exteroceptive (visual, tactile, olfactory, auditory) cues as well as some interoceptive information (e.g., visceral nociception, and nausea). In humans, the determination of what constitutes a threat relies increasingly on cortical mechanisms. In many psychiatric disorders the perceived threat may not be real. Anxiety results from inappropriate activation of the emergency response mechanisms. By contrast, lesions in the region of the preoptic area produce a state of abulia, a condition in which the patient fails to respond to stimuli in the environment. Whether this is due to destruction of preoptic area mechanisms involved in the regulation of responses to stress or to the interruption of ascending pathways to cerebral cortex remains to be determined.

The autonomic output associated with the hypothalamic emergency response involves a variety of cardiovascular and other adjustments necessary to ready the individual for fight or flight. Inotropic and chronotropic cardiac influences combine with vasoconstriction to increase cardiac output and blood pressure. Pupillary dilatation, dry mouth, and decreased bowel motility occur. Lipolysis and gluconeogenesis make increased reserves of energy substrate available. Endocrine responses include the increased output of cortisol and epinephrine by the adrenal gland, the former under ACTH and the latter under autonomic control. The most important responses to threat, however, are behavioral. There is an immediate increase in cortical arousal, and responses to environmental stimuli are made more quickly.

Much of the emergency response depends on the integrity of the posterior lateral hypothalamus. Lesions here may produce a hypersomnolent, hypothermic, hypometabolic and bradycardic state, from which it may not be possible to arouse the patient.

DISORDERS OF INTEGRATIVE FUNCTIONS OF THE BRAINSTEM

The brainstem (midbrain, pons, and medulla) is the phylogenetically oldest part of the brain and is directly responsible for the neural activity sustaining all vital functions. Whereas lesions in the hypothalamus can produce alterations in the coordination of autonomic, endocrine, and behavioral responses, lesions in the brainstem may affect these response individually.

Brainstem physiology: basic mechanisms

The brainstem is the site of termination for primary and most secondary autonomic afferents in the nucleus of the solitary tract and parabrachial nucleus. In addition, many parasympathetic pre-ganglionic neurons are located in the brainstem along with pathways that regulate the sympathetic preganglionic neurons in the spinal cord. The maintenance of baseline autonomic functions, called tonic responses, requires an intact brainstem. Phasic responses, the moment to moment changes in function imposed by responding to the environment are largely superimposed on the brainstem from activity in the hypothalamus and above. However, certain basic reflexes are intrinsic to brainstem. One example is the baroreceptor reflex neurons in the medulla; these cause a decrease in heart rate and blood pressure when an increase in blood pressure activates carotid or aortic pressure receptors. Important tonic brainstem responses control pupillary, cardiovascular, and respiratory function. These are discussed later.

Endocrine regulation by the brainstem is limited to its afferent influence on hypothalamic endocrine nuclei and its efferent innervation of endocrine tissues. Direct innervation of hypothalamic nuclei involved in neuroendocrine control by the nucleus of the solitary tract and its relay, the parabrachial nucleus has been demonstrated. Such inputs have been implicated in the regulation of secretion of various hormones, including ACTH and ADH. Little is known, however, about clinical endocrine dysfunction with brainstem lesions.

Brainstem participation in behavioral regulation primarily involves two types of mechanisms. First, somatomotor automatisms seem to be organized at a brainstem level, involving mainly the midbrain reticular formation. A variety of automatic stereotyped behaviors occur in animals or patients with impaired forebrain function. These include laughing, crying, sucking, grasping, and withdrawal responses. Anencephalic infants, completely lacking a forebrain, can often perform all of these tasks quite well. Electrical stimulation of the midbrain reticular formation after midbrain-diencephalic transection in

animals can even produce locomotor behavior such as treadmill walking in cats.
Second, the brainstem contains the origin
of a potent arousal system responsible for
tonic and phasic activation of the forebrain. In the absence of such inputs, the
forebrain falls into a sleep-like state called
coma, in which it responds only weakly
and transiently to sensory stimuli. The
arousal system takes origin in the rostral
pons and travels through the paramedian
reticular formation ventrolateral to the
central gray matter to the midbrain–diencephalic junction, where it splits into two
branches. The more dorsal branch innervates the intralaminar nuclei of the thalamus, which in turn provide a diffuse innervation of cerebral cortex. Electrical
stimulation of the intralaminar nuclei
causes diffuse cortical activation. The second, more ventral branch of the activating
system has been less well studied, but recent work indicates that it innervates the
hypothalamus, and the basal forebrain,
(both of which project diffusely to the
cortex) as well as providing some afferents to the cerebral cortex directly. Bilateral lesions in the posterior lateral hypothalamus, or along the course of the
ascending activating pathway in the
brainstem, produce coma.

Brainstem pathophysiology

The brainstem is less well protected from
insult than the hypothalamus and is subject to a great many focal and diffuse processes. Direct brainstem trauma is usually
lethal. Vascular lesions, on the other hand,
can be quite small and cause restricted deficits in sensation and movement secondary to circumscribed infarction of specific fiber tracts or nuclei (see Chap. 15).

Compression of the brainstem by adjacent areas of injured brain is not uncommon and may have a fatal outcome (Fig.
10–7). Three types of brainstem compression are seen. (i) Central herniation occurs
when a mass lesion of the forebrain causes
symmetric downward displacement of the

diencephalon through the tentorial notch
(see Fig. 10–7B). As the brainstem is compressed in a rostral to caudal direction,
small vessels tethering the brainstem to the
underlying basilar artery become stretched.
The resulting brainstem ischemia causes
edema, which may contribute to compression of lower portions of the brainstem. If
the small penetrating arteries are torn by
the strain, small slit-like hemorrhages into
the brainstem (Duret hemorrhages) may
occur. The rostrocaudal deterioration of
brainstem function is characteristic and is
described later in terms of disruption of
specific autonomic and motor responses.
(ii) In uncal herniation, the asymmetric
displacement of the forebrain by a mass
lesion causes herniation of one uncus
through the tentorial notch ahead of the
diencephalon (see Fig. 10–7C). Compression of the oculomotor nerve as it crosses
through the tentorial notch gives rise to
the classic sign of an ipsilateral dilated
pupil. Pupillomotor fibers are located along
the dorsomedial surface of the oculomotor nerve and are therefore most vulnerable to compression by the uncus.
Compression of the cerebral peduncles
(ipsilateral by the herniating uncus and
contralateral by the mass effect pressing
the opposite peduncle against the contralateral tentorial edge) may produce pyramidal motor signs on either side. As the
uncus herniates further, rostrocaudal
brainstem compression occurs. (iii) Cerebellar swelling, usually due to edema, tumor, or hemorrhage in the cerebellum,
causes direct compression of the brainstem, particularly the pons. In addition, the
fourth ventricle is compressed, and cerebrospinal fluid drainage from the lateral
and third ventricles becomes blocked resulting in acute hydrocephalus.

**Autonomic dysfunction with brainstem
lesions**

Although respiration is a somatic motor
function, in the absence of other pyramidal or extrapyramidal activity it proceeds

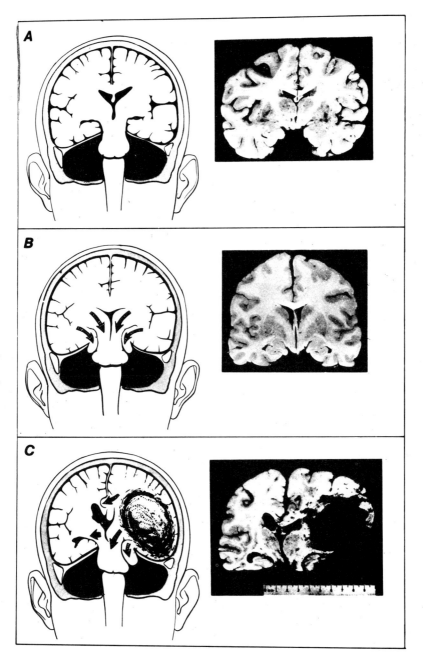

Fig. 10–7. **A.** Drawing of a coronal section through the normal cranium and contents on left, with a photomicrograph of a similar brain section on right. **B.** Central herniation syndrome. Cerebral edema has forced the diencephalon downward through the tentorial opening. Note the vertical elongation of the hypothalamus and third ventricle in the photomicrograph. **C.** Uncal herniation syndrome. A massive hemorrhagic infarct in one hemisphere has caused the ipsilateral medial temporal lobe (uncus) to herniate through the tentorial opening. (From *Stupor and Coma*, F. Plum and J. B. Posner, (eds.). F. A. Davis, Philadelphia, 1980. Reproduced by permission of the publisher.)

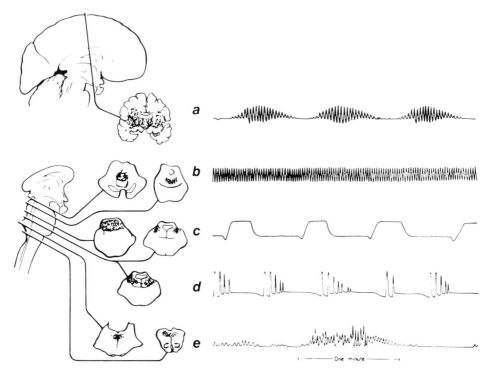

Fig. 10–8. A diagram of characteristic abnormal respiratory patterns associated with lesions (stippling) at various levels of the brain. **A.** Cheyne-Stokes respiration is seen with depression of forebrain control of breathing. **B.** Central neurogenic hyperventilation, which has rarely been reported in cases of midbrain damage, should generally be considered a sign of metabolic encephalopathy (accompanying, e.g., metabolic acidosis, sepsis, or hepatic failure). **C.** The apneustic pattern, with prolonged inspiratory cramp, is seen when lesions affect the region of the parabrachial nucleus in the rostral pons. **D.** Cluster breathing may occur with lesions affecting the medulla in the region of the nucleus of the solitary tract and nucleus ambiguous and may presage complete respiratory failure. **E.** ataxic breathing. (From *Stupor and Coma*, F. Plum and J. B. Posner (eds.). F. A. Davis, Philadelphia, 1980. Reproduced by permission of the publisher.)

automatically (see Fig. 10–8). Respiration is also under visceral afferent control (e.g., carotid body chemoreceptors), and its rhythmicity is generated by circuitry involving the nucleus of the solitary tract and other autonomic structures.

The highest levels of respiratory control are in the forebrain, where respiratory activity is generated independent of the need for gas exchange in the intact individual. An example of this is the posthyperventilation apnea test: After taking five rapid, deep breaths the pCO_2 is so low and

the pO_2 so high that there is no autonomic drive to breathe. A normal individual will continue to take shallow breaths in any case, but a person with depressed forebrain function will be apneic until sufficient chemosensory respiratory drive is reestablished. A similar respiratory pattern that consists of periodic hyperventilation followed by apnea, called Cheyne-Stokes respiration, occurs in patients with forebrain impairment. During rostrocaudal deterioration, the rostral pons is the next highest brainstem level at which impairment of respiration is seen. Neurons in the area of the parabrachial nucleus constitute a pneumotaxic mechanism responsible for maintaining normal respiratory rhythmicity. Bilateral lesions involving this area produce apneustic breathing in which inspiratory cramps occur (the respiratory muscles remain fixed at full inspiration for a significant portion of the cycle). More caudal lesions, involving the medulla, produce irregular, ataxic breathing in which the rhythmicity of respiration is lost. When the respiratory rhythm generators in the nucleus of the solitary tract and nucleus ambiguus are destroyed, respiratory arrest occurs. Lesions that spare the brainstem but damage the ventrolateral funiculi of the spinal cord may interrupt communication between the respiratory rhythm generators of the brainstem and the spinal respiratory afferent (thoracic, pulmonary, and chest wall sensation) and efferent (cervical phrenic nerve motor neurons) cell populations. When this occurs patients lose automatic control over breathing and have to be continuously reminded to take a breath, a condition called "Ondine's curse."

The cardiovascular system makes many adjustments in anticipation of and during various behaviors. These are presumably organized by forebrain structures such as the hypothalamus and amygdala. In the absence of phasic influences, the maintenance of baseline cardiovascular function appears to depend only on the integrity of tonic cardiac and vasomotor mechanisms in the lower medulla. Lesions of the nucleus of the solitary tract destroy baroreceptor afferent inputs and result in severe hypertension in animals, and perhaps also in humans. Injury to this area also induces changes in the pulmonary circulation that may cause pulmonary edema. Destructive lesions of the ventrolateral medulla at the same level can cause hypotension due to loss of vasomotor tone. However, it should be stressed that in the vast majority of patients with neurological deficits and hy-

potension, the decreased blood pressure has caused the neurological dysfunction, and not vice versa.

Pupillary control depends on the interaction of parasympathetic tone generated by preganglionic neurons in the region of the Edinger-Westphal nucleus in the midbrain and sympathetic tone originating in the sympathetic preganglionic intermediolateral column and associated cell groups in the upper thoracic spinal cord. The integrity of the parasympathetic pupilloconstrictor pathway is checked clinically by shining a light on the retina (pupillary light reflex). Certain retinal ganglion cells send axons to the pretectal area, from which fibers relay the light input to preganglionic neurons bilaterally. These cells send axons through the oculomotor nerve to the ciliary ganglion, from which fibers emerge to innervate the pupillary constrictor muscle. The integrity of the sympathetic pathway may be evaluated by pinching the skin of the neck (ciliospinal reflex). Afferent pain fibers reflexly stimulate upper thoracic sympathetic preganglionic neurons, whose axons exit in the ventral roots and join the sympathetic chain to innervate superior cervical ganglion neurons. Postganglionic fibers follow the internal carotid artery and ophthalmic division of the trigeminal nerve to the orbit, where they innervate the pupillary dilator muscle. The forebrain normally maintains a tonic pupillary dilator tone; depression of the forebrain or lesions in the hypothalamic origin of the descending pupillodilator pathway result in small but reactive pupils (see Fig. 10–9). Lesions of the ventral midbrain (Edinger-Westphal region or oculomotor nerves) release the pupil from preganglionic constrictor tone, causing maximal, fixed dilatation. Dorsal midbrain lesions leaving the pupilloconstrictor preganglionic neurons intact, but damaging the pretectal pupilloconstrictor reflex area, produce a midposition-fixed pupil. Lesions of the pons leave both sets of preganglionic neurons intact, but the

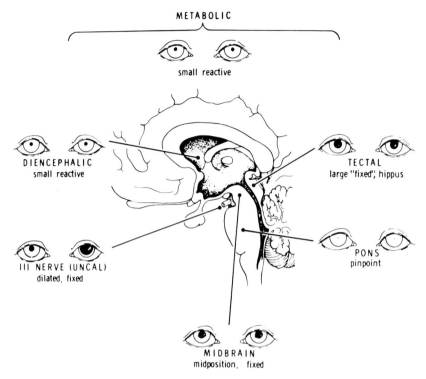

Fig. 10–9. A schematic summary of the typical pupillary findings in patients with lesions involving different portions of the brain. (From *Stupor and Coma*, F. Plum and J. B. Posner (eds.). F. A. Davis, Philadelphia, 1980. Reproduced by permission of the publisher.)

tonic descending sympathetic drive is lost. At the same time, ascending spinal and medullary pathways that inhibit the parasympathetic preganglionic neurons are destroyed. Consequently, unopposed pupilloconstrictor tone takes over, resulting in maximal pupilloconstriction. Lateral medullary lesions may interrupt the descending sympathetic pathway, but do not impair the ascending brainstem pathway that inhibits the parasympathetic preganglionic neurons; as a result a small, reactive pupil is seen on the side of the lesion, along with ptosis (eyelid droop) and anhydrosis (loss of sweating) on the ipsilateral side of the body—other signs of loss of sympathetic tone. During rostrocaudal brainstem deterioration, the pupils start out small but reactive (due to forebrain depression), then pass to midposition and

fixed as both the preganglionic parasympathetic neurons and the descending pupillodilator tract are completely disabled.

Somatic and ocular motor dysfunction with brainstem lesions

Characteristic oculomotor dysfunction is seen with lesions at different brainstem levels and the oculomotor function is consequently often of great value in localizing brainstem lesions. This material is discussed in some detail in Chapter 8.

Brainstem lesions also produce characteristic impairment of somatic motor function (see Fig. 10–10). Depression of forebrain function causes increased motor tone and the emergence of a variety of reflex movements organized at a brainstem or spinal level, such as grasping, sucking,

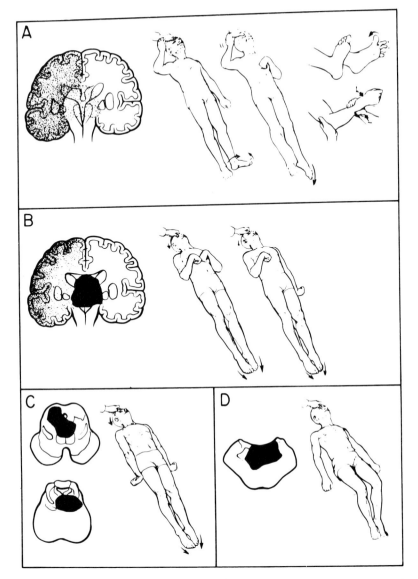

Fig. 10–10. A summary diagram of the characteristic motor responses seen in patients with lesions (shading) at various levels of the brain. **A.** Localizing responses with increased motor tone are seen with forebrain lesions. The plantar response may be extensor bilaterally, or if the lesion injures the motor system more in one hemisphere a contralateral hemiparesis is seen. If the lesion involves the midbrain unilaterally, contralateral decorticate (upper extremity flexor, lower extremity extensor) posturing may be seen. **B.** A lesion involving the midbrain bilaterally produces bilateral decorticate posturing. **C.** A lesion involving the caudal midbrain or rostral pons causes bilateral decerebrate (upper and lower extremity extensor) posturing. **D.** A lesion of the rostral medulla may produce lower extremity flaccidity or flexion in association with upper extremity extension. More caudal lesions cause a flaccid paralysis.

and the extensor plantar reflex (extension of the big toe on stroking the plantar surface of the foot). During rostrocaudal deterioration, lesions involving the rostral midbrain tend to produce flexor posturing of the arms sometimes associated with extensor posturing of the legs. More caudal midbrain lesions usually cause extensor posturing of all limbs. Lesions that involve the causal pons may elicit extensor posturing of the arms with flaccidity or weak flexion movements of the legs.

The detection of more subtle changes in motor function with less complete lesions is usually obscured by the overall depression of spontaneous behavior due to impairment of the ascending arousal system. Bilateral lesions involving its origin in the dorsal rostral pontine tegmentum, or any point along the ascending arousal pathway through the midbrain reticular formation, produce states of stupor or coma. Interestingly, lesions of the caudal brainstem, which leave the ascending activating system intact, do not impair consciousness, although they may disrupt all motor function except vertical eye movements and blinking. Such unfortunate de-efferented patients have been termed "locked in."

Although establishing a diagnosis in patients who are in coma is often a complex process, the problem is greatly simplified by an understanding of the pathophysiology. Unless there is generalized brain dysfunction due to toxic or metabolic processes, depressed level of consciousness implies structural injury to either the brainstem ascending arousal system or its connections in the forebrain (bilateral diencephalon or cerebral hemisphere injury). Examination of pupils, breathing pattern, eye movements, and the motor system helps localize the process within the brainstem.

GENERAL REFERENCES

Krieger, D. T., and J. C. Hughes. *Neuroendocrinology.* Sunderland, Mass., Sinauer, 1980.

Nauta, W. J. H., W. Haymaker, and E. Anderson (eds.). *The Hypothalamus.* Springfield, Ill., Thomas, 1969.

Plum, F., and J. B. Posner (eds.). *Stupor and Coma,* 3d ed. Philadelphia, Davis, 1980.

Reichlin, S., R. J. Baldessarini, and J. B. Martin. *The Hypothalamus.* New York, Raven Press, 1978.

11.

Cerebral Cortex

ROBERT C. COLLINS

In the last 20 years there has been a rapid increase in our knowledge of the cerebral cortex. Anatomical experiments have provided a refined analysis of cortical circuits in studies of connections between and within separate histological zones. Physiological experiments are identifying the receptive field properties of neurons within those zones, that is, the particular aspects of sensation and movement that correlate with neuronal firing in these areas. Metabolic experiments using intravenous injections of radioactive substrates hold promise for identifying widely distributed circuits in cortex and brain that become active during complex behaviors. From the clinical perspective, these advances in neuroscience give insight into the goal of localizing complex behavioral functions in the human brain. Experiments of nature, chiefly cortical lesions caused by stroke, trauma, and tumor, are considerably less precise than animal experiments and far more difficult to analyze. Nevertheless, patients suffering such lesions provide the only opportunity to study those unique aspects of human behavior associated with language and cognition. The history of neurology and neurosurgery is rich with well-studied examples of behavioral dysfunction following cortical lesions. Phenomenology is clear. The interpretation of phenomenology—the pathophysiological explanation of complex behavioral signs and symptoms—is constantly being revised as new principles of cortical function are discovered.

ANATOMY AND PHYSIOLOGY

The cerebral cortex is the largest subdivision of the human central nervous system, representing the greatest anatomical expansion in the evolution of the mammalian brain (Fig. 11–1). Of the three divisions of cerebral cortex, the *neo*cortex has accounted for most of this development by its infolding into fissures and sulci, thus greatly expanding its surface area. *Archi*cortex, chiefly the hippocampus and dentate gyrus, maintains a medial position in the human brain, becoming folded into the lateral ventricle in the medial aspect of the temporal lobe. *Paleo*cortex (the pyriform area or olfactory cortex) remains as a narrow, transitional zone between neocortex and archicortex. Posteriorly, this is called the entorhinal area (Brodmann's area 28,

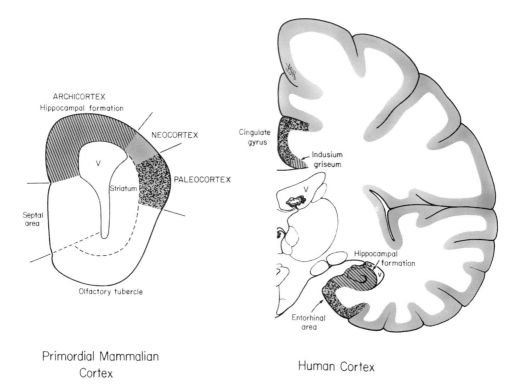

Primordial Mammalian
Cortex

Human Cortex

Fig. 11–1. The evolution of mammalian cortex is schematically summarized by comparing a cross section of a hypothetical promammalian brain with a human brain. The promammalian brain is based on studies of comparative neuroanatomy, particularly reptiles and marsupials (Elliot Smith 1910). Both archicortex (the hippocampal formation: subiculum, dentate gyrus, hippocampus) and paleocortex (pyriform-olfactory cortex) attain a medial position in human brain, remaining relatively undeveloped compared to the great expansion and infolding of neocortex. In advanced mammalian brains the archicortex and paleocortex form a crescent of cortex around the corpus callosum on the medial surface, constituting Broca's "limbic lobe." Evidence today suggests that paleocortex—defined broadly as the entorhinal area—parahippocampal gyrus ventrally and the cingulate gyrus dorsally, function as transitional zones, relaying activity from neocortex into the hippocampus and limbic system.

Fig. 11–4D)—an important zone where activity in neocortex is relayed into the hippocampus and limbic system.

The neocortex can be further divided into anatomical areas according to reciprocal corticothalamic connections (Fig. 11–2). These in turn imply functional subdivisions with regard to sensation: visual cortex-lateral geniculate nucleus; auditory cortex-medial geniculate nucleus; somatosensory cortex-ventral posterior thalamus. Motor cortex is defined by its low stimulation threshold for causing muscle contraction and movement. Both primary sensory cortex and motor cortex can easily be identified histologically. Sensory areas show a dense band of small granular (nonpyramidal) neurons in layer IV, which is the principle receiving zone for specific thalamocortical axonal endings (Fig. 11–3A). This granular cortex (called koniocortex) also characterizes large areas of frontal lobe that have reciprocal connections with the mediodorsal nucleus of

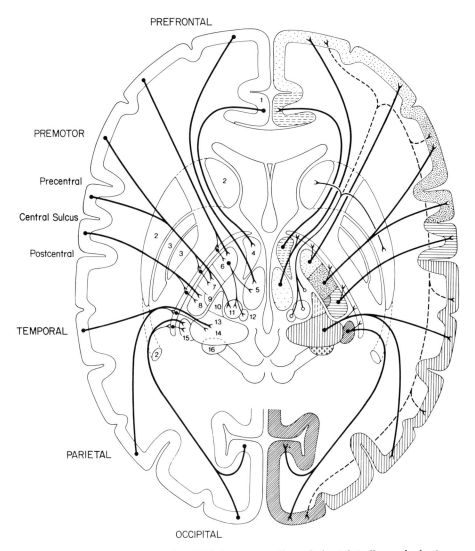

PREFRONTAL

PREMOTOR

Precentral

Central Sulcus

Postcentral

TEMPORAL

PARIETAL

OCCIPITAL

Fig. 11–2. Neocortex can be divided anatomically and physiolgically on the basis of corticothalamic (left) and thalamocortical (right) relationships. Note the relatively small size of cortical zones devoted to primary sensory afferents (ventral posterior nucleus [8] ↔ somatosensory cortex; lateral geniculate nucleus [15] ↔ visual cortex) compared to the large expanse of so-called association cortex (lateral posterior-pulvinar [13–14] ↔ temporoparietal cortex). The frontal lobe is the largest subdivision of neocortex (see Fig. 11–11). Its prefrontal, granular cortex has a reciprocal relationship with the mediodorsal nucleus (4) whose exact function is unknown. 1, cingulate; 2, corpus striatum; 3, globus pallidus; 4, n. anterior; 5, n. mediodorsal; 6, n. ventral-anterior; 7, n. ventralis; 8, n. ventral posterior; 9, n. ventroposterior, parvocellular; 10, n. lateral dorsal; 11, n. centromedian; 12, n. parafascicularis; 13, n. lateralis posterior; 14, pulvinar; 15, lateral geniculate; 16, medial geniculate. (Modified from R. Nieuwenhuys, J. Voogd, and C. Van Huijzen, *The Human Central Nervous System.* New York, Springer-Verlag, 1978, Fig. 121.)

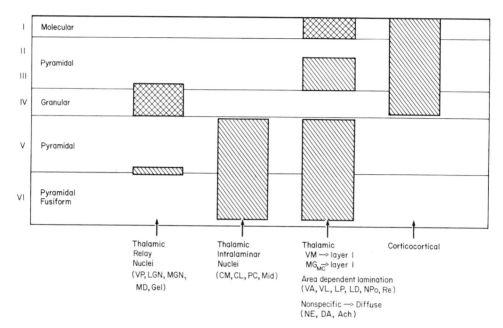

Fig. 11-3. Anatomical studies of neocortex have found that differences in lamination between zones are largely determined by three factors: thalamic input, intrinsic connectivity, and efferent (pyramidal) cell bodies. The number of neurons in any one vertical column of cortex is the same for all cortical areas and all mammals studied, except in the striate cortex of cat and primate, where the neuronal density is doubled. Mixtures of pyramidal neurons of layers II and III and V and VI and nonpyramidal (stellate) interneurons are different for columns in each area, but the total number is held constant. **A.** A schema is shown for different patterns of cortical afferents from thalamus (rat) and cortex (monkey, somatosensory). Patterns are area and species dependent. Ach, acetylcholine projections; CM, centromedial n.; CL, centrolateral n.; DA, dopamine projections; Gel, gelatinosus n.; LD, lateral dorsal n.; LGN, lateral geniculate nucleus; LP, lateral posterior n; MD, mediodorsal n.; MGN, medial geniculate nucleus; MG_{mc}, medial geniculate, magnocellular part; Mid, midbrain; NE, norepinephrine projections; NPo, nucleus posterior; PC, paracentral n.; Re, reuniens; VA, ventral anterior n.; VL, ventral lateral n.; VM, ventral medial n.; VP, ventral posterior n. **B.** Intrinsic connections of cortex are highly complex, with many different anatomical classes of neurons. Spiny stellate cells (prominent dendritic spines) characterize layer IV of primary sensory cortex and are thought to relay excitatory activity vertically through cortex. Many classes of nonspiny, or smooth, stellate cells contain the enzyme glutamic acid decarboxylase, indicating they are likely GABAergic and inhibitory. A large basket cell is shown forming axosomatic synapses on pyramidal neurons in a horizontal inhibitory network. Thalamic afferents ending in layer IV form synapses with both spiny and smooth stellate neurons as well as pyramidal dendrites passing into or through this layer. This fact, plus the recent identification of intrinsic peptidergic and cholinergic interneurons, makes the unraveling of intrinsic columnar input-output circuits exceedingly difficult. **C.** The destiny of corticofugal, or pyramidal neuron projections can be inferred from the laminar site of the cell body. (For details, see E. G. Jones, Anatomy of the cerebral cortex: Columnar input-output organization. In *The Organization of the Cerebral Cortex.* F. O. Schmitt et al. (eds.) Cambridge, Mass., MIT Press, 1981, pp. 199–236.)

B   Intrinsic Systems

Excitatory — Spiny Stellate (?)   Inhibitory — Nonspiny / Gabaergic

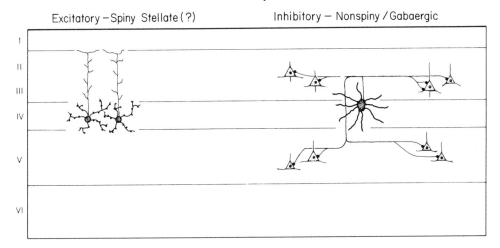

C   Cortical Efferent Systems

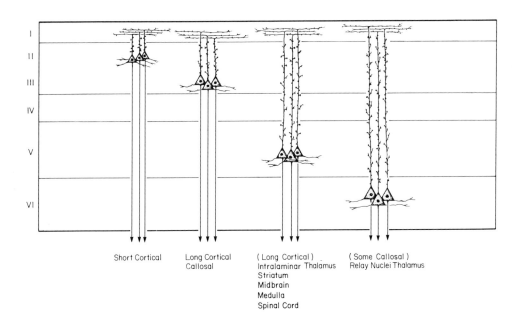

Short Cortical   Long Cortical   (Long Cortical)   (Some Callosal)
                   Callosal   Intralaminar Thalamus   Relay Nuclei Thalamus
                                        Striatum
                                        Midbrain
                                        Medulla
                                        Spinal Cord

thalamus. By contrast, motor cortex lacks a well-developed granular layer IV, receiving its thalamic afferents into layers III and V, principally from the ventral lateral nucleus. There are giant pyramidal cells (Betz cells) in layer V that distinguish motor cortex histologically from other areas. These neurons comprise some of the upper motor neurons whose axons travel in the pyramidal tract to form synapses on lower motor neurons in the anterior horn of the spinal cord (see Chap. 9).

Relative differences in cell morphology and density within different layers of neocortex have been used to define different architectonic zones (Fig. 11–4). Many maps of these zones were produced in the early part of this century, but fell into dis-

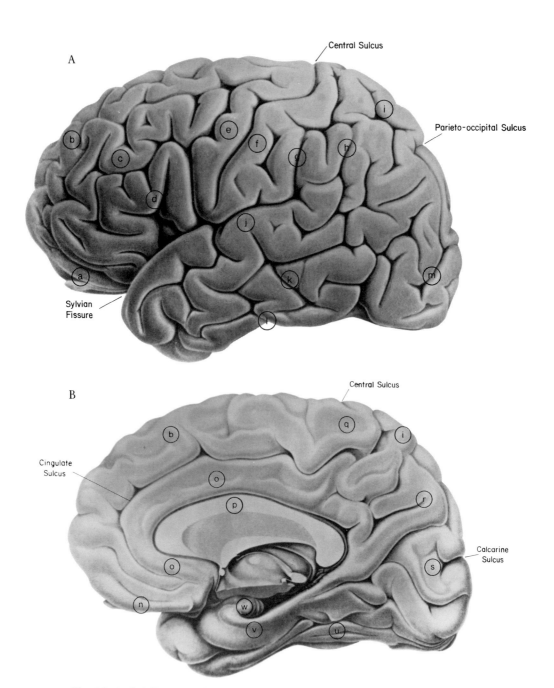

Fig. 11–4. Subdivisions of cerebral cortex based on major gyri and sulci, **A** and **B**; and on histological zones, or cytoarchitectonics, **C** and **D** (Brodmann 1909). Determination of boundaries between gyri and histological zones is somewhat variable among brains. Note also that histological zones do not adhere strictly to sulcal and gyral pattern. Major gyri: a, orbital; b, superior frontal; c, middle frontal; d, inferior frontal (the posterior third, or opercular part, area 44, is Broca's area); e, precentral (area 4, motor); f, postcentral (areas 3, 1, 2, somatosensory); g, supramarginal; h, angular; i, superior parietal lobule; j, superior temporal gyrus (Heschl's gyrus, the primary auditory cortex, extends medially into the insula, with the planum temporale, Wernicke's area, posterior to this); k, middle temporal; l, inferior temporal; m, occipital; n, rectus; o, cingulate; p,

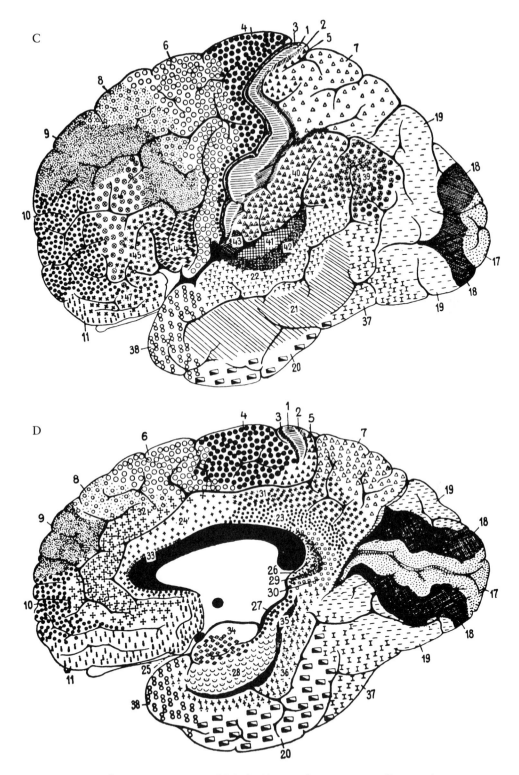

C

D

corpus callosum; q, paracentral lobule (the supplementary area lies anterior to this); r, precuneus; s, cuneus; t, medial occipitotemporal; u, lateral occipitotemporal; v, parahippocampal (entorhinal cortex, area 28, see Fig. 11–1); w, amygdala.

favor when different workers could not agree on exact boundaries, and when lesioning experiments failed to confirm that histological zones signified clear functional differences.

Today there is renewed interest in the study of architectonics for two reasons. Tract-tracing experiments have found that each zone can be characterized by a distinct pattern of thalamocortical input. Thus, architectonics imply connectivity. Second, each zone contains neurons with similar receptive field properties. For example, zone 1 in somatosensory cortex contains neurons that respond to superficial cutaneous stimulation, whereas adjacent zone 2 neurons respond primarily to deep stimulation (Fig. 11–5). In addition, within each architectonic zone in the sensory areas there is a receptive field map (Fig. 11–5c; see also the retinotopic map of visual cortex, area 17, Chap. 7; and the tonotopic map of auditory cortex, Chap. 6). Studies of primary sensory areas have also led to the hypothesis that there is a fundamental vertical structure-function unit of cortex called a "column." Lorente de Nó first drew attention to the vertical organization in neocortex when he described apical dendrites from deep pyramidal cells ascending to the surface in groups or bundles. Recent anatomical experiments have found that thalamocortical and corticocortical inputs occur within "columns" measuring 0.3–0.6 mm in diameter, although some also have longer anteroposterior dimensions and resemble "strips" or "bands" (see Fig. 7–10). Further, studies of cells and connections within cortex suggest that excitatory input is relayed vertically within a column between layers by spiny stellate interneurons and is inhibited on edges from spreading laterally through cortex by nonspiny GABAergic interneurons (Fig. 11–3B). Excitatory activity relayed through intrinsic cortical neurons can add to direct afferent excitation of pyramidal cell den-

drites and convert an input column into an output column. Pyramidal neurons comprise the efferent system of cortex and relay activity to other cortical areas or to subcortical sites (Fig. 11–3C).

Physiological studies of cortex were the first to suggest that columnar organization was important functionally. Mountcastle and his colleagues found that neurons in somatosensory cortex of cat that responded to a simple sensation (touch of skin, movement of joint) were organized in vertical columns (Fig. 11–5B). This organization preserved principles of subcortical sensory pathways where neurons and tracts were anatomically segregated by modality (a dedicated line) and place (somatotopic, retinotopic, etc.) and were physiologically sharpened by surround inhibition. Sensory stimulation also increases metabolism in cortex in a columnar pattern (Fig. 11–6; see also Fig. 7–10). Columns in cortex defined physiologically or metabolically are approximately the same size as anatomical columns. In addition, columns are approximately the same size in most areas of cortex and in most mammals studied. This suggests that evolution has simply added on more columns with the expansion of neocortex, rather than elaborated an entirely new pattern of cortical organization. Confirmation of columnar organization has been obtained in humans with stains for mitochondrial enzymes in visual cortex. In a series of patients who had lost one eye during life, ocular dominance columns were found in area 17 post mortem.

What is the relationship between the columnar organization of cortex and complex human behavior? The answer to this question is unknown. Although many detailed studies support the concept that columns are fundamental units or "functional modules" of cortex, there are few data at present teaching us how these interrelate across cortex over time. Nevertheless, it is clear that both short (e.g., Fig.

11–5D) and long corticocortical circuits (e.g., Fig. 11–5E and 11–11) would be active during even relatively simple behaviors, such as reaching out and grasping an object. Such a behavior might be envisioned as a transient and changing collection of widely distributed columns in different states of afferent-efferent excitability. Evidence suggests that such space-time configurations of activity would not only be influenced by momentary physiological adjustments, but would also be modified anatomically by learning and experience.

Although motor and primary sensory cortex have been well studied, these comprise only a small portion of the total area of neocortex (Fig. 11–4). Structure-function relationships for most of parietal and temporal cortex are less well known. Histologically these areas are characterized by a relatively even distribution of cells, making identification of individual architectonic zones and boundaries difficult. Subcortical connections are with the lateral nucleus and the pulvinar of the thalamus. Traditionally these areas of parietal and temporal cortex have been called association cortex. Since they receive projections from primary sensory zones they were thought to play a role in the elaboration of sensations into perceptions, or in the association of two or more different sensations into a conceptual whole.

Clinicians at the turn of the century suggested that perceptions, learned behaviors, or "engrams" became localized within particular association gyri, an idea historically derived from phrenology and the early schools of localizationists. Stated this way, association cortex was thought to be at a "higher level" of cortical function than primary sensory cortex. This *hierarchical* scheme of brain function was first formulated in the 19th century (Jackson 1874) and spoke to the complexity of behavioral dysfunction that occurs in humans following damage to, or epileptic

discharges from, different areas of cortex (see later discussion). It became accepted that simple sensations were processed serially through corticocortical connections until areas were reached whose function was the formation and storage of perceptions, or abstract psychological principles. This hypothesis has not been proved. To the contrary, many recent anatomical and physiological experiments point out that association cortex also receives sensory information directly from thalamus. For example, the pulvinar nucleus receives visual, auditory, and somatosensory input from midbrain tectum and projects widely to parietal and temporal cortex (Fig. 11–2). These facts underlie a scheme of brain functioning in which different aspects of sensation (and movement) are thought to be processed in *parallel* and not through a linear sequence of hierarchical stations. In addition, recent studies of cortex in non-human primates have discovered multiple maps of sensation in parietal and temporal cortex so that "pure" association cortex may be very small (Fig. 11–7).

These schemes of *hierarchical* and *parallel* processing are briefly introduced to emphasize the difficulty in understanding cortical functions and their relationship to human behavior. To a considerable degree, both schemes often place undue emphasis on cerebral cortex, ignoring the contribution of simultaneous physiological activity in other areas in brain. Recognizing this, Mountcastle has emphasized that behavior is the momentary expression of functional activity in widely distributed circuits throughout brain. It is thought that each anatomical area that is active during a particular behavior adds a unique physiological contribution that modulates the activity within the entire functional circuit. At the cortical level this idea means that physiological columns within widely separated architectonic fields can be very closely associated as functionally active units. These con-

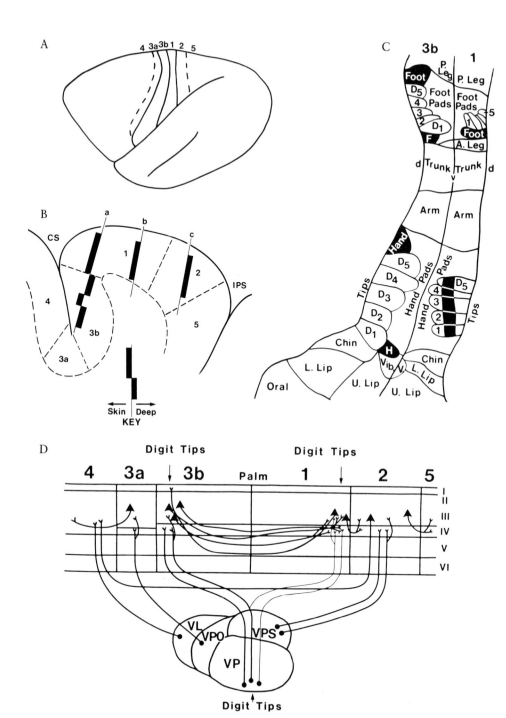

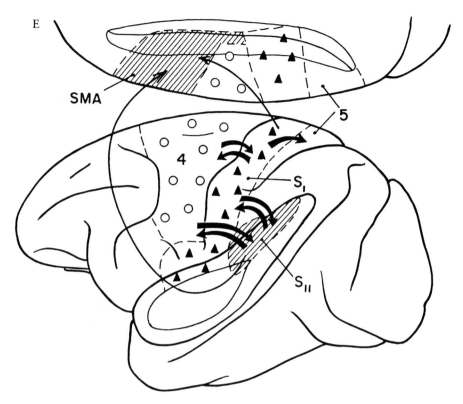

Fig. 11–5. Schema of structure-function relationships of sensorimotor cortex. **A.** Cytoarchitectonic zones are indicated on the lateral surface of an owl monkey's cortex. **B.** Sagittal section (anterior is left) across central sulcus. Three recording electrodes (a, b, c) indicate an increase in the firing rate of cortical neurons to either superficial stimulation of skin (e.g., camel's hair brush) or deep stimulation (e.g., electrical pulses through deep needles). Note the change in the response of neurons to the type of stimulus when the electrode crosses cytoarchitectonic boundaries, as along the electrode track in a. **C.** Separate somatotopic maps exist in varying degrees of resolution for each somatosensory architectonic zone. (From Kaas, *Physiol. Rev.* 63:206–31, 1983, Fig. 1.) **D.** Thalamocortical and short corticocortical relationships for sensorimotor cortex (from Kaas, Fig. 2.) VL, ventral lateral n.; VP, ventral posterior n.; VPO, ventral posterior n., pars oralis; VPS, ventral posterior n., pars superior. **E.** Long corticocortical projections of monkey sensorimotor cortex. S_1, primary somatosensory cortex; S_{II}, secondary somatosensory cortex in the parietal insula; SMA, supplementary motor area on the medial aspect of the frontal lobe. (From E. G. Jones and T. P. S. Powell, Connections of the somatic sensory cortex of the rhesus monkey. *Brain* 92:477–502, 1969, Fig. 15).

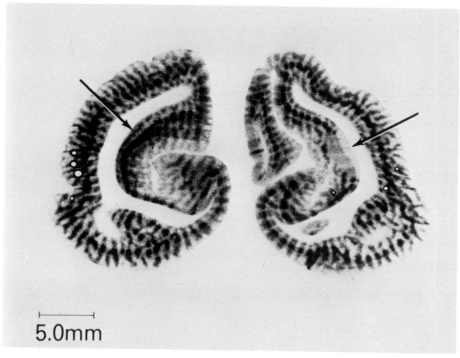

Fig. 11–6. Autoradiograph of a coronal brain section of a monkey at the level of the striate cortex of the occipital poles. The right eye has been occluded and the left eye visually stimulated. With the ¹⁴C-deoxyglucose technique functional labeling occurs in alternate cortical columns (dark and light bands) indicating the ocular dominance pattern (see Chap. 7). The columns run the full thickness of cortex, with preferential labeling in layer IV, the lamina receiving afferents from the lateral geniculate nucleus (see Fig. 11–3A). The arrows indicate the presence (left) or absence (right) of continuous labeling in layer IV, the cortical representations of the retinal blind spots. (From C. Kennedy, M. H. Des Rosiers, O. Sakurada, M. Shinohara, M. Reivich, J. W. Jehle, and L. Sokoloff, *Proc. Nat. Acad. Sci. USA* 73:4320–4, 1976, Fig. 4c.)

cepts, although still evolving, should be kept in mind as we try to understand the pathophysiology of behavioral syndromes that follow focal cortical lesions in humans.

PHYSIOLOGIC AND METABOLIC "LESIONS" OF CORTEX

Focal abnormalities

Certain diseases express their symptoms by involving cortical circuits in an abnormal way. Epilepsy and migraine are two ex-

amples. In both of these conditions patients are entirely normal until the process starts. With focal seizures (see Chap. 12) the first site of abnormal motor convulsion or sensation, such as a hand or foot, indicates the site of the epileptic focus in the cortex. Occasionally, seizures spread slowly across the cortex (Jacksonian march) with the progression of symptoms indicating the somatotopic organization of the cortex. For example, convulsive jerking can begin in one hand and then progressively involve the arm, shoulder, and leg as it spreads medially over the sensory-

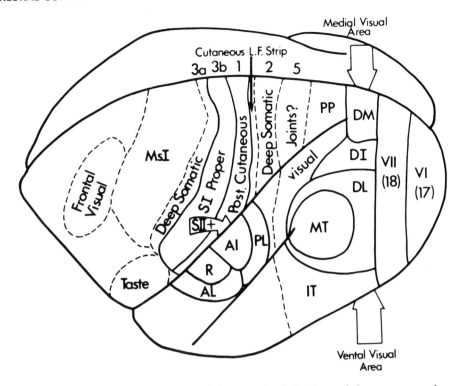

Fig. 11–7. Schematic summary of functional subdivisions of the neocortex of the New World monkey. The discovery of multiple somatosensory (SI, SII, areas 1, 2, 5), visual (VI, VII, DM, DI, DL, MT, IT, PP), and auditory (A1, R, AL, PL) maps has been responsible for reducing the area of cortex thought to be purely "associational." (From Merzenich and Kass, *Prog. in Psychobiol. and Physiol. Psych.* 9:1–42, 1980, Fig. 4.)

motor strip (Fig. 11–5C). It can also "skip" from a patient's hand to his face when the process spreads laterally toward the sylvian fissure. Such symptoms probably represent abnormal spread through intrinsic cortical pathways when circuits responsible for lateral inhibition break down. A similar process may occur during migrainous scotoma, although the evolution of symptoms is much slower, commonly lasting 20 minutes as compared to 1 to 2 minutes for Jacksonian seizures. In classic migraine, flashing lights begin near the center of the visual field. The progressive enlargement and lateral movement of this "scintillating scotoma" suggest that a wave of excitation-depolarization travels across the retinotopic field in visual cortex (see Fig. 7–11). The scintillating bars and spots

suggest that spread may occur abnormally through adjacent columns. It has been postulated that a wave of spreading excitation-depression is carried contiguously through extracellular space by high concentrations of potassium. This can be produced in experimental animals and is called the spreading depression of Leao. But since animals cannot tell us about "scintillating scotomas," and since spreading depression has not been studied in human cortex, the exact pathophysiological mechanisms for migraine remain inferential (Chap. 7).

Diffuse abnormalities

Diffuse physiological abnormalities of cortex probably play a role in several con-

Table 11–1. Common definitions of terms

Aphasia: Loss of the capacity for spoken language
    Expressive aphasia: More difficulty speaking than comprehending. (Synonyms: Broca's, motor, nonfluent.)
    Receptive aphasia: More difficulty comprehending than speaking. (Synonyms: Wernicke's, sensory, fluent.)
    Conduction aphasia: Relatively normal comprehension and spontaneous speech, but difficulty with repetition.
    Global aphasia: Difficulty with comprehension, repetition, and speech.
Agraphia: Loss of the capacity to write.
Alexia: Loss of the capacity to read.
Apraxia: Loss of the capacity to perform skilled or learned tasks with the hands although sensation, muscle power, and speech are relatively normal.
    Ideomotor apraxia: Loss of the ability to perform intransitive or imaginary gestures.
    Ideational apraxia: Loss of the ability to demonstrate the use of real objects.
    Constructional apraxia: Loss of the ability to draw or construct objects.
    Dressing apraxia: Loss of the ability to orient one's body to clothes necessary for dressing.
Agnosia: Loss of the ability to recognize objects within one sensory system. Correct identification by another sensory system demonstrates normal memory and naming.
    Auditory agnosia: Inability to recognize sounds.
    Tactile agnosia: Inability to recognize objects felt by the hand. (Synonym: astereognosis.)
    Visual agnosia: Inability to recognize objects by sight. (Synonyms: cortical blindness, psychic blindness.)
    Prosapagnosia: Inability to recognize familiar faces.
    Anosagnosia: Denial of deficit or illness

---

ditions in humans. For example, some evidence suggests that the cholinergic input from basal forebrain to cerebral cortex may be preferentially destroyed in Alzheimer's disease (Chap. 13). It is thought that this would remove a diffuse modulatory system necessary for maintaining normal cortical (and intellectual) functions. Psychiatric syndromes such as affective disorder (depression) may preferentially involve catecholamine neurotransmission, diffusely affecting cortex and other brain areas. The generalized epilepsies may also represent an abnormality of diffuse innervation of cortex (Fig. 12–8). At present, these are interesting but largely unproven hypotheses.

As discussed in Chapter 16, systemic metabolic disorders such as hypoxemia, hypoglycemia, and liver failure commonly disrupt mental functions as the first abnormality. Symptoms are usually nonspecific and nonlocalizing: difficulty with abstract thinking, poor attention span, poor memory functions, slowness, perseveration, and difficulty naming and writing. These symptoms disappear with correction of metabolic abnormalities. They also occur, however, with very large or widespread structural lesions of cortex, and in

these cases usually reflect the size of the lesion rather than its location.

FOCAL STRUCTURAL LESIONS OF CORTEX

Focal lesions of human cortex commonly produce characteristic behavioral symptoms and syndromes. The phenomena have been well studied clinically and are often so characteristic that observation of a patient's abnormal behavior is sufficient to localize the site of a cortical lesion. When hemiparesis and hemianopsia are present it is obvious there is a lesion of the contralateral hemisphere. When abnormalities occur in language functions (aphasia, Table 11–1) or in spatial orientation, the behavioral syndrome can be complex, but also highly localizing. The reason for this is quite interesting: Brain is not functionally symmetric. Humans are unique among primates in this regard, a fact that probably reflects the appearance of language and motor dominance as a late step in evolution. In 90% of right-handed individuals language function is localized to the left hemisphere. In 75% of left-handed individuals speech production is localized to the left side. Speech comprehension, however, is more equally localized between the hemispheres in left-handers. It should be noted that specialized language studies of patients whose corpus callosum has been surgically divided indicate that the right hemisphere in right-handed individuals has at least a latent childhood capacity for language comprehension, but little or no ability to produce spoken or written language.

The source of this functional asymmetry of human cortex is unknown. Anatomical studies have found a larger *planum temporale* (auditory association cortex) on the superior aspect of the left temporal lobe in 65% of cases, on the right in 11%. The possible relationship of this anatomical asymmetry to language function is intriguing since the Wernicke area for speech comprehension (discussed later) is located in the left planum temporale.

The behavioral abnormalities that result from focal cortical lesions depend on several factors in addition to the site of lesions. The patient's age, intellectual capacity, personality, and handedness are all important factors. The pathology of the lesion is critical. Sudden but localized infarcts produced by stroke are often associated with dramatic and obvious behavioral abnormalities. By contrast, patients with lesions of similar size and location caused by slow-growing tumors often require special testing to document behavioral dysfunction. In these patients the deficits are often dynamic and fluctuate with time, depending on such factors as the patient's fatigue, distractions in the environment, or the speed and complexity of the task at hand. Fixed deficits and stereotyped dysfunction—the rule for lesions of muscle, nerve, and most subcortical sites—are less common with cortical lesions.

Lesions of the left hemisphere

Aphasia. Lesions of the left hemisphere disrupt language functions in 70% of all individuals. The process usually involves cortex around the sylvian fissure in an area

traditionally called the zone for language (Fig. 11–8): auditory association cortex in the temporal lobe, inferior parietal lobule (supramarginal and angular gyrus), the inferior portion of the precentral gyrus, the third frontal gyrus, and the arcuate fasciculus that connects the temporal to the frontal lobes around the sylvian fissure. All of these structures are supplied by the left middle cerebral artery, making stroke within the distribution of this vessel the most common cause of aphasia. Two points should be noted in passing. Lesions in this area do not influence vocalization in nonhuman primates. In these species vocalization conveys only emotion, a function that is primarily localized bilaterally in limbic structures (cingulate, septum, amygdala, preoptic area, hypothalamus, and midbrain reticular formulation). Bilateral lesions in these areas in humans—most commonly of the basal forebrain and hypothalamic area—result in mutism and a general depression of behavioral activity (see later discussion and Chap. 10). Second, infarction of the supplementary motor cortex on the medial aspect of the frontal lobe (anterior cerebral artery, see Fig. 15–2) commonly causes a transient disruption of language. The deficit is more obvious in speech production than speech comprehension.

Students of language and aphasia have traditionally tried to classify the phenomenology of aphasia. This was originally done to determine if different brain areas within the left hemisphere controlled different aspects of language. Wernicke (1874) proposed the first scheme with two areas, one for speech reception in the temporal lobe-auditory association area and the other for speech production anteriorly in the frontal lobe, an area originally localized by Broca (1861) at the posterior third (opercular part) of the inferior frontal convolution. Wernicke described two aphasia syndromes coinciding with lesions in these two areas: sensory-receptive vs. motor-expressive (discussed later), and suggested a third syndrome would appear

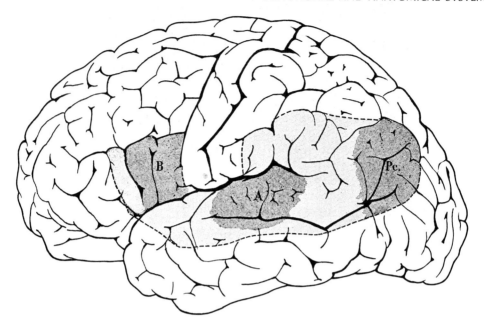

Zone of Language

Fig. 11–8. The "Zone of Language" was proposed by Dejerine *(Semiologie des affections du Systeme Nerveux,* Library of the Academy of Medicine, Paris 1914, Fig. 1). Lesions within this zone (dashed line) cause aphasia by impinging on Broca's area, B ("center for motor images of articulation"), or Wernicke's area, A ("center for auditory images of words"), or the parieto-occipital cortex, Pc. ("center for visual images of words"). See also horizontal section in Figure 11–9.

when a lesion occurred between these two areas and separated them. This localizationist scheme of aphasia was popularized by Dejerine (1914) and more recently by Geschwind and his colleagues. Simply stated it says that different aspects of language are the products of distinct areas of brain such that damage to these areas or between them (called disconnection syndromes) will cause characteristic abnormalities in language. This scheme has been criticized from the beginning, Pierre Marie (1926) among others claiming that language functions could not be localized to particular brain centers. Today the latter argument consists of two major points: First, most observers emphasize that *pure* aphasic syndromes are exceedingly rare. For example, patients with anterior frontal lesions and "expressive aphasia" can always be found to have difficulty with language comprehension ("receptive aphasia") if they are tested properly. Second, even when a small lesion causing aphasia occurs within one part of the language zone that is anatomically separate from other parts it is never physiologically separate, i.e., it always disrupts activity within synaptic reach. These arguments propose that language is a dynamic function reflecting fluctuations in physiological activity within interconnecting circuits. Damage at any point will cause more or less the same type of aphasic syndrome. These two schools of aphasiology—the localizationists and nonlocalizationists—form two ways of analyzing the complex symptomatology of language disorders.

Two developments are adding new insights into studies of aphasia. Advances in radiology (computerized tomography, positron emission tomography, nuclear magnetic resonance imaging) make possible a degree of anatomical localization *in vivo* not previously possible. Second, students of linguistics are bringing their discipline to bear on the problems of aphasia to learn more about the rules that govern the relationships between sound and meaning. Phoemic, semantic, and syntactic errors in aphasia are analyzed in detail, adding further complexity to schemes of classification. For a student who first encounters an aphasic patient these concerns will likely seem somewhat abstract, if not arbitrary. Aphasic patients are severely incapacitated. Their problems often overwhelm naive observers. Disruption of language destroys our most characteristic function. What follows in this chapter is a partial classification of the phenomenology that provides a clinically useful outline for the localization of lesions and empirical guidelines for prognosis for recovery.

Expressive Aphasia (Synonyms: Broca's, Motor, Anterior). Patients have disproportionate difficulty in speaking and writing while comprehension of language is relatively well preserved. They can follow multiple-step commands, but speech is slow, nonfluent, strained, and composed mostly of nouns and verbs, lacking phrases, clauses, or sentences (agrammatism). Spontaneous speech is markedly reduced, and some patients are totally aphonic at the onset. Broca's original patient could only utter "tan, tan, tan." Curiously, in the presence of a severe incapacity for propositional speech, many patients can count, recite the days of the week, or sing overlearned songs, like "Happy birthday." Lesions usually involve cortex of the third frontal convolution, adjacent motor strip and/or the subadjacent white matter. Patients commonly have weakness (or complete paralysis) of the right side of the face and right arm and considerable difficulty with willed movements of lips, tongue, and palate independent of speech. Partial syndromes occur with small lesions. Two additional points are important. Patients are almost always aware of their language dysfunction, in contradistinction to patients with receptive aphasia. Second, prognosis for recovery of spoken language is generally good, although this can require three months or longer. Although most patients will eventually communicate effectively, they only rarely regain full skills of articulation.

Receptive Aphasia (Synonyms: Wernicke's, Sensory, Posterior). Small lesions of the temporal-parietal area of the dominant hemisphere cause a complex behavioral syndrome. Close relatives of such patients often conclude a "mental breakdown" has occurred. Not uncommonly, patients with strokes or tumors in this area are first referred to psychiatric hospitals. Patients themselves often have no awareness of their difficulty. If the lesion is restricted to this zone, there is no weakness or sensory complaint. Speech is usually spontaneous, fluent, and often quite rapid, with an abundance of phrases and clauses. The problem is that the speech makes little or no sense. The patient's response to a question is usually long and circumlocutious, adding tangential phrases that lead farther and farther from the target. Speech is full of prepositional constructions but is usually deficient in verbs, proper nouns, and complete sentences. In addition, there are occasionally substitutions of sounds or words when others are intended, called verbal or literal paraphasias. Patients with this syndrome cannot read, write, spell, or calculate normally, and control of the hands in complex gestures is occasionally impaired (see apraxias, discussed later). The hallmark of the syndrome is a severe deficit in speech comprehension, including an inability to follow even simple commands.

In contrast to patients with frontal lesions who are aware of their deficit and are frustrated by it, these patients lack awareness and are often quite jocular. In addition, although many factors are involved in recovery, most observers have found that prognosis for regaining skills of verbal comprehension with receptive aphasia is not good. Patients rarely regain full participation in the world of human discourse.

Global aphasia. This is a term used when there is clear and usually profound dysfunction in both speech reception and expression. Often the lesion is large, such as follows occlusion of the left middle cerebral artery, and contralateral hemiparesis is invariably present. Patients are severely impaired, as loss of language leaves them functionally demented. The prognosis depends primarily on the pathological cause, but is usually poor. Two exceptions are important. Symptoms caused by external compression from a subdural hematoma are often relieved following surgery. Physiological disruption of language caused by focal epileptic discharges can usually be brought under control with anticonvulsants.

Conduction Aphasia. Pure examples of this syndrome are rare. Speech comprehension and expression are relatively preserved, but there is disproportionate difficulty in repeating an examiner's phrase. Spontaneous language can be nearly normal in flow and content, but attempts to repeat what is heard result in numerous paraphasias (substitutions of words and sounds) and blocking. Reading aloud is mildly affected and writing is always abnormal. The syndrome is crucial for localizationist schemes of aphasia since the hypothesis (Wernicke) states the lesion should occur within the arcuate fasciculus. This would disconnect Wernicke's area from Broca's area, theoretically leaving spontaneous speech reception and expression normal, but interrupting language trans-

mission from ear to cortex to tongue during repetition. At present, too few patients with this syndrome have been studied in detail to resolve all of the anatomical and pathophysiological issues.

Several additional aphasic syndromes have been described by categorizing symptoms: transcortical motor, transcortical sensory, isolated speech, anomic-amnesic. At present there are insufficient anatomical and physiological data to warrant a highly fractionated nosology. To a certain degree, differences in phenomenology will reflect the individual patient's education and verbal achievement, factors that are difficult to quantitate and analyze. Two additional features of the aphasia syndromes deserve emphasis. It is now recognized that difficulty with writing has no localizing value. It always occurs as part of aphasia and is affected in proportion to the disruption of spoken language. Second, difficulty with naming is also poorly localized. For reasons that are not known, both of these language functions are quite fragile, occurring as early manifestations of aphasia, or even as symptoms of diffuse encephalopathy.

Alexia. Difficulty with reading commonly occurs as part of the syndrome of receptive aphasia as a consequence of lesions in the dominant temporal-parietal-occipital region. Of note, however, is that alexia can occur *without* any aphasia. It is also striking that the patient with this syndrome is able to write to dictation, but is unable to read what he has written. In this situation there is usually a lesion in the left occipital-parietal junction, or in the left visual cortex (medial occipital lobe) *and* the posterior third (splenium) of the corpus callosum (Fig. 11–9). A right homonymous hemianopsia is usually present. One explanation for this syndrome is that the unaffected left visual field conveys written material normally to the right visual cortex but this information cannot be subsequently sent to the language centers in the left temporal lobe because of de-

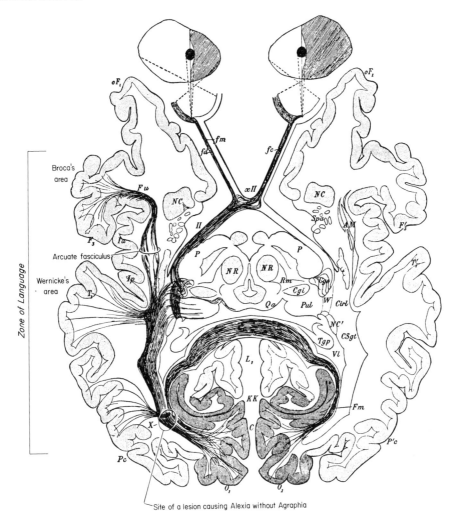

Site of a lesion causing Alexia without Agraphia

Fig. 11–9. Horizontal section through the Zone of Language (from Dejerine, *Semiologie du Systeme Nerveux,* 1914, Fig. 5). The visual fields are shown in front of the retina to indicate a right homonymous hemianopsia. The lesion causing this visual deficit is indicated in the left parietooccipital area by X. This lesion destroys the left optic radiation and also prevents fibers from the right visual cortex from reaching the "Zone of Language." This is thought to be one anatomical explanation for why patients with this lesion cannot read (alexia) although they can still speak (no aphasia) and write (no agraphia).

struction of the visual pathways in the left parietooccipital junction or the corpus callosum. These abnormalities are well documented and constitute the best example of a disconnection syndrome. The cause is usually occlusion of the left posterior cerebral artery.

Three additional features are sometimes present in the alexia syndrome. Often

patients have difficulty in naming colors, but are able to point correctly to colors when they are named for them and are able to make correct color matches. This deficit is called color anomia or dysnomia. Less commonly, patients have difficulty in recognizing objects (visual agnosia) or identifying faces (prosopagnosia). In visual agnosia, objects held in the hand and manipulated are readily identified. Similarly, when a patient with prosopagnosia hears the voice of a familiar person he cannot visually recognize he knows the person immediately. The term *agnosia* (Freud 1891) is used to describe these syndromes and means failure of recognition. The abnormal phenomena are usually confined to a single sensory channel in any one patient (visual, auditory, or tactile agnosia). Usually there is relatively mild disruption of primary sensation compared to the deficit in recognizing the stimulus. Although these behavioral abnormalities are complex, they at least imply difficulty in relating information seen with uninvolved portions of the visual fields to circuits involved with language and memory.

Apraxia. Apraxia is broadly defined as difficulty in performing skilled motor acts with the hands. In pure forms of apraxia there is no disturbance in sensation, comprehension, strength, or coordination. This is rare. More commonly, what strikes the examiner is the disproportionate difficulty a patient has with skilled movements relative to mild sensory loss, aphasia, or motor system impairment. Since Liepmann's (1905) first description of apraxia many different categories have been proposed that attempt to formulate the pathophysiology of this type of dysfunction. Most schemes remain bound to original ideas that motor "engrams" (kinesthetic memories) for skilled movement reside in areas within association cortex. Destruction of these areas, or lesions disconnecting them from the efferent motor system, is proposed to account for the loss of skilled movement. Such hypotheses remain unproven; they rely heavily on the historical proposition that symptoms that result from damage of a part indicate the function of the part when it is undamaged. Whereas many observers think apraxia is highly localized, others conclude it is primarily a nonspecific concomitant of aphasia. Two forms of apraxia commonly occur with left-hemisphere damage.

1. *Ideomotor apraxia:* Patients have difficulty performing intransitive or imaginary gestures that convey ideas, such as waving goodbye, praying, saluting, or making the victory sign with the fingers. Patients are unable to obey verbal instructions to perform these gestures or even copy the maneuvers after demonstration by the examiner.

2. *Ideational apraxia:* Patients are said to have this disorder when they are unable to demonstrate the use of objects placed in their hands. The examiner provides instructions and examples; objects commonly used include toothbrush, key and lock, nut and bolt, scissors, and hammer.

These two types of apraxia usually occur with lesions of the left parietal area. Often they are present together, although some investigators think ideomotor apraxia is more common. They suggest that the more abstract the movement, the more susceptible it is to disease processes. In this sense, apraxia is thought to occur on a continuum, with ideational apraxia (use of objects) being a more severe manifestation of ideomotor apraxia (difficulty with abstract gestures). Other investigators try to separate these two apraxic behaviors on anatomical and theoretical grounds. From a different perspective, however, the important pathophysiological point is that they most commonly occur along with some impairment in language.

Since motor dominance and language have apparently evolved together, it is likely that there are neural mechanisms basic to both skilled hand movements and speech. Investigators have suggested that these mechanisms may involve the speed and sequencing of short, rapid physiological events necessary for gesture, communication, and verbally guided (learned) hand movements. In addition, there are apparently mechanisms for "summarizing" or "recognizing" characteristic strings of physiological events. For example, it is now known that human speech can be processed ("comprehended") faster than any other sequence of sensory data, suggesting that there are learned mechanisms for spanning or abstracting strings of phonemes or words rather than processing each one individually. Patients with mild aphasia or apraxia often perform normally when instructions are presented simply and slowly. Deficits become manifest when rapid sequencing is required in speech reception or in the skilled motor performance of speech or hand movement. In addition, it should be emphasized that deficits are always more obvious when a behavioral response is requested by an examiner compared to when the behavior is evoked spontaneously. It is not uncommon for an apraxic patient to be unable to obey the request to mimic the act of drinking a glass of water, or demonstrate the use of a real glass of water, yet when one arrives on his dinner tray and he is alone, the water is quickly and smoothly down the hatch.

A final example of dominant hemisphere dysfunction emphasizes the effect of lesions on verbally learned behavior. As children we are taught the names of our fingers, to count on our fingers, to divide the world into right and left sides as we distinguish our right and left hands. Damage to the left parietal lobe can cause mild receptive aphasia and Gerstmann's syndrome (1925): finger agnosia (inability to name or indicate fingers), acalculia (inability to calculate), and right-left confusion.

Right hemisphere

Damage to the right hemisphere, the nondominant or "minor" hemisphere in right-handed people, has no appreciable effect on language function. By contrast, lesions in the right temporal-parietal-occipital "association" cortex commonly result in a distinct behavioral abnormality in visual-spatial orientation. This syndrome is known by many names, including nondominant parietal lobe syndrome, the minor hemisphere syndrome, and visuospatial agnosia. Many characteristic abnormalities can be present; the basic feature can be broadly defined as difficulty in recognizing and using the left side of the body and orienting toward the left side of the world.

Abnormalities in sensation are usually present. If the lesion involves primary sensory cortex for the hand (areas 3, 2, and 1; Figs. 11–4, 11–5) there are deficits in *passive* touch (touch thresholds, pressure sensation, two-point discrimination, joint movement sensation) and *active* touch (discrimination of size, shape, and texture). In addition, finger movements are stiff, slow, and awkward. Primary somatosensory cortex is tightly integrated with the motor strip so that it is useful to think of this area of cortex as sensorimotor. During operations for epilepsy, Penfield stimulated each side of the central sulcus and found considerable overlap in sensation and movement. The hand normally functions as a unified, feeling-moving, tactile-kinesthetic apparatus; lesions of the central sulcus almost always impair both sensation and fine fractionated movements.

A lesion posterior to the central sulcus in the parietal cortex usually does not disturb primary sensations. Examination of the patient's left hand will demonstrate relatively normal responses to pain, temperature, and passive touch. Detection of joint movement may be mildly impaired. By contrast, abnormalities in stereognosis are usually obvious: The patient is slow and often unable to identify common objects placed in the left hand. This is called astereognosis, which is essentially synonymous with the term *tactile agnosia*. In addition, there is often difficulty with comparisons of the texture and weights of different objects. These lost functions are euphemistically called *cortical sensations* in that they require elaboration and comparison of primary sensations delivered to the cortex along separate pathways, or dedicated lines. Precise judgments on abnormalities of primary sensations in the left hand are complicated, however, by a curious finding. If both of the patient's hands are touched simultaneously while the eyes are closed, the left hand stimulus is frequently not reported. This is called *neglect*. In severe cases neglect extends to the entire left side of the body and occurs for noxious stimuli as well as light touch. With large lesions, left hemiparesis occurs in addition to the parietal lobe syndrome. In these instances, patients may neglect or deny their hemiparesis and even fail to identify their own paralyzed limbs. This behavior is called anosognosia, or denial of deficit. The pathophysiological explanation for these neglect phenomena is not clear. Although careful testing often reveals slight elevation of tactile thresholds even in mild cases, the severity of the concomitant neglect indicates that mechanisms in addition to sensory impairment are involved.

Visual neglect may also occur with right parietal lesions. In this situation patients commonly fail to report left-sided visual stimuli. This neglect can be severe when associated with a left homonymous hemianopsia that results from parietal lesions involving the optic radiations. Of note, however, is that left visual neglect can occur with normal visual fields, and conversely, complete left homonymous hemianopsia from an occipital lesion can occur without causing behavioral neglect.

Several investigators have reported examples of neglect in patients with lesions in the frontal cortex, cingulum, thalamus, or reticular system of the brainstem. In some circumstances patients appear not to notice contralateral tactile, visual, or even auditory stimuli. This has been called sensory neglect. Other patients do not attend to, orient toward, or reach for contralateral stimuli, suggesting a syndrome of motor neglect. As there are usually signs of motor system damage (unilateral increased reflexes, Babinski sign, slow movement) in the latter condition, it becomes a semantic point whether to call such behavior motor neglect or just a mild up-

per motor neuron syndrome. Asymmetrical orienting behavior can be produced in animals by small lesions in many cortical and subcortical sites, suggesting that the pathophysiology of neglect is somewhat nonspecific. Unilateral lesions in sensory, motor, limbic, or associational pathways somehow upset a dynamic left-right balance within systems necessary for animals to sense and respond equally to both sides of the world. In humans the abnormality is usually transient, lasting only a few weeks after a lesion in most patients. Full recovery from neglect is expected except in very severe cases.

When left-sided visual and tactile neglect are present from right parietal lesions other behavioral abnormalities also occur. When patients are asked to draw a clock from memory they will leave out of the numbers on the left side, or squeeze them all to the right. This occurs using either hand. Such patients are unable to copy flat geometrical designs from drawings or to use blocks to copy a pattern or build a simple structure (Fig. 11–10). Taken together these abnormalities are called *constructional apraxia*. The term is used to emphasize that primary abnormalities in visual or tactile sensation and movement are relatively mild while complex visual-spatial behavior is markedly abnormal. In addition, patients may be unable to find their way around in familiar environments, or to indicate routes to be taken on maps. They may also have difficulty with spatial relationships on their own body, being unable to localize the site where they are touched (somototopagnosia). Putting on clothes may be particularly difficult unless garments are aligned and ready to slip into (dressing apraxia).

How do we understand this behavior? The nondominant parietal lobe syndrome is a second example of the fact that the human cerebral hemispheres are functionally asymmetric. A right-sided lesion can disrupt orientation toward space. Although errors are made predominately on

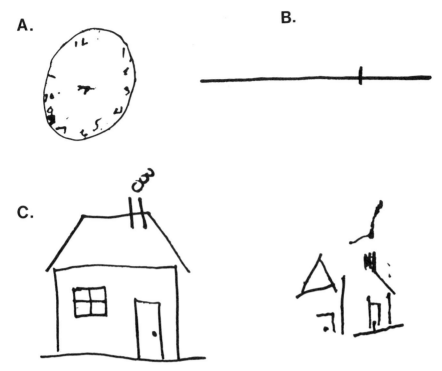

Fig. 11–10. Constructional apraxia and the nondominant parietal lobe syndrome. A 67-year-old man suffered a hemorrhagic infarction of the right parietal lobe. Two weeks after his stroke he denied any complaints. He walked about the ward with a decreased left arm swing, usually without wearing his left shoe. His visual fields were full when each eye was tested individually, but he consistently neglected left visual stimuli with both eyes open during double simultaneous stimulation. He was unable to identify objects placed in his left hand. **A.** The result when asked to draw the face of a clock at 9:15. **B.** The result when asked to mark the horizontal line in its middle. **C.** The result when asked to copy the drawing of a house. The patient could point to and name all the parts, but attempts at reconstruction resulted in reduplication of the right side.

the left side, they occur when either the left or right hand is used for exploration. The reason for this is unclear. It has been suggested that a component of spatial orientation was "pushed out" of the left hemisphere and into the right with the development of cerebral dominance and language on the left. This is conjectural and teaches little of basic physiological mechanisms. Recently, electrophysiological studies of the parietal lobe in monkeys (areas 5 and 7, the superior parietal lobule) have found populations of neurons with complex sensorimotor receptive field properties. Such neurons increase their rate of firing when the animal reaches toward and examines objects in contralateral space. The parietal lobe receives cortical and subcortical polysensory input and has a major cortical projection anteriorly to premotor cortex and medially to limbic cortex. These may constitute part of a physiological circuit important in turning eyes (see Chap. 8), body, and attention toward a contralateral object for closer visual and tactile examination. This parietal lobe function is bilaterally symmetric in nonhuman primates. In humans it is probable but not certain that a small component of this function exists in the left hemisphere. Our lack of certainty on this point arises because it is hazardous to conclude that subtle defects in visuospatial orientation are present when a receptive aphasia interferes with a patient's ability to understand the instructions for behavioral tests.

Patients with lesions of the right temporoparietal area are similar to those with homologous left-sided lesions in being unaware of their deficit. As patients with receptive aphasia continue to speak unabashedly with little sense, so patients with visuospatial disorientation often fail to dress the left side of their body and often make only right turns at each corner. They are blandly unaware of the half of the world they have lost. Literally speaking, in both cases they do not know how much they miss. This raises difficult questions concerning human self-awareness and the organization of consciousness in the brain. Patients with lesions in motor or primary sensory zones know or can be taught the nature of their deficit. This is usually not true following lesions in parietal, temporal, or frontal cortex. Disruption of learned behavior following lesions in these areas also removes knowledge of the behavior, its object, and goals. In addition, evidence from studies of the effects of rehabilitation suggest that reteaching has little impact on recovery of cognitive behavior.

FRONTAL LOBES

The frontal lobes constitute the largest subdivision of neocortex (Fig. 11–11), yet their functions are the least understood. A few zones are related to the motor system, including the supplementary motor area on the medial surface, and the field for contraversive eye movements (area 8) in the dorsolateral convexity in premotor cortex (see Chap. 8). The latter area receives extensive cortical input from parietooccipital cortex, and lesions here can cause a transient syndrome of contralateral "mo-

tor" neglect (discussed earlier). More anterior lesions of prefrontal cortex produce no obvious deficits in simple motor, sensory, or language functions.

There are only a few good clues as to how best to describe the role of frontal cortical areas in human behavior. One clue comes from studies of lesions of the dorsolateral convexity in nonhuman primates. Small bilateral lesions involving the posterior aspects of the sulcus principalis disrupt delayed response behavior. These deficits are demonstrated by placing the monkey in a restraining chair (arms free) facing two small wells. Food is placed in one well and then an opaque screen is lowered to remove the wells from sight. After a delay of 4 seconds or longer the screen is raised and the monkey is allowed to retrieve the food. Monkeys with lesions perform no better than if they arbitrarily chose a well. This is called a delayed response deficit. Bilateral lesions in adjacent areas of frontal lobe or other areas of cortex (sensory, motor, limbic) do not cause delayed response deficits, but frontocortical efferent pathways through caudate nucleus are critical since bilateral lesions here also disrupt this behavior. In addition, animals who have delayed response deficits perform normally on visual discrimination tasks, suggesting that short-term memory processes per se are normal. Thus the abnormal behavior is best interpreted as a deficit in spatial memory.

A second clue regarding frontal lobe function comes from neuropsychological studies of patients following surgical removal of a frontal lobe. Removal of the left frontal lobe (anterior to premotor cortex and Broca's area) causes only a mild deficit in language function, manifested primarily as a decrease in verbal fluency. By contrast, removal of either frontal lobe causes a more obvious deficit in obeying serial instructions. The deficit was discovered by Milner, who tested patients by asking them to sort a deck of cards with four different symbols in four different

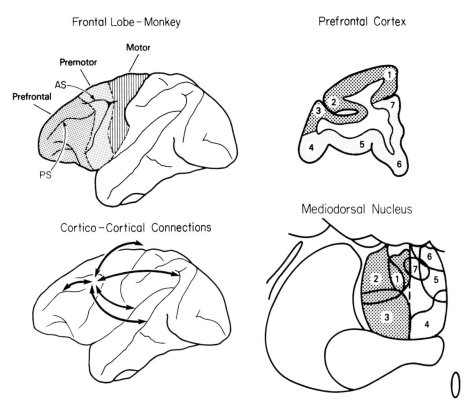

Fig. 11–11. The frontal lobe of the rhesus monkey has three major subdivisions: motor, premotor, and prefrontal. Prefrontal cortex is granular (spiny stellate neurons in layers III–IV) and has reciprocal connections with the thalamic mediodorsal nucleus. In addition, there are extensive long corticocortical connections from dorsolateral frontal cortex to other cortical zones in parietal, insular, temporal, and limbic (medial) areas. AS, arcuate sulcus. PS, principal sulcus. (From P. S. Goldman-Rakic, Development and plasticity of primate frontal association cortex. In Schmitt et al. (eds.), pp. 69–100, Figs. 1 and 2.)

colors on their faces. The patient must first sort by one criterion, (e.g., color) and then shift to another criterion. Patients with frontal lobe lesions or removals do very poorly on this test. They tend to perseverate, that is, to stick to one choice for sorting, and have great difficulty in shifting to new strategies when old ones become incorrect. Curiously, patients are often able to verbalize the correct choice but continue to perseverate in their motor response. Some observers suggest this dissociation between cognition (knowing the error and the correct strategy) and subsequent goal-directed behavior (i.e., taking advantage of the error and following a new plan) is characteristic of frontal lobe dysfunction in humans.

A third body of evidence bearing on frontal lobe function comes from examinations of patients with lesions in the thalamus. Lesions in thalamic nuclei that relay directly to cortex produce dysfunction that has features similar to the dysfunction that results from lesions of the cortical areas that receive the relay. This emphasizes that brain functions are distributed physiologically through connecting circuits rather than being the sole property of specific loci. Lesions in the left posterior thalamus (pulvinar) disrupt language, whereas lesions in the right thalamus can disrupt visuospatial perception. Two types of thalamic lesions bear upon frontal lobe functions. First, bilateral lesions of the dorsomedial nuclei (trauma; Korsakoff's psychosis, see Chap. 13) cause impairment in short-term memory functions. Similarly, patients with bilateral prefrontal cortical lesions in zones of dorsomedial projections are often quite forgetful. Memory dysfunction is more severe with thalamic than cortical lesions, however. Second, bilateral lesions of basal forebrain result in severe behavior retardation. These patients are either abulic (i.e., they fail to initiate any meaningful behavior) or akinetic and mute. This probably results in part from disruption of ascending projections to medial frontal cortex (particularly dopamine projections in the medial forebrain bundle) and/or disruption of reciprocal projections between orbitofrontal cortex and temporal lobe-amygdala (uncinate fasciculus). Patients with large bilateral frontal lesions that impinge on medial and orbital frontal cortex usually show a generalized decrease in behavior, with a lack of initiative and spontaneity, slow movements, and a flat emotional affect. Such a clinical picture often suggests dementia, but standard intelligence testing discloses normal or only slightly impaired cognitive functions.

How do we interpret these different observations regarding frontal lobe functions: delayed response deficits, perseveration, forgetfulness, and blunting of affect and behavior? First, it should be emphasized that the frontal lobes are so large it would be unwise to try to assign one basic physiological or behavioral function to the entire area. Similarly, there is considerable variation between patients with frontal lobe lesions so that there is no one "frontal lobe syndrome." Second, although there has been a considerable advance in anatomical studies of frontal lobe, electrophysiological studies of neurons during sensory stimulation, movement, or complex behavior are difficult to interpret. Only a small proportion of frontal lobe neurons ever respond during a task, and the change in firing rate is not robust. It seems likely that new experimental strategies will be required to probe frontal areas. Finally, because a lack of hard data has never retarded speculation, students of human behavior have offered many hypotheses regarding the essential role of frontal lobes. Most of those speak to our ability to gather data, form abstractions, generate a plan of action, learn from mistakes, and work toward meaningful goals that inspire enthusiastic action and promise future pleasures, both imaginary and real.

CONCLUSION

Lesions of cerebral cortex in humans can cause characteristic syndromes of abnormal linguistic and cognitive behavior. Although such syndromes are complex, they are of clinical value in localizing damage to one hemisphere, or even to a part of one hemisphere. Localization of symptoms, however, is not synonymous with either a precise or an exclusive localization of function. Results from animal experiments emphasize that complex behavior is highly fractionated and widely distributed through interconnecting anatomical circuits throughout the brain. Summarized simply, the pathophysiology of behavioral dysfunction following cortical lesions can be viewed as disruption of but one part of a complex machine. For truly human behavior, however, cerebral cortex is *the* critical part, the most recent and unique experiment of evolution.

GENERAL REFERENCES

Critchley, M. *The Parietal Lobes*. London, Edward Arnold, 1953.

Diamond, I. T. The subdivisions of neocortex: A proposal to revise the traditional view of sensory, motor, and association areas. *Prog. in Psychobiol. and Physiol. Psych.* 8:1–43, 1979.

Gazzaniga, M. S. (ed.). *Neuropsychology: Handbook of Behavioral Neurology,* vol. 2. New York, Plenum Press, 1979.

Geschwind, N., and W. Levitsky. Human brain: Left-right asymmetries in temporal speech region. *Science* 161:186–7, 1968.

Heilman, K. M., and E. Valenstein (eds.). *Clinical Neuropsychology.* New York, Oxford University Press, 1979.

Horton, J. C., and E. T. Hedley-White. Mapping of cytochrome oxidase patches and ocular dominance columns in human visual cortex. *Philosoph. Trans. Roy. Soc.,* Ser. B. 304:255–272, 1984.

Kaas, J. H. What, if anything, is SI? Organization of first somatosensory area of cortex. *Physiol. Rev.* 63:206–31, 1983.

Kojima, S., M. Kojima, and P. S. Goldman-Rakic. Operant behavioral analysis of memory loss in monkeys with prefrontal lesions. *Brain Res.* 248:51–9, 1982.

Lorente de Nó, R. Cerebral cortex: Architecture, intracortical connections, motor projections. In *Physiology of the Nervous System.* G. Fulton (ed.). London, Oxford University Press, 1943, pp. 274–313.

Merzenich, M. M., and J. H. Kaas. Principles of organization of sensory-perceptual systems in mammals. *Prog. in Psychobiol. and Physiol. Psych.* 9:1–42, 1980.

Mountcastle, V. B. An organizing principle for cerebral function: the unit module and the distributed system. In *The Mindful Brain,* G. M. Edelman and V. B. Mountcastle (eds.) Cambridge, M.I.T. Press, 1978.

Passonneau, J. V., R. A. Hawkins, W. D. Lust, and F. A. Welsh. *Cerebral Metabolism and Neural Function.* Baltimore, Williams & Wilkins, 1980.

Powell, T. P. S., and V. B. Mountcastle. Some aspects of the functional organization of the cortex of the postcentral gyrus of the monkey: A correlation of findings obtained in a single unit analysis with cytoarchitecture. *Bull. Johns Hopkins Hosp.* 105:133–62, 1959.

Schmitt, F. O., F. G. Worden, G. Adelman, and S. G. Dennis (eds.). *The Organization of the Cerebral Cortex.* Cambridge, Mass., MIT Press, 1981.

Smith, G. Elliot. Some problems relating to the evolution of the brain. *Lancet* 1:1–6, 147–53, 221–7, 1910.

Sperry, R. Some effects of disconnecting the cerebral hemispheres. *Science* 217:1223–6, 1982.

PART TWO

Disease Processes

12.

Seizures

ERIC W. LOTHMAN and ROBERT C. COLLINS

Seizures are among the most common neurological disorders in clinical medicine. It is important to recognize that a seizure is a symptom of dysfunction in the gray matter of the brain rather than a disease itself. Because there are many causes of seizures (Table 12–1), a primary task of the physician is to determine whether a specific etiology for the patient's seizures can be identified. If this cannot be done and seizures recur, a diagnosis of idiopathic epilepsy is made. In every instance seizures arise because of an abnormal, excessive, paroxysmal, synchronous discharge in a population of neurons. The pathophysiological events in a seizure are both transient and readily differentiated from the normal background activity of the brain, features encompassed by the term *paroxysmal.* Because of their sudden nature, seizures are sometimes described as *ictal events,* from the Latin *ictus,* to strike. Seizures rarely last longer than 1 or 2 minutes and are commonly followed by a depression of neurological function lasting minutes or hours that is called the postictal state. Seizures may result in positive symptoms such as jerking of a limb, or negative symptoms such as interruption of

Table 12–1. Causes of seizures

Congenital
  Maldevelopment
  Inborn metabolic errors
Perinatal
  Immediate: hypoxemia, hemorrhage, trauma
  Latent: temporal lobe sclerosis
Metabolic
  Hypocalcemia
  Hyponatremia
  Hypoglycemia
Infectious
  Simple febrile convulsions
  Encephalitis
  Meningitis
Neoplastic
  Primary
  Metastatic
Vascular
  Arteriovenous malformation
  Postinfarction
  Posthemorrhage
Trauma
  Penetrating wounds
  Closed head injuries
Toxins
  Drug abuse
  Withdrawal from alcohol and sedative drugs

normal behavior with brief amnesia. The clinical manifestations depend on which neuroanatomical regions are involved.

The clinical and EEG manifestations of seizures can be classified in either of two

Table 12–2. Classification of seizures

1. **Partial (focus, or local) seizures**
   A. Simple partial seizures. There is no impairment of consciousness. The EEG shows epileptic activity localized in surface leads, arising from paroxysmal discharges in neocortical cells.
      1. Focal motor seizures, with localized jerking (face or extremity), or Jacksonian march, or tonic contralateral postural change.
      2. Focal sensory seizures, such as somatosensory, visual, auditory, olfactory, gustatory, or vertiginous.
      3. Dysphasic/aphasic seizures.
   B. Complex partial seizures. Alteration or loss of consciousness occurs. The EEG shows localized, or bilaterally asymmetric discharges over temporal, or frontotemporal areas. Depth electrodes show discharges in hippocampus and amygdala.
      1. Psychic aura only. Brief altered states of emotion, cognition, or memory. Patients usually retain some awareness.
      2. Loss of consciousness with or without preceding aura. Blank stare and/or automatisms occur.

2. **Generalized seizures**
   A. Nonconvulsive. Occur predominately in children. There is impairment of consciousness, but little or no convulsive movement.
      1. Absence seizures (petit mal). Abrupt onset and cessation of 3-Hz, symmetric spike and wave EEG discharges.
      2. Atypical absence. More varied EEG and clinical features, such as tonic posturing.
   B. Convulsive. Occur at all ages. Bilateral motor convulsions from the start.
      1. Tonic-clonic (grand mal). EEG shows bilateral rhythm at 10–20 Hz. Tonic and clonic phases may occur independently, or as isolated manifestations.
      2. Myoclonic seizures. Single or repetitive jerks of muscles. Metabolic or degenerative disease is usually present.

broad categories, *partial seizures* or *generalized seizures* (Table 12–2). Partial seizures are those that begin in a discrete cortical area, called a seizure focus, and have restricted or asymmetric clinical manifestations. *Simple partial seizures* affect the motor or sensory functions without disrupting consciousness. Common examples of this type of seizure are jerking of a single extremity or flashing lights in a visual field. *Complex partial seizures* is a term synonymous with psychomotor, temporal-lobe, or limbic system seizures. These often begin with a conscious awareness of a brief abnormal sensation such as a strange odor, intense fear, or a rising feeling in the abdomen. This part of the seizure is called an *aura* and is usually followed by loss of contact with the environment. In this phase patients are unconscious, remain immobile, and show nothing more than a blank stare. Others exhibit *automatisms,* which are stereotyped, involuntary motor activities such as lip smacking or fumbling with clothes. These "behavioral" seizures can last up to a minute or two and are commonly followed by a period of confusion. It should be noted that both simple and complex partial seizures can spread from a focus bilaterally through the brain and cause a secondarily generalized motor convulsion.

Generalized seizures are those that are bilaterally symmetric in the brain from the onset. They can be further classified into convulsive and nonconvulsive types, depending on whether they have motor manifestations. The nonconvulsive type is called an absence seizure, often referred to by the older name *petit mal epilepsy.* They occur in children and adolescents and are characterized by brief, 2–10-second attacks of impaired consciousness associated with rolling up of the eyes, blinking, and occasionally mild clonic or atonic components. Absense seizures are associated with a three per second spike and wave EEG abnormality (Fig. 12–1). The most common form of generalized convulsive seizure is referred to as *grand mal* or tonic-clonic seizure. Such convulsions often begin with a loud cry when a sudden con-

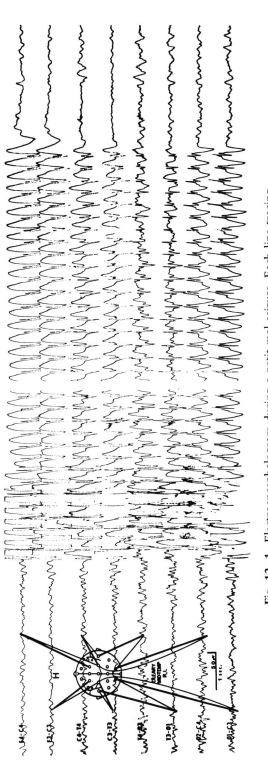

Fig. 12–1. Electroencephalogram during a petit mal seizure. Each line tracing denotes the difference in electrical potential between two electrodes on the scalp. These are indicated on the dorsal view of the head (nose anterior) called the EEG montage. Note the sudden eruption and cessation of three per second spike and wave discharge pattern distributed synchronously throughout all leads. The clinical correlate in this 12-year-old boy was staring with occasional eye blinks. During the discharge he was unresponsive to questions. Discontinuity in record denotes removal of 3 seconds of tracing.

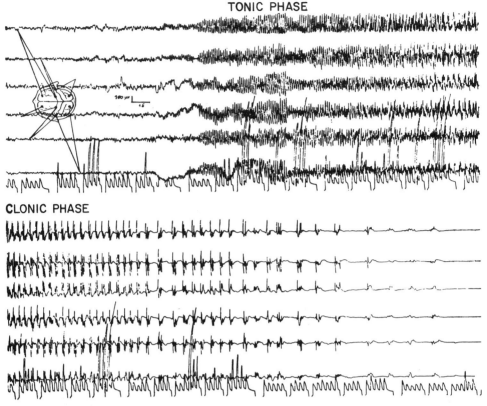

Fig. 12–2. Electroencephalogram of generalized seizure associated with a tonic-clonic convulsion. Top six traces are recordings led from eight electrodes positioned as shown in the inset montage. Bottom trace is continuous display of frequency analysis of EEG activity. Seizure begins with a rhythmic, high-frequency discharge, followed by multiple, closely grouped spikes of variable amplitude and wave form (tonic phase), and ends with distinct polyspikes separated by isoelectric intervals (clonic phase). (Reprinted from *Epileptic Seizures*, H. Gastaut and R. Broughton, Springfield, Ill., Charles C. Thomas, 1972, with permission.)

traction of the thorax forces out air against a partially closed glottis. Patients fall to the ground in rigid extension for 15–20 seconds, become cyanotic, salivate, and frequently lose bladder and bowel control. The tonic phase blends into a clonic phase of rhythmic limb contractions for an additional 20 to 30 seconds. The EEG shows high amplitude, 10–20 cycles/sec activity during the tonic phase and grouped polyspikes separated by quiet intervals during the clonic phase (Fig. 12–2). The EEG is often flattened or slow in the post-

ictal phase. After a grand mal seizure the patient slowly regains consciousness over several minutes, but remains sleepy for several hours. Postictal headache and muscle soreness are common.

This classification provides a practical clinical guide for determining which of the many anticonvulsant drugs now available would be best suited for an individual patient. However, the reader should be aware that knowledge about the pathophysiology of epilepsy, although increasing, is incomplete and that classifications are con-

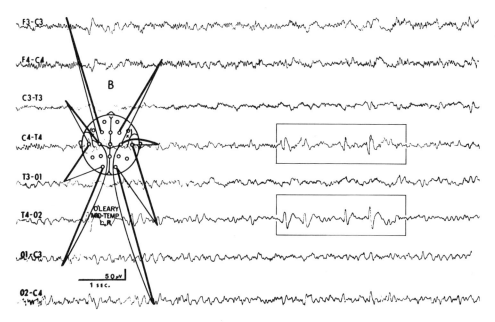

Fig. 12–3. Focal interictal paroxysms. Four sharp waves (enclosed in boxes) localized to the right temporal area disturb normal background activity.

tinually being modified. The ultimate goal in studying seizures is to understand the genetic, physiologic, metabolic, and anatomic substrates so as to prevent causal pathology or to design optimal treatment. Recently, there have been substantial advances in three areas of epilepsy research: (1) the basic cellular mechanisms behind paroxysmal discharges; (2) the functional anatomy of seizures; and (3) the pathophysiology of damage to the brain with prolonged or recurrent seizures.

PATHOPHYSIOLOGIC CORRELATES OF PAROXYSMAL DISCHARGES

The electroencephalogram (EEG) of a patient with focal epilepsy characteristically contains distinctive spikes or sharp waves (Fig. 12–3). Since these occur without any clinical abnormality and are interspersed between fully developed seizures or ictal events, they are called *interictal discharges*. Compared to the normal background pattern of the EEG, interictal discharges have a large amplitude (up to

several millivolts), but are of short duration (less than 80 msec for a spike and 200 msec for a sharp wave). Since the EEG recorded at a particular location is a reflection of electrical activity in neurons near the recording electrode, spikes or sharp waves that appear only in some channels of the EEG localize the cortical zone where interictal discharges arise. In the case shown in Figure 12–3, the seizure focus is in the right temporal lobe. Interictal spikes cause no clinical abnormality, but when a seizure occurs here and spreads to motor cortex convulsions begin on the contralateral size of the body.

Neuroscientists have long been interested in basic aspects of the focal seizure process. By applying chemicals or stimulating electrically at discrete sites, investigators have been successful in producing focal epilepsy in experimental animals. Using such models, researchers have extensively studied mechanisms underlying interictal discharges as well as the transition between a relatively harmless interictal spike and a full-blown seizure.

A. INTERICTAL DISCHARGE

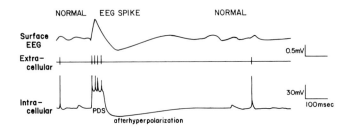

B. SEIZURE DISCHARGE

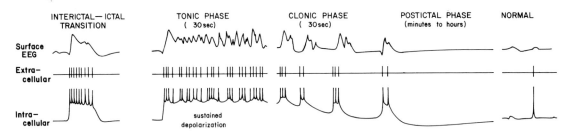

Fig. 12–4. Neuronal correlates of paroxysmal discharges. **A.** Normal activity is interrupted by an interictal spike on the surface EEG. This signal indicates that a local population of neurons has undergone a paroxysmal depolarization shift (PDS, intracellular trace). This is followed by a long-lasting hyperpolarization of neurons during which the EEG trace is relatively flat. A high-frequency discharge (burst) of action potentials occurs on the crest of the PDS and accounts for the volley of action potentials registered by the extracellular microelectrode (middle trace). **B.** During the interictal to ictal transition (left-hand side) the afterhyperpolarization is replaced with an afterdepolarization. This results in an increased number of action potentials. The surface EEG changes from a simple spike to a complex, polyphasic spike. A fully developed seizure (right-hand side) is initiated with a tonic phase seen on the surface EEG as rhythmic, high-frequency discharges (see Fig. 12–2). This occurs when neurons undergo sustained depolarization with generation of protracted trains of action potentials. Subsequently the seizure begins to abate during the clonic phase. This is characterized by groups of polyspikes on the EEG, reflecting periodic neuronal depolarization and grouped discharge of action potentials. Seizure activity stops (postictal phase) as neurons become hyperpolarized below resting level. Subsequently, neuronal membrane potential returns to resting level, but normal neuronal activity and function are altered for a variable period.

Intracellular recordings in the focus reveal that during an interictal discharge on the EEG, a compact population of neurons displays a stereotyped abnormality that is called a *paroxysmal depolarization shift* or *PDS* (Fig. 12–4). These PDSs are characterized by a sudden, large amplitude (about 30 mV) and sustained (70–150 msec) depolarization that is synchronized in many neurons. Multiple, high-frequency action potentials are superimposed on the crest of the slow membrane depolarization, accounting for the burst of action potentials seen in extracellular traces. The PDS and EEG spikes can occur spontaneously or be triggered by afferent stimuli, which excite neurons in the focus. A PDS is followed by a potent (10–20 mV below resting membrane potential) and long-lasting (up to 700 msec) hyperpolarization. During this *afterhyperpolarization* neurons are silent and even resistant to stimulation delivered through afferent pathways.

The cycle of PDS and afterhyperpolarization is related to a complex sequence of events (Fig. 12–5). At the most fundamental level, the changes in membrane potential arise from imbalances in inward (depolarizing) and outward (hyperpolarizing) ionic currents. These currents are the result of conductance increases that allow specific ions, driven by electrochemical gradients, to move across the membrane through various channels. These channels can be activated or opened by two types of mechanisms. First, some channels are voltage dependent and are activated by changes in membrane potential. Second, other channels are chemically activated by ions such as Ca^{2+} or neurotransmitters such as GABA.

The mechanisms underlying the depolarization–afterhyperpolarization sequence in a single epileptic neuron relate primarily to two ionic channels. The depolarization is produced when voltage-sensitive Ca^{2+} channels are opened and $g_{Ca^{2+}}$ (calcium conductance) increases. The magnitude of $g_{Ca^{2+}}$ is dependent on the membrane potential in that it is activated when the cell is depolarized above a certain threshold level (an all or none phenomenon) and increases in proportion to the amount of depolarization. A positive feedback occurs where calcium ions move from the extracellular to intracellular space depolarizing the neuron and causing further activation of the channel and further increases in $g_{Ca^{2+}}$ (Fig. 12–5C). At the same time, however, the increase in concentration of calcium inside the neuron activates a second, chemically dependent channel, $g_{K^+Ca^{2+}}$. This channel allows potassium ions to move out of the cell,

which produces a hyperpolarizing influence. As the membrane potential is returned to resting level, $g_{Ca^{2+}}$ is decreased and the PDS is terminated. This whole sequence is regenerative once an adequate triggering event occurs (Fig. 12–5B). At the conclusion of the cycle metabolic pumping reestablishes the normal concentrations of ions in the intra- and extracellular spaces.

Experimental studies in animals indicate that these membrane-ionic events are characteristic of neurons during seizure discharges. They do not occur in normal neurons. For example, when a small depolarizing current is introduced into a normal neuron (Fig. 12–5C) the membrane potential rapidly returns to normal. If the same current depolarizes an "epileptic neuron" above a certain threshold, then the entire PDS-afterhyperpolarization sequence occurs. Although this all or none feature might seem similar to the generation of action potentials in normal neurons it is entirely different. It is slower, lasts longer, involves different conductances, and causes bursts of high-frequency potentials.

This schema provides some understanding of the epileptiform discharge that occurs in a single neuron. However, it does not explain the synchronization of the event that occurs with a local population of many neurons. Synchronization must occur at the cellular level for an interictal spike to be evident on the EEG. Such synchronization is dependent on synaptic connections as diagramed in Figure 12–6. For example, when a PDS occurs in the soma of an "epileptic neuron," cell A, a burst of high-frequency action potentials travels to its axon terminals. After a brief delay, cell B is recruited into an epileptic discharge by excitatory synaptic connections from cell A. The brief, synchronized discharge of many such synaptically coupled cells results in a spike in the EEG lead overlying this area. The number of neurons necessary to produce an EEG spike is not re-

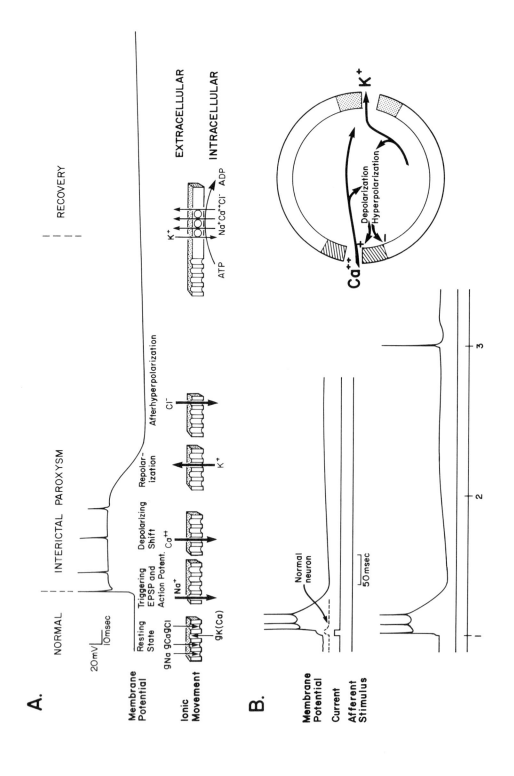

Fig. 12–5. Pathophysiology of "epileptic neurons." **A.** Ionic conductances underlying interictal spike. Before the onset of the PDS (shown at top) conductance channels for major ions are in their resting state (indicated by narrow lines). When a PDS is triggered with an initial EPSP (excitatory postsynaptic potential) and an action potential, g_{Na^+} increases, allowing sodium ions to move into the cell (shown by heavy line). The resultant depolarization is above threshold for activation of $g_{Ca^{2+}}$ so that calcium ions move into the cell and cause a prolonged depolarizing phase. This activates multiple sodium and calcium action potentials. The accumulation of calcium ions subsequently activates $g_{K^+(Ca^{2+})}$, which serves to repolarize the cell and turn off $g_{Ca^{2+}}$ (see **C**). The persistence of $g_{K^+(Ca^{2+})}$, together with the movement of chloride ions inward through channels opened by the inhibitory neurotransmitter GABA, causes the phase of afterhyperpolarization. Finally, ions are translocated by metabolic pumps to reestablish normal, resting transmembrane potential. **B.** Characteristic features of epileptic neurons. In the top tracings a PDS is initiated by passing a depolarizing current pulse into an epileptic neuron. Note that the active, regenerative response outlasts the initiating pulse and contrasts to the smaller, symmetrical response in the normal neuron. In the bottom tracings an epileptic response is triggered by stimulating afferents that impinge on an epileptic cell (stimulus 1, lowermost line). After an initial EPSP, a PDS identical to the PDS shown above develops. Immediately thereafter the cell is refractory, failing to respond to a second afferent stimulation, but develops a normal EPSP-action potential sequence on the third stimulus. Subsequent stimuli would provoke another PDS. **C.** Calcium-potassium conductance system responsible for slow depolarization and afterhyperpolarization sequence during epileptic paroxysm. Calcium channels (slashed area) are opened by depolarization and closed by hyperpolarization of the membrane potential. When open they permit calcium to flow into the cell, leading to further depolarization and an activation of potassium channels (stippled area). The opening of potassium channels allows potassium ions to move out of the cell, thereby hyperpolarizing the cell and inactivating g_{Ca}.

solved. In experimental animals a seizure focus with a surface area of 0.5 mm² is sufficient.

The summated output of abnormal neurons like A and B can result in further spread of epileptic activity. In this sense they can be considered "pacemaker" cells that can recruit normal neurons or "follower" cells into epileptic activity in the focus and at distant sites. Inhibitory synaptic connections keep this from happening. As diagrammed in Figure 12–6, the discharges from cell A would also excite local inhibitory interneurons. These feed back onto cell A, release GABA and help shut down epileptic firing. Such recurrent inhibition plays a role in the temporal containment of discharges. In addition, inhibitory interneurons send axons horizontally

through cortex to inhibit neurons at the edge of the focus (Fig. 12–6, cell C). This arrangement serves to spatially contain epileptic discharges. This ring of inhibition around a focus is called the "inhibitory surround." It should be appreciated that this is primarily a physiological definition and that the size of a focus is in large part dynamic, i.e., dependent on the moment to moment interplay of excitatory and inhibitory activity.

What happens when an interictal spike changes into a seizure? Neurophysiological studies have shown that there is a failure of membrane repolarization during the epileptic paroxysm (Fig. 12–4B). The membrane stays in a depolarized state and initiates nearly continuous high-frequency discharges over many seconds. These pro-

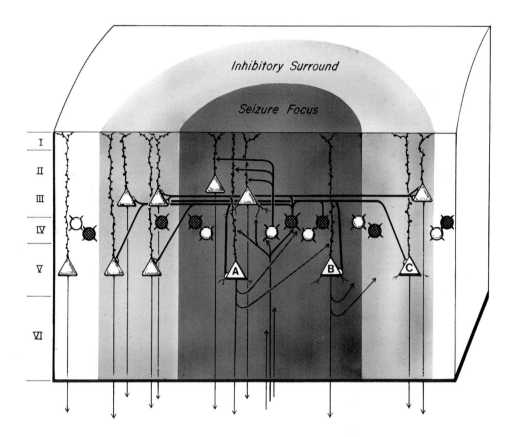

Fig. 12–6. Organization of a neocortical seizure focus. The spatial and temporal organization of a seizure focus reflects the dynamic interaction of excitatory and inhibitory synaptic activity. If cell A is an epileptic neuron its continuous discharge will tend to capture cell B into activity via excitatory recurrent collateral connections. When many cells like A and B fire synchronously (PDS), an epileptic spike appears on the EEG. Inhibitory interneurons (dark round cells) become activated and turn off cells A and B (temporal containment) as well as prevent neurons in contiguous cortex (cell C) from firing at all. Thus inhibitory interneurons (GABAergic) activated within the focus reach out horizontally and create the inhibitory surround (spatial containment). Activity within a neocortical focus can be triggered and increased by afferent activity from thalamus (ascending arrows). Excitatory connections impinge on pyramidal dendrites, as well as excitatory interneurons (light round cells). These may serve to capture and pace additional pyramidal neurons.

tracted discharges are very potent in enlarging the focus and spreading synaptically to distant areas in cortex, brainstem, and spinal cord (Fig. 12–7). Hence, there is almost always a clinical convulsion associated with this type of discharge. The prolonged cellular depolarization that occurs in the seizure focus seems to be the

end result of several local factors. First, intense discharges promote a failure in inhibitory mechanisms, either within the inhibitory interneurons themselves, or postsynaptically at GABA receptors. Second, prolonged depolarization could arise because of changes in dendritic structure and function caused by repeated interictal discharges. Third, local changes in ions in the extracellular milieu contribute to ictal discharges. Studies with ion probes have found that there are changes in the concentrations of cations in the extracellular space during a seizure, with calcium falling and potassium rising. These changes would favor membrane depolarization (Fig. 12–5). Finally, distant circuits may play a role, as a cortical seizure focus causes both orthodromic and antidromic firing into thalamus, which in turn sends the paroxysms back into the focus, causing further excitation.

Although experimental studies have gone far in describing the events of a seizure, the exact cause of these discharges in humans remains less certain. There are three hypotheses. First, there could be loss of inhibition in a seizure focus. In principle, a decrease in the effectiveness of inhibitory postsynaptic potentials (ipsp) would allow for PDS formation and propagation. As a result of experimental studies, such disinhibition has long been advocated as a primary cause of epilepsy. Many convulsant agents used to study epilepsy, such as penicillin, picrotoxin, and bicuculline, have been shown to diminish GABA-mediated inhibition. As this occurs PDS discharges emerge. Additional support for this hypothesis comes from immunohistochemical studies that have found a loss of GABAergic neurons and terminals in chronic experimental seizure foci.

Second, large pyramidal neurons themselves may become damaged. Morphological changes have been found in dendrites of pyramidal neurons in seizure foci of neocortex and hippocampus. Initially they become swollen and distorted. With time there is atrophy and shrinking. These changes may make them more prone to abnormal burst firing.

The third hypothesis addresses the issue of timing. What causes a seizure to occur at any particular moment? It is thought that afferent excitatory circuits from the thalamus or distant areas of cortex may play a role in initiating seizure discharges.

A well-timed volley of excitatory activity may serve to synchronize a population of cortical neurons into a burst epileptic discharge, perhaps much like a tendon jerk causes a synchronized discharge of spinal motor neurons and the reflex contraction of muscle. For example, certain patients with epilepsy are abnormally sensitive to photic stimulation and will have a seizure when they are confronted by flashing or patterned light. This phenomenon is called reflex epilepsy. By contrast, some patients have seizures only during sleep. In this case it is thought that the removal of the highly asynchronous activity present in waking cortex allows the intrinsic synchrony of the seizure focus to take over and capture normal follower neurons into abnormal activity. Other patients with epilepsy commonly have seizures from a lack of normal sleep, or as a result of minor changes in salt and water balance as occurs with menstruation. How these factors trigger discharges in a seizure focus in humans is unknown.

FUNCTIONAL ANATOMY OF EPILEPSY

Neocortical Seizures

Focal seizures cause symptoms by spreading through the brain and disrupting normal function and by passing through motor pathways in brainstem and spinal cord to activate motoneurons and muscles, thereby causing convulsions. During interictal spikes there are no symptoms since the seizure process remains tightly contained within a small focus as described earlier (Fig. 12–6). When a full-blown seizure occurs, the focus becomes much larger as the local inhibitory surround breaks down. A large number of pyramidal neurons in layers II–III and V–VI then fire synchronously into distant sites, either in other cortical areas or in subcortical regions. The site of distant projections is not random; rather, the amount of seizure activity in distant synaptic fields reflects the strength of the anatomic connection with

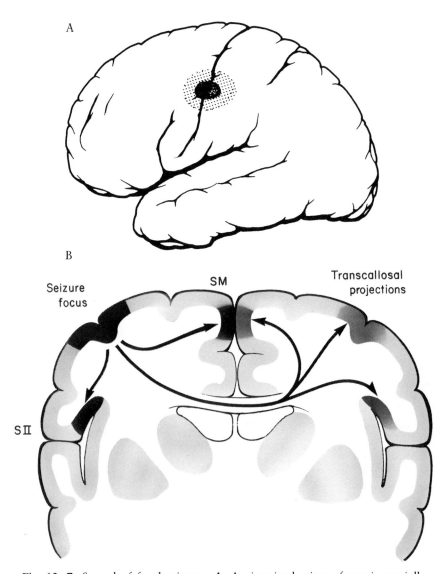

Fig. 12–7. Spread of focal seizures. **A.** An interictal seizure focus is spatially contained (see Fig. 12–6) in the hand area of the sensorimotor cortex. **B.** Cortical spread of a seizure occurs through specific pathways, here from primary sensorimotor cortex to supplementary motor cortex (SM), to secondary sensory cortex (SII) and to the homotopic sites transcallosal to the focus. **C.** (next page) Subcortical spread occurs to first order (solid line) and polysynaptic sites (broken line). Note that activity can be projected back into the seizure focus from distant sites. 1, Caudate; 2, putamen; 3, globus pallidus; 4, ventral lateral and anterior thalamus; 5, medial thalamus; 6, intralaminar nuclei; 7, midbrain tectum; 8, subthalamic nucleus; 9, parvocellular; and 10, magnocellular red nucleus; 11, pontine nuclei; 12, cerebellar nuclei; and 13, cortex. Only ipsilateral pathways are emphasized but a direct contralateral projection from a sensorimotor seizure focus to caudate/putamen would also play a role in the functional anatomy of seizure spread.

C

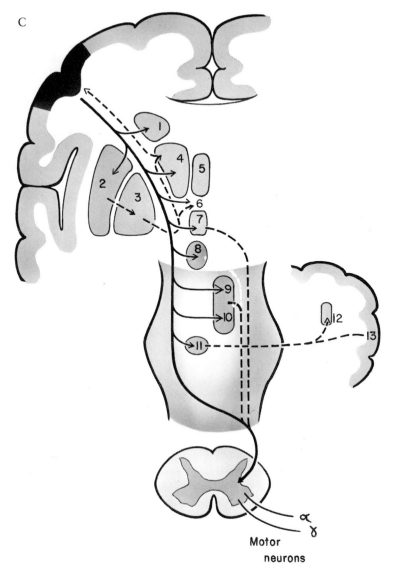

Motor
neurons

the primary focus. Distant sites connected to the focus seem to behave in an all or none fashion. That is, once a focal seizure begins there is rapid, full, and complete projection into synaptically coupled sites in thalamic, extrapyramidal, midbrain, and spinal cord circuits rather than a slow sequential traverse through these sites (Fig. 12–7). The reason for this is that each cortical point sufficiently large to constitute a seizure focus contains projection neurons to all these areas and all fire in unison. In the motor system this results in a crude and stereotyped jerking of muscles (usually flexion in the upper extremity and extension in the lower) in marked contrast to the case of smooth, delicate physiological movements. The particular muscles activated in any one patient depend on the somatotopic site of the focus in the cortex and on the capture of local and long circuits. Usually each patient has the same seizure manifestations on each separate occasion. Seizure foci in sensory cortex cause brief attacks of crude, elementary sensory symptoms such as tingling in a hand, or flashing lights in a homonymous visual field.

During a strong focal seizure other cortical fields become induced by the focus to fire subcortically, increasing ipsilateral then bilateral epileptic projection into spinal cord. This sequence can occur quite rapidly, a condition classified as a focal seizure with secondary generalization. The spread can also occur quite slowly, with the progression from hand to face or leg, and then to contralateral musculature taking up to a minute or longer. This is called the Jacksonian march, after Hughlings Jackson, who first described it in 1876. Exact pathophysiologic mechanisms of spread in this situation are unknown. The neocortex is physiologically and anatomically organized to maintain homotopic boundaries such as the separation of individual fingers from each other and from the face. A Jacksonian march breaks through these boundaries and spreads contiguously across cortex. Local cortical as well as reciprocal corticothalamic circuits probably play a role in this process.

Generalized seizures and Jacksonian seizures often occur secondarily in patients after many years of restricted focal seizures. It is thought that each focal seizure process causes a minor but permanent change in excitability within seizure pathways. Over time the size, distribution, and ease of spread within these seizure pathways increase. A mild focal seizure process ultimately "learns" to spread quickly and widely through brain circuits. This phenomenon can be reproduced quite easily using electrical seizures in animals and is called "kindling." Electrical stimulation in the limbic system is the most effective means for causing kindling. A single, brief stimulus (30–60 Hz; 1–10 seconds) that initiates a local afterdischarge at first causes no behavioral manifestations. When the same stimulus is repeated once a day the afterdischarge gradually becomes longer, spreads to other limbic areas, and eventually (after 20–70 days) causes the animals to have motor convulsions. At this point a permanent change has occurred in the seizure pathways. For example, animals given several months' rest following kindling will have a full motor convulsion when restimulated. There are probably many mechanisms underlying this phenomena, including transynaptic changes in distant sites. For example, if the primary stimulus site— the focus—is removed from fully kindled animals, stimulation in distant sites will also cause the motor convulsion. This phenomenon is called "transference" and is thought to underlie the creation of secondary or "mirror" seizure foci. Whereas these events can be produced quite readily in amphibians and lower mammals, not all of the phenomena are fully manifest in primates. For example, electrical recordings from neurons in a transcallosal homotopic "mirror" focus in monkey have found that epileptic discharges are all driven from the primary focus and do not originate independently. In addition, when a pathological seizure focus is removed surgically from a patient with epilepsy the seizures stop. Other distant sites do not continue or emerge as in lower mammals.

Limbic system

The clinical consequences of seizures in the hippocampus and the amygdala are quite different from those with focal neocortical seizures. Instead of causing stereotyped jerking of muscles or primary sensory sensations, limbic system seizures cause complex experiential phenomena or changes in behavior. Much of our knowledge in this area has come from studies of patients with intractable epilepsy who have had recording electrodes inserted into deep limbic structures for diagnostic studies prior to surgery. These studies have indicated that unilateral discharges can be associated with brief emotional states, such as fear or shame, or can evoke brief fragments of memory, such as a visual scene from a past experience. For some patients these are quite specific and recur exactly the same way each time. Other patients are unable to give precise descriptions but recognize the experience as an abnormal mental or emotional state, such as an intense feeling of familiarity (*déjà vu*, already seen) or dissociation from the environment (*jamais vu*, never seen).

When a focal limbic seizure spreads to contralateral limbic cortex and bilaterally through subcortical circuits (septum, midline thalamus, nucleus accumbens, substantia nigra, and hypothalamus), patients lose conscious contact with the environment. Such patients commonly show a blank stare or an expression of fear. They fail to respond to conversation and often exhibit stereotyped automatisms, such as lip smacking, chewing, swallowing, and fumbling with clothes. This stage lasts 30–60 seconds and is followed by a brief period of confusion. The patient forms no memory during this "spell" and often has no awareness of having had a seizure. The patient gradually reorients to his circumstances and then carries on in a normal manner. Often such spells are very brief, only a few seconds of time are lost, forming brief holes in the stream of consciousness. Naive observers often do not recognize such abnormal behavior, or consider it to be part of the patient's personality or just an odd mannerism.

There is some evidence suggesting that long-term limbic system seizures have a determinant effect on interictal behavior. Initially, some observers concluded that these seizures could be a cause of schizophrenia. More recently, detailed psychological studies suggest that an accentuation of certain personality traits occurs, such as religiosity, circumstantiality, hu-

morless sobriety, and hyposexuality. The appearance of these interictal behavioral phenomena is thought to correlate with the chronicity of the limbic seizure focus.

Generalized seizures

The anatomic substrates involved in generalized seizures remain largely unknown. Chemicals that cause generalized convulsions when given systemically or intraventricularly in animals either interfere diffusely with GABAergic inhibition (bicuculline, penicillin, picrotoxin), or act through excitatory glutamergic synapses (kainic acid) or opiate receptors (β endorphin, enkephalin). However, at present there is no convincing evidence for abnormalities within these systems in patients with generalized epilepsy.

Early experimental work in generalized epilepsy suggested the existence of an anatomic system in upper brainstem and diencephalon that was responsible for generalized seizures. This was called the "centrencephalon" by Penfield and Jasper in the 1940s and was suggested as a functional system rather than an anatomic substrate with strict boundaries. In particular, it was discovered that low-frequency stimulation of deep midline, interlaminar, or reticular nuclei of the thalamus could reproduce the spike and wave abnormality seen in petit mal epilepsy. This suggested that seizures originating in such bilaterally diffusely projecting thalamic systems might cause generalized seizures. As these systems were known to play a role in mechanisms of arousal and consciousness, seizures originating or spreading into this centrencephalic system would explain loss of consciousness with these seizures. To date there has been no direct evidence supporting this hypothesis in humans. Stimulation of the midline thalamus in a few patients with a generalized seizure disorder failed to cause convulsive discharges. By contrast, medial frontal cor-

A

MODULATORY SYSTEMS   RECRUITING SYSTEMS

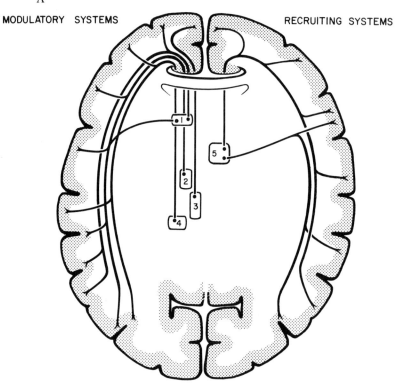

1. Basal nucleus – acetylcholine   5. Anterior, intralaminar and
2. A-10 mesolimbic – dopamine   midline thalamic nuclei
3. Raphe nuclei – serotonin   • central medial, paracentral, central lateral
4. Locus coeruleus –noradrenergic   • reuniens
                                             • ventral anterior
                                             • ventral medial

B   SPIKE   WAVE

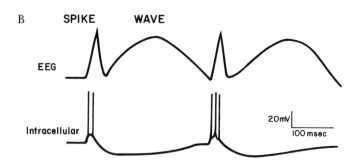

EEG

Intracellular

20mV
100 msec

                  1. Neuronal burst firing
                  2. Widespread and synchronous
        SPIKE   3. Anterior > posterior
                  4. (?) Thalamic exitatory recruitment
                  5. (?) Loss inhibitory modulation

                  1. Neuronal inhibition
        WAVE   2. Local inhibitory circuits
                  3. (?) Disynaptic thalamic inhibition

tex has a very low stimulus threshold for causing generalized seizures in these patients. This suggests that the anatomic substrates of generalized seizures may lie within corticothalamic systems, rather than purely in thalamus or cortex.

Further evidence in support of this hypothesis has come from studies in cats given systemic injections of large doses of penicillin as a convulsant. In this model brief spike-wave discharges occur diffusely over cortex while the animals exhibit staring and myoclonic facial twitches. Such discharges can be easily invoked by stimulation of the midline and anterior thalamic nuclei and striatum, but not by stimulation of specific sensory nuclei (medial geniculate, lateral geniculate, ventral posterior nucleus). The cortical spike discharge itself was found to be due to synchronized burst discharge of cortical neurons, while the wave was caused by summated inhibitory potentials elaborated within cortical inhibitory circuits (Fig. 12–8). This model is attractive since it suggests how thalamus and cortex interact in elaboration of diffuse spike-wave abnormalities. Both neocortex and limbic cortex could be involved. Finally, there are several diffusely projecting systems that may play a modulatory role in generalized epilepsy. Neurotransmitters involved in these systems (acetylcholine, dopamine, norepinephrine, serotonin) cause relatively prolonged shifts in membrane potential. Should one of these systems become abnormally active (or inactive), wide areas of brain might discharge synchronously.

METABOLIC AND PATHOLOGICAL CONSEQUENCE OF SEIZURES

Seizure discharges cause a marked increase in brain energy metabolism (Fig. 12–9). This is caused when large fluxes in Na^+, K^+, and Ca^{2+} stimulate ATP-dependent membrane enzymes. In addition, there is a marked increase in energy-dependent neurotransmitter metabolism consequent to release, reuptake, and synthesis. Brain has the capacity to maintain energy balance near normal during seizures as long as cerebral blood flow increases and blood oxygen remains normal. During focal seizures there is a 1.5- to 3-fold increase in glucose utilization in the focus and its pathways and a modest rise in tissue lactate with a fall in pH. Oxygen utilization is also increased and there is an oxidative shift in mitochondrial enzymes during seizures (Fig. 12–10). The result of these changes is to keep the levels of ATP essentially normal.

Recurrent focal seizures that last several hours in animals have been found to cause pathological changes in synapses. There is swelling of dendrites in the seizure focus and at synapses in distant pathways. Thalamic neurons projecting into the focus show marked dilation of axon terminals. There are several possible causes of these changes. The marked shift in cations during seizures results in an obligate, passive flux of water from the extracellular to the intracellular space. Second, there is a large increase in arachidonic acid dur-

Fig. 12–8. Functional anatomy of generalized seizures. **A.** Anatomic circuits responsible for causing generalized seizures are unknown. Since they begin suddenly and diffusely many investigators think that subcortical-cortical modulatory and/or recruiting systems may be involved. **B.** The spike and wave EEG pattern has been produced experimentally by giving large injections of penicillin to cats. In this model the spike discharge seems to reflect synchronous discharge of widely distributed cortical neurons driven from below. The wave reflects activity in local inhibitory circuits within the cortex.

ENERGY BALANCE IN BRAIN

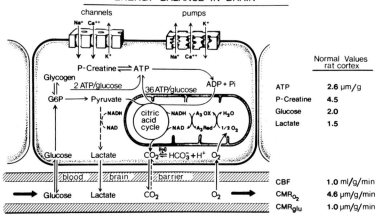

Normal Values rat cortex	
ATP	2.6 µm/g
P-Creatine	4.5
Glucose	2.0
Lactate	1.5

CBF	1.0 ml/g/min
CMR_{O_2}	4.6 µm/g/min
CMR_{glu}	1.0 µm/g/min

FOCAL SEIZURES

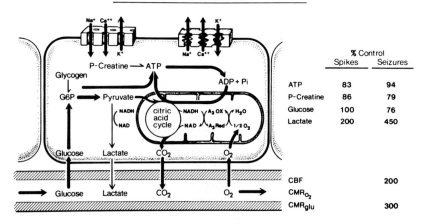

	% Control	
	Spikes	Seizures
ATP	83	94
P-Creatine	86	79
Glucose	100	76
Lactate	200	450

CBF		200
CMR_{O_2}		
CMR_{glu}		300

GENERALIZED SEIZURES - HYPOXEMIA

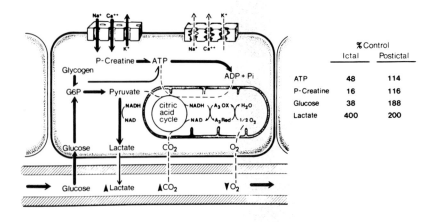

	% Control	
	Ictal	Postictal
ATP	48	114
P-Creatine	16	116
Glucose	38	188
Lactate	400	200

ing seizures, indicating an increase in turnover of membrane lipids. Disruption in membrane synthesis or recycling of membranes during neurotransmission may occur. Finally, excessive release and/or delayed reuptake of excitatory neurotransmitters such as glutamate and aspartate could have a direct toxic effect at postsynaptic sites on dendrites and cause them to swell. One consequence of all these actions seems to be a predilection for pathological changes in local interneurons, probably since they receive both afferent and recurrent excitatory input. Destruction and loss of inhibitory interneurons are thought to be one mechanism whereby seizures become stronger over long periods of time.

Generalized convulsive seizures interrupt ventilation and cause hypoxemia, CO_2 retention, and severe systemic acidosis. Oxygen deficiency in the face of severe metabolic demands results in depletion of brain energy metabolites during generalized seizures. Following the cessation of convulsions, hyperventilation rapidly corrects blood gases and brain energy metabolites return to normal or even become slightly increased during the postictal phase. The latter finding in experimental animals suggests that the postictal state in humans is not a result of metabolic exhaustion. Rather, it is thought that neurological abnormalities in this period are a reflection of synaptic dysfunction, but direct evidence is lacking.

Generalized seizures that recur rapidly without the resumption of consciousness are called *status epilepticus*. In addition to marked disruption of brain energy metabolism, there are often superimposed pathophysiological insults from systemic hypoxemia, acidosis, and hyperthermia. Hypoglycemia and hypotension can result as well. All these changes add further metabolic insult to the brain, resulting in widespread neuronal damage in neocortex, hippocampus, cerebellum, and scattered areas in the thalamus. Status epilepticus carries a high incidence of morbidity and mortality if patients are not treated promptly.

Fig. 12–9. Energy balance in brain is shown in the normal state, inside a seizure focus, and in cortex during a generalized convulsion. By comparing to the normal state (upper figure), focal seizures (middle figure) cause a marked increase in glucose and oxygen consumption (heavy lines). This occurs when the seizure causes a shift in ions that stimulate membrane pumps, leading to a breakdown in ATP to ADP and Pi. These metabolites greatly stimulate glycolytic and mitochondrial enzymes to synthesize more ATP, thus using more glucose and oxygen and producing more lactate and CO_2. The rise in these products causes local vasodilation (this is called metabolic autoregulation) and blood flow increases. As long as blood oxygen tension remains normal the brain energy state remains near normal. When generalized seizures occur and ventilation is interrupted, then blood oxygen falls. In this state a profound depletion of energy substrates occurs along with a lactic acidosis. Energy balance is restored after a single generalized convulsion, but if status epilepticus occurs, energy depletion, acidosis, and ion and water shifts cause permanent damage.

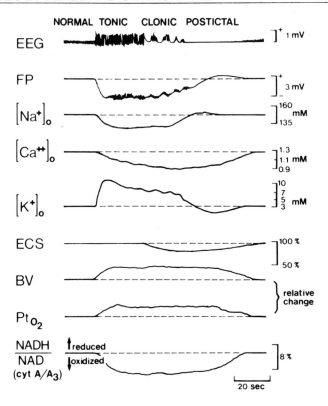

Fig. 12–10. Changes in cortical metabolism with seizures. Coincident with discharges on the EEG there is a drop in the cortical DC field potential (FP). Neurons release potassium into the extracellular space (fifth trace) and sodium and calcium (third and fourth traces) fall. Some studies indicate a drop in extracellular volume with strong seizures (ECS, extracellular space, sixth trace), suggesting movement of water intracellularly. There is a prompt increase in blood flow to the focus with seizures (reflected here as blood volume, BV, seventh trace) with increase delivery of oxygen (increased tissue oxygen tension, Pt_{O_2}) and an oxidative shift in mitochondrial enzymes as metabolism accelerates to provide ATP for cation pumping (see Figs. 12–5, and 12–9).

GENERAL REFERENCES

Delgado-Escueta, A. V., C. G., Wasterlain, D. M. Treiman, and R. J. Porter. *Status Epilepticus, Mechanisms of Brain Damage and Treatment.* New York, Raven Press, 1983.

Glaser, G. H., J. K. Penry, and D. M. Woodbury (eds.). *Antiepileptic Drugs, Mechanisms of Action.* New York, Raven Press, 1980.

Gloor, P. Generalized epilepsy with spike-and-wave discharge: A reinterpretation of its electrographic and clinical manifestations. *Epilepsia* 20:571–88, 1978.

Laidlaw, J., and A. Richens. *A Textbook of Epilepsy.* New York, Churchill Livingstone, 1976.

Prince, D. A. Neurophysiology of epilepsy. *Ann. Rev. Neurosci.* 1:395–415, 1978.

Schwartzkroin, P. A., and A. R. Wyler. Mechanisms underlying epileptiform burst discharge. *Ann. Neurol.* 7:95–107, 1979.

Ward, A. A., J. K. Penry, and D. Purpura (eds.). *Epilepsy.* New York, Raven Press, 1983.

13.

Aging and Dementia

LEONARD BERG

Students of the human brain and of human behavior must attend to issues of the intellectual, adaptive, and integrative behaviors that distinguish us from other species. Dementia, a clinical syndrome that represents the loss of those behaviors, is at once a fruitful area for research in neuroscience and a public health problem of enormous importance. There is a linkage with the neurobiology of aging, since the incidence of dementia increases dramatically with age from the sixth decade onward, and since aging itself implies gradual erosion of the vigor and adaptive capabilities of cell, tissue, organ, and total organism.

IMPLICATIONS OF "THE GRAYING OF AMERICA"

The elderly are increasing, both in absolute and in relative numbers. At present, persons over age 65 constitute 11%–12% of the population in the United States. There are approximately 26 million persons in that age group, about 10% of whom are demented. Those over age 75 constitute the most rapidly growing segment of our population and also represent the age group with the highest prevalence of dementia, 20%–25%. It is estimated that the 1982 national budget for the care of persons in nursing homes was $21 billion and that more than half of the nursing home residents were there because of dementia. The current national cost of nursing home maintenance of demented persons is therefore well over $10 billion!

Consider the national prospects for the year 2030. Estimates from the census bureau predict that 17% of the population, or 51 million persons, will be over age 65. More than five million elderly will be demented (at least twice the present numbers) if current trends continue. Alzheimer's disease, the principal cause of the syndrome of dementia, has been called "the disease of the century."

THE WEALTH OF HUMAN BEHAVIOR

Both survival and quality of life depend on sets of integrative functions that build on the simpler behaviors of attention, perception, recognition, learning, memory, and association. The term *integrative* is used not only to mean the synthesis of parts to make a whole, but also to imply that the linking of separate functions of the brain results in new, more elaborate functions, not mere combinations of simple elements.

These integrative functions include pursuit of biological needs, language, emotion, curiosity, and pursuit of knowledge. There are also the goal-directed behaviors of abstraction, calculation, planning skilled actions, vigilance, judgment, creativity, and appropriate inhibition. Effective adaptive techniques are essential, as is the capacity to persevere and maintain organization under stress.

Unfortunately, there is an enormous gap between recognition of the importance of these intellectual and integrative behaviors and understanding the underlying human neurophysiology. In many ways we are not much farther along the road to understanding the relationship of mind and brain than was Hippocrates 2,300 years ago when he recognized that, "with the brain we think, we reason, and we see and hear, and recognize good and bad, and we rave and become alienated."

We assume, with reasonable evidence, that the cerebral cortex plays the dominant role in the synthesis and integration of human behavior, although there is still much to be learned about the contribution of various subcortical regions to behavior. Studies of the results of injury or focal disease of the brain have told us that impairment of integrative functions and emotion occurs with lesions of the frontal lobes and that loss of memory results from destruction of both medial temporal lobes. The enormous difficulties in understanding the complexities of the full range of human intellectual and integrative functions have led current-day neurobiologists to isolate and study somewhat "simpler" behaviors, such as perception, learning, and memory. These psychological processes were once left largely to psychologists, who, of necessity, often viewed the nervous system simply as a "black box."

EXPERIMENTAL APPROACHES TO THE NEUROBIOLOGY OF MEMORY

It was once thought that brain events responsible for long-term memory were represented by continuous activity in reverberating neuronal circuits. However, deep general anesthesia halts neuronal electrical activity without abolishing stored memories. On the other hand, short-term memory, with a duration of seconds to 1 minute, might be explained by continual neuronal activity, such as excitatory feedback connections. There have been attempts to discover neurophysiological changes of longer duration that might help to explain memory storage lasting longer than a few minutes. Following brief trains of high-frequency stimulation delivered via monosynaptic pathways into the mammalian hippocampus, the amplitude of evoked potentials is increased for several hours or days. This phenomenon, known as long-term potentiation, is being studied as one example of long-lasting changes in neuronal physiology that may have a bearing on memory.

In studies of the simpler nervous system of the snail, *Aplysia,* Kandel and his associates have demonstrated that basic forms of learning (habituation, sensitization, and classical conditioning) can be induced in the gill withdrawal reflex and last for days to weeks. Changes in the synaptic efficiency of certain specific neurons are responsible. The mechanisms responsible include alterations in membrane function, such as changes in potassium ion currents, altered influx of calcium ions, and phosphorylation of specific protein kinases responsible for closing potassium ion channels. Serotonin has been demonstrated to participate in some of these processes.

In contrast to these approaches based on synaptic efficiency there is the demonstration of the proliferation of dendrites and synapses that accompanies the learning of birdsong each year in the canary. Proliferation of the dendritic arborization in the cerebral nuclei responsible for bird-song has been demonstrated during spring when the song is learned, followed by loss of dendritic arborization and shrinkage of the nuclei in the fall. In the canary, new neurons also proliferate during that learning process, but mammalian brains do not have that luxury!

Even though there have been these demonstrations of striking changes in neuronal connectivity and in synaptic efficiency that can be correlated with elementary learning and memory, our understanding of the neurobiology underlying human integrative behavior is only primitive.

POPULAR MISCONCEPTIONS ABOUT THE ELDERLY

Prejudice toward the elderly and failure to study their problems have led to many misconceptions. There is the notion that older people are usually feebleminded, irritable, depressed, rigid, apathetic, and asexual. A corollary follows that serious mental deterioration in the elderly ("senility") is "just due to old age." Furthermore, one hears that both normal aging and senility result from "hardening of the arteries" or loss of blood supply to the brain. Pessimism and misinformation promote the propositions that dementia is always progressive and irreversible, and that irreversible brain disease is present when computed tomography demonstrates shrinkage of the brain.

These misconceptions will be addressed in successive sections of this chapter. Here we point out that most of the elderly (about 90% of those over age 65 and about 75% of those over age 75) are not demented. Most of them are not depressed. Major impairment of intellect in the elderly results from disease, not "just aging." True, many abilities decline with normal aging, but the elderly can usually compensate. They vary more in physio-

logical measures, and they tolerate stress less well than do their younger cohorts.

There are distinctive changes in the structure, function, chemistry, and pharmacology of the aging brain. These should be recognized in order to provide an approach to delirium and dementia, both of which occur much more frequently in the elderly than in young adults. (Note that the very young and the elderly are both predisposed to the development of delirium under metabolic stress.) A caution to be scrupulously observed in all aging research is that subjects must be screened carefully to be certain one is studying the effects of aging, not those of superimposed disease.

NORMAL AGING

Clinical Neurology

There still are only inadequate normative data on changes in structure and function of the human nervous system with aging, and on the clinical reflections of those changes. Confounding that study is the fact that many elderly are known to have hypertension, diabetes mellitus, peripheral atherosclerosis, and aging changes in muscles, tendons, and joints, all of which may influence the testing of neurological function. For those reasons and others, one still finds divergent opinions on the prevalence of neurological abnormalities in the healthy elderly. Nevertheless there is agreement that with increasing age beyond 65, progressively greater percentages of the apparently healthy elderly show neurological signs considered abnormal in younger adults.

Motor signs of aging include stooped posture, slowness of movement, shortening of stride, and decreased swing of the arms. Muscle tone is often mildly increased. These motor signs resemble mild parkinsonism, yet most of the individuals described here, if studied post mortem, will be found to have normal-appearing neurons in the substantia nigra. Declining function of the dopaminergic system has been postulated.

Impairment of tandem gait and mild impairment of coordination are often present. Healthy 80-year-old subjects often cannot stand on one leg alone and may therefore report trouble pulling on their pants. Many of the elderly have wasting of the small muscles in the hands but strength remains preserved.

Tendon reflexes are well preserved in the elderly, except that the ankle jerks may be weak or absent. Some neurologists contend that aging is an insufficient cause for loss of the ankle jerks and that their loss reflects an unrecognized peripheral neuropathy. Plantar reflexes remain normal in uncomplicated aging, but several "pathological" or "primitive" reflexes may appear. The incidence of these abnormal reflexes in the healthy elderly is still subject to debate, but they include the snout and palmomental reflexes.

Among the sensory functions, perception of vibration in the distal lower extremities has most consistently been found impaired with advancing age in the apparent absence of disease. There are conflicting reports on impairment or preservation of sensation to touch and pin.

Diminution in the special senses is uniformly found with normal aging. Mild reductions in corrected visual acuity are found even when cataracts and retinal disease are absent. Visual accommodation is regularly impaired and the frequency at which flicker fusion occurs is reduced. A particularly good example of the general principle of aging changes (mild impairment of baseline function and greater impairment under stress) is the effect on hearing. There is a mild decline in auditory acuity for pure sounds with advancing age, but the more complex the task (e.g., divided attention, dichotic listening, masked or filtered sounds), the greater the

impairment in aging. Decreases in the senses of taste and smell have also been documented. Additional changes in cranial nerve function in the healthy elderly include slowing of the pupillary reflexes, loss of upgaze and ocular convergence, slowing of smooth ocular pursuit, and appearance of saccadic (cogwheel) tracking.

Psychometric testing in healthy aging

Mental functions also change with aging but fundamental problems remain in their interpretation. The importance of this issue is that clinicians must determine whether the behavior of an elderly person represents normal aging or the early stage of a dementing illness. For example, in comparing the psychometric performance of healthy older and young adults one finds major unresolved issues of methodology that still lead to discrepant opinions in the literature. Most current neuropsychological tests are based on the performances of younger adults. Active older persons who appear healthy annd function well in the community may score in the abnormal range on psychometric tests standardized on younger adults. They may be "impaired" on neuropsychological tasks and yet perform daily activities well that require the same abilities. Even when norms for the elderly are available, it is often unclear whether the subjects used in the normative sample were truly healthy or whether some had chronic diseases. It has become increasingly clear that the presence of a wide variety of chronic illnesses may affect intellectual function.

Most age-corrected norms have been derived from cross-sectional studies (comparing young adults with older adults) and therefore may be cohort specific. It is not known whether age norms based on subjects who were 70 or 80 years old in 1960 are applicable to the study of 70- or 80-year-old persons at present. These groups differ in educational achievement and health status and may well differ in other measures, such as motivation, methods of problem solving, and response to testing situations. Data derived from longitudinal studies of middle-aged and older adults are subject to other criticisms, such as the likelihood of selective subject dropout.

Other issues in the interpretation of psychometric test results on older adults include concerns regarding greater anxiety, motivational differences, greater caution, lower expectations of performance, greater susceptibility to fatigue, aging changes in sensory and motor functions, and prolonged reaction times. Studies of age differences have almost always been conducted in the context of a specific problem or in the setting of a specific experimental model and therefore cannot be generalized.

Short-term memory is a temporary storage system ("scratch-pad memory") that has the capacity to retain about five to seven "chunks" of information for about 1 minute. These chunks must be rehearsed and processed before they are committed to long-term memory. Many experiments have suggested that age differences in short-term memory are minimal, but even that general conclusion is still being challenged. Older subjects are especially penalized in divided-attention situations that give less opportunity for rehearsal and processing. Furthermore the elderly have disproportionate difficulty when the material to be stored must be reorganized. Therefore, to the extent that the experimental (or real-life) situation requires manipulation and reorganization of the input, short-term memory deficits may contribute to poorer performance of older subjects on some tasks.

Most workers have consistently found a deficit of long-term memory in the elderly, whether tested by verbal or nonverbal means. Age differences are found even under self-paced conditions when speed is not a consideration. Clearly, rate is not the only factor limiting the performance of the aged. It appears that the processes of transfer into and retrieval from long-term memory are both impaired. On the other hand, there is no good evidence that older subjects exhibit more rapid loss of material from storage, either through decay or interference.

With respect to intellectual function other than memory, there is still reason to ask the question, Does intelligence decline in old age? It appears from both cross-sectional and longitudinal studies that persons who perform well when young will also perform well when old. Most authors conclude that a modest decline in intellectual ability is clearly a part of the aging process, but these declines may start later in life than many thought and may be small in magnitude. They may also include fewer of the many functions of which intelligence is composed. For instance, there is an age-related decline in "fluid" intelligence, which is concerned with new problem solving, adaptation to new situations, and the discrimination and identification of stimuli and appropriate responses. "Crystallized" intelligence depends on learned information and skills, such as vocabulary, and tends to show very little change throughout adulthood.

Despite its shortcomings, most clinicians still view the Wechsler Adult Intelligence Scale (WAIS) as a good measure of intelligence for use with the aged. There are eleven subtests: six verbal and five performance (Table 13–1). Scores on the

Table 13–1. The Wechsler Adult Intelligence Scale[1]

Verbal	Performance
Information	Digit symbol
Comprehension	Picture completion
Arithmetic	Block design
Similarities	Picture arrangement
Digit span	Object assembly
Vocabulary	

[1]Scores on the performance subtests tend to decline with aging and with dementia to a greater extent than do the verbal subtests.

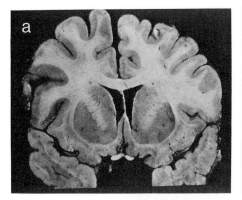
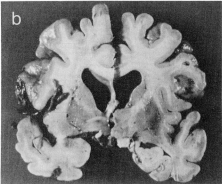
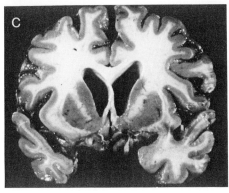

Fig. 13–1. Coronal sections of the brain in (**A**) healthy young adult, (**B**) healthy old adult, and (**C**) old adult with Alzheimer's disease. In both healthy aging and Alzheimer's disease there is shrinkage of the brain with dilatation of the ventricles, cortical sulci, and Sylvian fissures (compare Fig. 13–3). Whereas there is greater atrophy of the brain in a group of elderly subjects with Alzheimer's disease than in a group of healthy elderly persons, there is considerable overlap. The appearance of more severe atrophy in the brain of this nondemented aged individual (**B**) as compared with the specimen from a person with Alzheimer's disease (**C**) emphasizes the point that gross atrophy of the brain cannot be equated with dementia. (Specimens courtesy of Keith H. Fulling, M.D.)

six verbal tasks may be combined to form a verbal score from which a verbal intelligence quotient (IQ) can be derived by reference to an age-specific table. The same can be done for the performance subtests. Verbal and performance scores can be combined for a score from which a full-scale IQ is derived. WAIS verbal scores "hold" with aging but performance scores "don't hold."

Drawbacks of the WAIS include the fact that much time, effort, and attention are required of both the examiner and subject. Training is necessary for administration, scoring, and interpretation.

Changes in brain structure

Both in humans and in lower animals the brain shrinks with advancing age (Fig. 13–1). Cortex and white matter decrease in volume. Most likely there is some loss of neurons from the cortex with healthy aging, but quantification of the loss is still debatable. One must recognize the enormous technical difficulties of obtaining valid counts of the multitudes of neurons in human cortex. Some investigators remain skeptical of even the most advanced cell-counting techniques. With that reservation, there appear to be mild decreases in the number of cortical neurons with advancing age, to a degree that varies from region to region.

Aged neurons shrink in volume and pyramidal neurons become rounded. An earlier concept held that most aging neurons had shrinking dendritic trees, but more recent observations on human and lower animal brains indicate that expansion of the dendritic tree continues through middle and late adult life. This plasticity of the neuron well beyond the early life developmental period is an important principle. Note that dendritic proliferation has been reported to be increased by sensory stimulation and enriched environments. Ramón y Cajal predicted these discoveries in 1911 when he wrote: "One might suppose that cerebral exercise, since it cannot produce new cells, carries further than usual protoplasmic expansions and neural collaterals forcing the establishment of new and more extended intercortical connections."

The study of dendritic morphology depends at present on the Golgi technique of histology, a procedure that does not lend itself well to quantitative analysis. This method of neuronal impregnation discloses only a few of the many neurons in the cortex. Variations of Golgi methods lead to differing results in the number of dendritic branches and dendritic spines that are visualized. It is not surprising, therefore, that discrepant conclusions are available regarding the dendritic tree in normal aging and in disease. It appears that aging cortex contains some neurons in dendritic regression and some with still proliferating dendritic arborizations. The question of the relative numbers of each is still under investigation.

Old neurons accumulate "aging pig-ment" or lipofuscin. Despite many observations in lower animals and humans, it is still not clear whether lipofuscin represents a normal aging phenomenon, a reaction to stress and/or injury, or a protective mechanism. Neurons of the inferior olive, which accumulate great quantities of lipofuscin, do not decline in number even in advanced age. The next section of this chapter presents evidence that lipofuscin-laden neurons maintain a healthy response to stimulation.

Occasional cortical neurons in the brains of most healthy elderly people accumulate abnormal cytoplasmic inclusions, such as neurofibrillary tangles and granulovacuolar organelles. Sparse numbers of neuritic (senile) plaques also appear in the aging cortex. It must be emphasized that the tangles and plaques, which are the histological hallmark of Alzheimer's disease and which are found in profusion in that disorder, are found only in small numbers in the cortex (mainly the hippocampus) of the healthy elderly.

Other changes in the healthy elderly brain include fibrous astrocytic gliosis and a reported decrease in the extracellular space, but this latter change is reported from only limited observations on the extracellular space in aged lower animals.

The aged human brain also is marked by atherosclerosis of its major arteries, but present evidence is that atherosclerosis does not affect the brain unless infarction results. The brains of some healthy elderly persons, however, are found to contain a few small infarcts. These are clearly not the result of healthy aging, but rather are the effect of atherosclerotic or hypertensive changes in the brain's blood vessels. Irregularities, kinking, coiling, and complex distortions of the microvasculature can be seen, but it has not been possible to quantify these changes or to determine with certainty their relationship to disease as opposed to healthy aging. Further research is appropriate because of the obvious implications of microvascular changes for the nutrition and function of the adjacent brain parenchyma.

The physiology of the aging brain

Little is known of the effects of healthy aging on human cerebral physiology. Increased reaction times and increased latency of sensory evoked potentials indicate slowed CNS conduction times and perhaps other slowings in "central processing." Amplitudes of somatosensory evoked potentials are often increased, a finding which can be interpreted as compensatory or as an effect of loss of inhibitory influence. The significance of the mild slowing of EEG alpha activity with advancing age is not known. Increased beta activity and anterior temporal slow waves are found in EEGs of many healthy elderly individuals.

One valuable model is that of the cerebellar cortex in the aged rat. Purkinje cells decline in number and contain altered Nissl substance (rough endoplasmic reticulum), as judged by loss of its staining properties. In contrast to the Purkinje cells of young adult rats, these old neurons are better recognized by their lipofuscin than by the presence of Nissl substance. Some old Purkinje cells retain normal spontaneous firing rates, but others generate action potentials with abnormally long interspike intervals. Even those cells that have very slow spontaneous firing rates will respond normally to stimulatory volleys through climbing fibers derived from inferior olivary neurons. Volleys of impulses are conducted more slowly in the parallel fibers of the aged cerebellar cortex than in the young adult. Shrinkage of the dendritic arborization of the Purkinje cells, especially in the terminal branches, has been cited as partial explanation for declining abilities of the Purkinje cells to respond to stimulation by parallel-fiber volleys.

Older methods of estimating global and regional cerebral blood flow have indicated that there is a mild decline of that variable with aging. There has been disagreement on whether the decline is linear from early adulthood on, or whether it begins only in late adult life. It is clear that the decline is less evident the more carefully one chooses the elderly subjects to be free of disease. These problems of cerebral blood flow and metabolism in aging are just beginning to be addressed by positron emission transaxial tomography, from which more definitive conclusions may be available.

Chemical and pharmacological changes

There is still much to be learned about the chemistry of the aging brain, but one chemical change currently under scrutiny is the decline in activity of the cholinergic transmitter system, both in lower animals and in humans. This subject will be discussed later in this chapter.

Thus far there appears to be relative preservation of other neurotransmitter systems (catecholamine, dopamine, neuropeptides) in the aging brain, but data are still preliminary. Levels of brain monoamine oxidase activity appear to increase with aging.

There is only meager and conflicting evidence on whether the aging brain has altered receptor sensitivity to administered drugs. The well-known increased frequency of adverse drug effects on the elderly nervous system is largely explained by altered pharmacodynamics and pharmacokinetics with aging, in addition to the problems of multiple drug interactions.

Theories to explain neuronal aging

Putative causes of aging include complex interactions between intrinsic cellular genetic factors and extrinsic environmental agents. Since neurons are postmitotic cells that do not regenerate, certain considerations in other aging tissues are not applicable to aging neurons. These include changes in DNA synthesis and loss of proliferative capacity after a finite number of replications.

Among the postulated alterations programmed within the neuronal genome are age-related declines in DNA or RNA content per cell and loss of efficiency of DNA repair mechanisms for response to extrinsic insults. Some of these extrinsic factors are mutagens, such as toxins, irradiation, and viruses, as well as free radicals that accumulate as metabolic by-products. It has been suggested that impaired preservation of the genetic code would lead to errors in protein transcriptions and translations that might result in abnormal accumulation of proteins (neurofibrillary tangles) or to decreases in neurotransmitter enzyme activities, such as choline acetyltransferase. The list of possible mechanisms of neuronal aging also includes loss of trophic factors, altered immunological status, and changes in neuronoglial relationships, all of which may have both genetic and environmental bases.

DEMENTIA

The global loss of intellectual and integrative functions of the brain in an alert patient is termed *dementia*. This syndrome may be acute in onset and static, as after head injury, cerebral anoxia, or encephalitis. More often it is gradual in onset and progressive. It may be reversible, as with hypothyroidism, or irreversible (at present), as with Alzheimer's disease. Even when irreversible, dementia is treatable by palliative means, such as psychosocial support, attention to accompanying medical problems, and judicious trials of medication.

The term *delirium* refers to global impairment of intellectual function associated with impairment of consciousness or awareness of the environment. Delirium

Table 13–2. Imitators of dementia

Disorders of consciousness and attention: delirium, lethargy, stupor
Disorders of communication and language: mutism, aphasia
Sensory disorders: deafness, blindness, multimodal sensory deprivation
Mental retardation
Variation in intellectual performance resulting from social and/or cultural differences
Nonorganic psychiatric and psychological disorders: depression, schizophrenia, hysteria, boredom
Focal and multifocal brain dysfunction: aphasia, apraxia, agnosia, amnesia

tends to be acute in onset, fluctuating in degree, and often reversible. If not reversed, it may lead to dementia. Delirium is sometimes spoken of as confusional state or acute metabolic encephalopathy and is discussed further in Chapter 16. Both dementia and delirium can be subsumed under the general heading of organic mental disorder (psychiatric diagnostic terminology) or the useful term *brain failure,* which should evoke a response of appropriate investigation, differential diagnosis as to cause, and management. Brain failure is thus akin to heart failure and kidney failure. An apparently sudden onset or exacerbation of dementia occurs if metabolic stress superimposes a delirium upon a background of mild dementia.

It is well to remember that dementia, a global deterioration of intellectual function in an alert person, must be differentiated from many disorders (Table 13-2) with which it may be confused by the unwary. These may appear to represent progressive decline of intellectual function but careful clinical assessment will show their differences from dementia. (For instance, mental retardation is a nonprogressive failure of development of intellect dating to birth or infancy, not a loss of previously acquired intellect.)

While dementia can be considered as an accumulation of multiple focal cortical dysfunctions, it is important for the clinician and the neuroscientist to distinguish dementia, a generalized disorder of brain function, from disorders that reflect localized dysfunction of the brain. Some examples will be described briefly here: the syndrome of the frontal lobes, the syndrome of the dominant temporoparietal cortex, and the amnesic syndromes.

Frontal lobe lesions often cause personality changes, especially apathy, loss of initiative, neglect of personal cleanliness, loss of social inhibitions, and lack of insight. In contrast to dementing illnesses, however, frontal lobe lesions alone usually do not affect measured intelligence or memory.

Another syndrome that can be confused with dementia results from damage to the temporoparietal region of the dominant posterior hemisphere. These patients have fluent aphasia with poor comprehension, inability to read, write, or calculate, right-left disorientation, and difficulty naming fingers. These clinical features also occur with the diffuse cortical dysfunction of dementia. However, preservation of nonverbal memory and of spatial orientation helps to distinguish patients with this focal dominant hemisphere syndrome from those with dementia.

Amnesic syndromes result from damage to the medial temporal lobes (especially the hippocampus and amygdala) and/or diencephalic structures (dorsomedial thalamus and mamillary bodies) (Table 13-3). These patients have profound difficulty in learning new information and in remembering current everyday events, despite an intact immediate recall (digit span, for example) and normal intellectual capacities, such as the abilities to calculate, manipulate information, and form judgments. It is the preservation of these intellectual abilities that distinguishes amnesia from dementia, in which amnesia is accompanied by more widespread failure

Table 13-3. Differential diagnosis of amnesic syndromes

Bilateral medial temporal localization
Trauma
Herpes simplex encephalitis
Transient global amnesia (? ischemic)
Infarction from basilar or posterior cerebral artery occlusion

Midline-bilateral diencephalic localization
Trauma
Korsakoff's syndrome, usually secondary to thiamine deficiency in chronic alcoholics
Neoplasms around the third ventricle

of intellect. Two famous cases have been extensively studied and reported in the literature. "H.M." had the medial aspects of both temporal lobes removed to treat intractable epilepsy. "N.A." suffered an injury from a fencing foil to his dorsomedial thalamus. Both have severe permanent deficits in recent memory functions.

Amnesic patients usually have impaired memory for information acquired for a variable period of time before the onset of amnesia (retrograde amnesia). However, memory for information acquired in early life, such as social and language skills and general knowledge, is normal. A further point illustrating the complexity of memory function is that these amnesic patients retain the ability to learn and remember procedural skills.

Another state not to be confused with dementia is the mild decline in mental function of healthy aging. Forgetfulness, common at all ages, is most often not the result of disease. Much more often it results from factors such as inattention, poor motivation, distractability, and stimulus interference or "system overload."

Dementia is not part of normal aging. Although dementing syndromes and diseases are much more frequent in the elderly than they are in persons under the age of 60, dementia should be regarded at present as an age-related, not an age-induced disorder (See section on Reflections).

Table 13-4. Common causes of dementia [1]

Alzheimer's disease
Pick's disease
Huntington's disease
Parkinson's disease
Progressive supranuclear palsy
Spinocerebellar degenerations
Multiple sclerosis
Multi-infarct state
Infections: neurosyphilis, tuberculous or bacterial
   meningitis, cryptococcosis, acute virus encephali-
   tis, Jakob-Creutzfeldt disease, progressive multi-
   focal leukoencephalopathy
Intracranial neoplasms
Trauma, including subdural hematoma
Hydrocephalus
Metabolic disorders: hypothyroidism, vitamin B_{12}
   deficiency, renal dialysis
Toxic/nutritional disorders: alcoholism, chronic drug
   intoxication, malnutrition

[1] Since a complete list would include 100 or more disorders, those listed here represent the common causes and
illustrate the principle that dementia may result from many
categories of diseases, some confined to the nervous system
and some originating elsewhere with secondary effects of
the brain.

Causes of dementia

Alzheimer's disease is the prototype and the commonest cause of dementia, since it acounts for at least half of the instances of dementia in the elderly and contributes substantially to the dementia in another 15%–20%. Nevertheless, it is important to consider a long list of disorders that can lead to dementia. Some of these are found in Table 13-4.

Some authors have suggested a classification of dementias into cortical and subcortical varieties. The former, typified by Alzheimer's and Pick's diseases, cause marked mental changes, often with aphasia, apraxia, and visuospatial difficulties. Motor function and speed of responses are usually normal. By contrast, the "subcortical" dementias (Parkinson's and Huntington's diseases, hydrocephalus, some multi-infarct states) are characterized by preserved language and visuospatial orientation, but moderate impairment of motor functions, such as posture and gait, with slowness of thinking, verbal responses, and movements.

Other authorities reject the notion of two types of dementia (cortical vs. subcortical) and prefer the unitary concept of dementia alone, with a varying clinical spectrum depending on the number and degree of cortical dysfunctions (e.g., language) and on accompanying involvement of other neuronal systems, such as attentional and extrapyramidal mechanisms.

The most frequent dementing disorder after Alzheimer's disease is multi-infarct dementia, which, as its name implies, results from multiple small and/or large infarctions of the brain (Fig. 13–2). These occur at varying points in time and can be recognized by history and findings suggesting acute small or large focal cerebral lesions. Transient or persistent aphasia, dysarthria, dysphagia, visual field defects, hemiparesis or monoparesis, and emotional incontinence are common manifestations. The risk factors of hypertension, diabetes mellitus, and atherosclerosis are helpful in clinical identification. (Remember that "hardening of the arteries" does not cause dementia unless there is infarction of the brain.) The multi-infarct state only leads to dementia when sufficiently large volumes of brain have been destroyed, perhaps 50–100 ml. The question remains how much damage to which critical areas of the brain must occur in this multifocal disease before dementia results.

Alzheimer's disease

This is a disorder of unknown cause with specific abnormalities on histological examination of the brain and with profound effects on intellectual and other integrative functions. Although what we call Alzheimer's disease (AD) may prove to represent a group of heterogeneous disorders, it is still appropriate to view it as a single entity. The recent recognition that senile dementia is mainly the result of AD (senile dementia of the Alzheimer type) has rep-

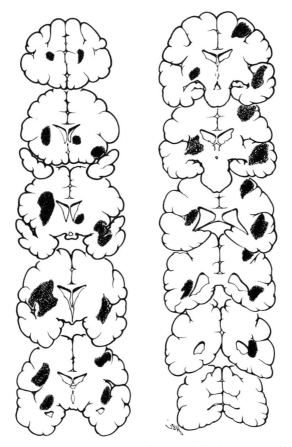

Fig. 13–2. Schematic representation of coronal brain sections from a patient with multi-infarct dementia. Regions of infarcted brain are finely cross-hatched. These gross lesions are often accompanied by many other infarctions too small to be seen grossly. The total volume of tissue infarcted approaches 100 ml. Such a patient has a history suggestive of multiple minor and major strokes, and step-wise progression of dementia. Signs of focal neurological dysfunction, abnormal gait, and dysarthria are evident.

resented a major step in understanding the problems of our aging population.

Clinical Picture. In the advanced stages, Alzheimer's disease leads to devastation of a human being from loss of the adaptive, integrative, and intellectual functions of the brain. Victims of the disease are eventually rendered totally helpless. However, the clinical picture in the early stages varies according to which of the many integrative behaviors are affected. The onset is often so subtle that it may be difficult to date and to describe, even by an observant witness, one of whom wrote: "Over the period that we worked together . . . I became gradually aware that the fine edge of his intellect was becoming dull. He was less clear in discussion and less quick to make the jump from a new piece of evidence to its possible significance. He spent more time over his work and achieved less. He tended also to become portentous and solemn about his subject. . . . The change was so slow as to be barely perceptible, and the signs vanished when I tried to pin them down. . . . The change was as yet mainly a loss of intellectual clarity and he remained himself, but a self that was subtly devitalized" (Anonymous. *Lancet* 1:1012, 1950; by permission of publisher).

Intellectual fatigue, impoverished language (before definite aphasia), and changes in mood or personality (e.g., depression, paranoia) may signal the onset. The illness begins only rarely with evidence of focal cortical dysfunction, such as aphasia, dressing apraxia, or spatial disorientation, when intellectual functions seem well preserved.

As the dementia progresses, defects become evident in memory, orientation, reasoning, judgment, and in the abilities to abstract, calculate, and use language. Routine activities may be handled reasonably well, but the patient fails at the task whenever new or altered principles are required. Patients tend to confabulate and to deny or hide their deficits. They may avoid answering routine questions or may respond with excited outbursts. Emotional changes such as depression, a fatuous euphoria, or a wide variety of changes in personality may dominate the clinical picture and may be the most distressing element. A common example is the angry accusation that others have stolen personal articles the patient has misplaced.

Primary physicians are often unaware of the development of dementia, especially in elderly patients. Early symptoms may often be overlooked by the family as well. A major problem is that mild changes in memory, learning, or judgment are difficult to identify with confidence, especially in the elderly. Notice how much more difficult it is to identify and to quantify changes in personality, behavior, and the other integrative functions mentioned. For all these reasons the early stages of AD may escape notice or may in error be interpreted as reactions to stress or to the common problems of aging, such as retirement or loss of jobs, friends, and relatives.

Social skills are retained by many patients with even more advanced Alzheimer's disease. Evidence of the disorder may not be apparent in ordinary encounters and on superficial interview, especially when support systems shield the patient from intellectual challenges.

Progressively, over months or a few years, the abilities to perform everyday duties and tasks are lost. Eventually there is deterioration of self-care. Some of the manifestations are slovenly appearance, neglect of hygiene, dressing with undergarments over outerwear, wandering into the cold without protection, getting lost, neglect of nutrition, and incontinence of urine and feces. A benign childlike behavior may develop with increasing dependence on the caretaker, punctuated by periodic restlessness and irritability. Primitive reflexes or frontal lobe release signs are frequently found. These include paratonia and the sucking, snout, rooting, and grasp reflexes. Only late in the disease does one find marked rigidity, seizures, myoclonus, dysphagia, or mutism.

The total clinical picture in dementia is influenced by the interactions of aging, other structural changes in the brain, metabolic disorder or disease elsewhere in the body, psychological reactions (both resulting from and independent of the dementia), and social problems. Fluctuations in the degree of disability in demented persons often depend on psychosocial or general medical factors. Therapeutic programs must include attention to depression, paranoia, inactivity, isolation, impaired hearing and sight, malnutrition, failure of other organ systems, and drug effects.

Psychometric Testing. On testing of patients with mild dementia there is general impairment on tasks of learning and memory, with only the span of immediate recall remaining intact. Defects appear in all stages of the memory process: encoding, storage, and retrieval. Tasks that require manipulation of information or of visuospatial relationships (performance subtests of the WAIS) may be particularly difficult for the mildly demented subject.

Impairment on the WAIS in dementia can be demonstrated most convincingly when the scores decline in a subject tested repeatedly over time. Methods have been proposed to assess impairment from a single WAIS. These include (1) a reduction in full-scale IQ from that predicted on the basis of past achievement in education and vocation; (2) a greater than normal spread between verbal and performance IQs; and (3) increased interest score variation with low scores on subtests (e.g., block design and digit symbol) considered to be particularly sensitive to brain dysfunction. However, questions arise repeatedly about the validity of the spread between verbal and performance IQs and the usefulness of comparing scores on "hold" and "don't hold" tests. Elderly depressed patients often give a pattern suggestive of dementia.

Psychological testing is properly used as an aid in clinical evaluation, not as a primary diagnostic instrument. Physicians unfamiliar with the testing procedures sometimes attribute unwarranted validity to them. Psychologists are likely to suggest the possibility (even the probability) of multiple interpretations.

Brain Structure. In persons who die of Alzheimer's disease under the age of 60, the brain is almost always atrophic when measured at autopsy or by computed tomography (CT) during life. However, normal aging leads to some atrophy of the brain over age 60. Neurologists recognize that one cannot diagnose brain atrophy of AD on CT of elderly patients, since the CT of a healthy elderly person and that of a patient with AD may well be identical in appearance. Recent quantitative studies of volumetric CT data suggest that there is more severe shrinkage of the brain in elderly subjects with AD, as evidenced by greater dilatation of the cerebral ventricles

and enlargement of the cerebral sulci and other subarachnoid spaces (Fig. 13–3, compare Fig. 13–1).

Loss of cortical neurons is probably one factor responsible for shrinkage of the brain in AD. With the caveat cited earlier regarding the counting of neurons, one notes reports of significant loss of larger cortical neurons (those over 90 μ^2 in cross section) in elderly subjects with AD compared with controls. Shrinkage of cell bodies of individual neurons and of their dendritic trees has also been observed and would contribute to loss of cortical volume.

Useful data on quantitative aspects of dendritic morphology in AD are still sparse because of the problems inherent to the Golgi technique discussed earlier. There are reports of diminished dendritic arborization that would imply failure of interneuronal communication and would help explain deterioration of cortical function.

The histological abnormalities of the cortex characteristic of AD are neurofibrillary tangles and neuritic (senile) plaques (Fig. 13–4). With silver stains the neurofibrillary tangles are seen as bundles of coarse argentophilic fibrils in the cytoplasm of neurons (Fig. 13–5, 13–6). They may fill the neuronal perikaryon, but even then one can detect healthy cytoplasmic organelles by electron microscopy. This technique also reveals the ultrastructure of the tangles, which are composed of paired filaments, each 10 nm in diameter, wound helically around each other with crossovers at 80-nm intervals. The term *paired helical filaments* is used to refer to these elements whose structure is unique to human neurons. Paried helical filaments (PHF) are found only in a limited group of disorders, including AD, Down's syndrome, postencephalitic parkinsonism, the parkinsonism-dementia complex on Guam, dementia of boxers (dementia pugilistica), and subacute sclerosing panencephalitis. A few neurons of most healthy elderly people contain paired helical filaments.

These abnormal filaments are proba-

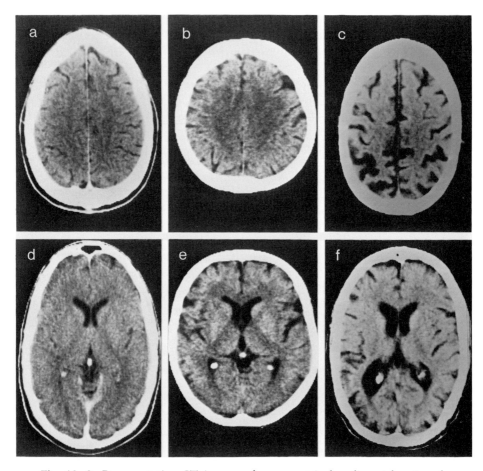

Fig. 13–3. Representative CT images of supraventricular slices (above) and midventricular-basal ganglial slices (below) from a healthy young adult (**A, D**), a healthy elderly adult (**B, E**), and an elderly AD patient (**C, F**). There is mild dilatation of the frontal horns of the ventricles and moderate dilatation of the subarachnoid spaces in this healthy elderly subject (**B, E**). These CT examples of atrophy are more marked in the elderly subject with Alzheimer's disease (**C, F**), but the CT cannot at present differentiate atrophy of aging from that of AD (compare Fig. 13–1). (CT scans courtesy of Mokhtar Gado, M.D.)

bly related to normal neuronal neurofilaments, that class of structural proteins known as intermediate filaments. Since neurofilaments act as a framework for intracellular space within axons, dendrites, and perikarya, they should be capable of multiple interactions with other cytoplasmic structures.

A remarkable insolubility has impeded understanding of the chemistry of paired helical filaments, but by immunochemical staining and preliminary chemical analyses they appear to contain many of the same protein components as normal neurofilaments. Neurofibrillary tangles have been produced in experimental animals by mitotic spindle inhibitors (colchicine, vincristine) and by aluminum salts, but the ultrastructure of human paired helical filaments has not been duplicated.

Fully developed neuritic (senile) plaques are found in the cortical neuropil and

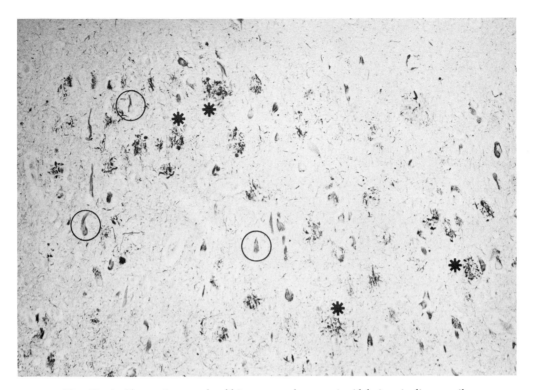

Fig. 13–4. Photomicrograph of hippocampal cortex in Alzheimer's disease, silver stain (Sevier), low magnification. Neuritic (senile) plaques (*) and neurons with neurofibrillary tangles (encircled) are abundant. (Figures 13–4 to 13–7, courtesy of Keith H. Fulling, M.D.)

measure 5–100 μm or more in diameter. They consist of a central core of amyloid and a peripheral collection of neuronal processes, both normal-appearing and altered neurites (Fig. 13–7, 13–8). Most of the dysmorphic neurites are axon terminals or preterminals. They contain altered cytoplasmic organelles and paired helical filaments identical to those that compose the neurofibrillary tangles. The periphery of a neuritic plaque also contains processes of fibrous astrocytes, microglial cells, and macrophages. Amyloid fibrils are also composed of paired helical filaments, but these are thicker than neurofilaments and have a periodicity (40 nm) different from that of the paired helical filaments of neurofibrillary tangles. Immunoglobulins are present in the amyloid core of neuritic plaques. Whether they are involved in the formation of the plaque or only represent a secondary phenomenon is not known, but their possible importance is weakened by the recognition that other serum proteins are also present. This finding has been cited as evidence for an altered blood-brain barrier in AD cortex.

There are conflicting hypotheses that the amyloid proteins are derived from neuronal cytoplasmic proteins and that they represent proteins of extraneuronal origin (possibly immunoproteins). A major difficulty in understanding the protein composition of plaque amyloid and neurofibrillary tangles (NFT) results from the realization that both of these structures have the capacity to trap and bind extraneous proteins that then appear in their analyses.

Small collections of altered neurites are

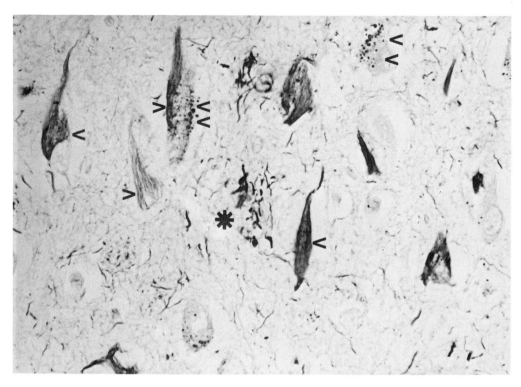

Fig. 13–5. Photomicrograph of hippocampal cortex in Alzheimer's disease, silver stain (Sevier), high magnification. Pyramidal neurons with neurofibrillary tangles are evident (>) as are neurons with lipofuscin granules (≳). A neuritic plaque is marked with an asterisk (*).

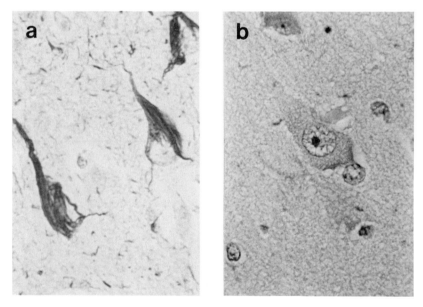

Fig. 13–6. Photomicrographs of hippocampal pyramidal neurons with coarse neurofibrillary tangles as seen (**A**) with silver stain (Sevier). Normal neurons are poorly stained by this technique, but the delicate reticulated appearance of their nucleus and cytoplasm is well shown by hematoxylin and eosin, as in (**B**).

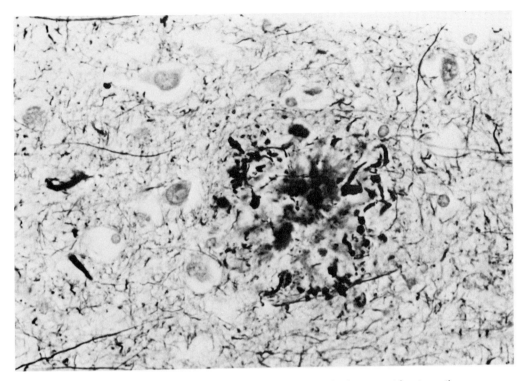

Fig. 13–7. Photomicrograph of a neuritic plaque at higher magnification, silver stain (Sevier). There is a central core of amyloid, surrounded by dysmorphic neurites.

found in AD cortex without associated amyloid and are thought to represent an early stage in the formation of the plaque. However, it is still possible that a few wisps of amyloid are deposited initially. The mature plaque contains both the amyloid core and the surrounding neurites, while an amyloid core without neurites is considered an end-stage or burned-out plaque.

Healthy-appearing synaptic elements are found in the membranes of even the abnormal plaque neurites. This finding, along with the presence of healthy-appearing organelles in neurons laden with neurofibrillary tangles, provides a basis for optimism that future therapies may improve neuronal dysfunction in AD.

Plaques and tangles in AD are found in the greatest concentration in hippocampal cortex, but they are also often found widespread through the neocortex.

Either plaques or tangles may be found in profusion without the other. This observation contradicts the theory that the altered neurites of a plaque represent terminal processes of neurons burdened with neurofibrillary tangles. There is no substantial evidence on the origin of, or the relationship between, plaques and tangles. Since both paired helical filaments and amyloid appear to originate from natural cellular proteins, both may result from a post-translational alteration in either the protein itself, in its reassembly, or in its degradative pathway. One clue, still to be developed, is the observation that both neurofibrillary tangles and amyloid exhibit green-red birefringence on staining with Congo red, which implies a particular configuration (β-pleated) of their proteins.

Other neuronal inclusions, such as

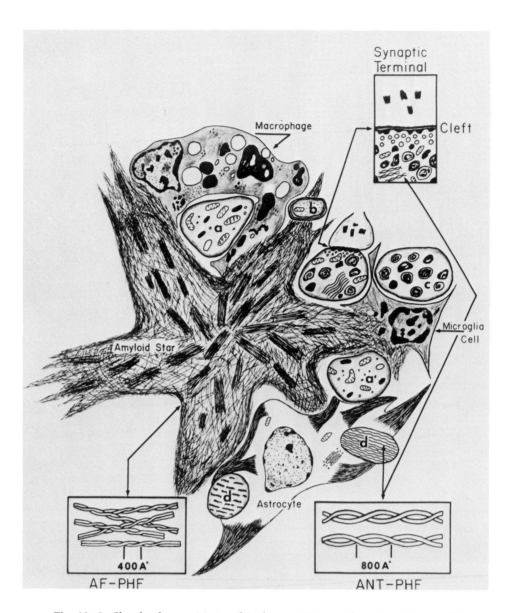

Fig. 13–8. Sketch of a neuritic (senile) plaque: **(A)** normal neurite; **(B)** normal axon; **(C)** altered neurite filled with electron-dense profiles; **(D)** altered neurite filled with PHF. AF-PHF, amyloid fibrils-paired helical filaments; ANT-PHF, Alzheimer neurofibrillary tangle-paired helical filaments. (Reprinted with permission from *Trends in Neuroscience,* courtesy of H. W. Wisniewski, M.D., Ph.D.)

granulovacuolar organelles and Hirano bodies, are found in neurons of patients with AD (and rarely in healthy elderly subjects), but little is known of their significance and most investigators believe they are secondary in importance to the plaques and tangles.

Congophilic material (amyloid) is also deposited in the walls of arterioles, capillaries, and venules in some AD brains. However, amyloidosis is not found in the rest of the body and there is no known link between systemic amyloidosis and AD. The congophilic angiopathy may lead to infarction and/or hemorrhage in the brain as a complicating feature in AD. The same angiopathy is seen in a smaller percentage of elderly people who do not have plaques and tangles.

At least two laboratories have reported that the frequency of plaques and tangles in the cortex is directly related to the degree of dementia in AD. Despite that observation, it is clear that we have little understanding regarding the mechanisms of either the impaired neuronal function or of the dementia. The list of speculations includes loss of neurons or of critical populations of neurons, clogging of neuronal machinery with neurofibrillary tangles, altered structure of neurites, loss of dendritic networks and synapses, and loss of neurotransmitter system(s).

Cholinergic hypothesis. From several lines of evidence, there has been derived the hypothesis that dimished cholinergic neurotransmitter function is at least one of the factors responsible for intellectual decline both in normal aging and in AD. There are modest reductions in chemical markers of presynaptic cholinergic systems in the cerebral cortex of healthy aged subjects and more profound reductions in the cortex of almost all patients with AD. The most striking abnormality is a decrease in activity of choline acetyltransferase, the presynaptic enzyme necessary for the synthesis of acetylcholine. The sparse data available suggest that the degree of choline acetyltransferase deficiency is related to the degree of intellectual impairment in AD.

Cholinergic blockade with scopolamine in young human subjects can reproduce memory loss similar to that found in aging and dementia. These scopolamine-induced memory deficits are partially reversed by physostigmine (which potentiates acetylcholine action by inhibiting acetylcholinesterase) but not by CNS stimulants, such as methylphenidate or amphetamine. Similar memory deficits are not produced by analogous blockade of dopamine or β-adrenergic receptors.

Agents that promote central cholinergic transmitter function (physostigmine, choline, lecithin, arecoline) have sometimes slightly improved cognitive impairment in aged humans and other animals. Furthermore, hippocampal neurons of old animals are less responsive than those of younger animals to stimulation with acetylcholine, but age differences are not apparent in responses of these neurons to glutamic acid. One notes that the seeming importance of the cholinergic system to memory and cognition may mean an effect on some alerting mechanism rather than on a specific cognitive system. Further caution in response to the cholinergic hypothesis is suggested by the observation that benzodiazepines can induce memory deficits in experimental animals similar to that produced by scopolamine.

The cholinergic input to the cerebral cortex is derived mainly from basal forebrain neurons whose cell bodies are located in a group of nuclei that measures 3–4 cm in length and that lies between the anterior commissure and the optic chiasm. The group includes the basal nucleus of Meynert, providing cholinergic innervation of the neocortex, and both the medial septal nucleus and the nucleus of the diagonal band of Broca, which provide cholinergic supply to the hippocampus (Fig. 13–9). Striking loss of neurons from these

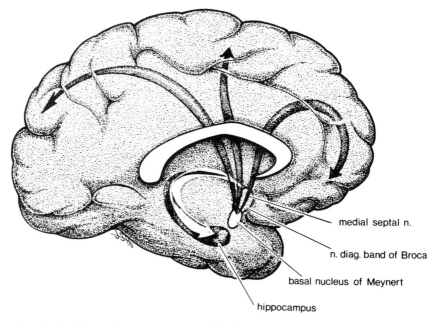

medial septal n.

n. diag. band of Broca

basal nucleus of Meynert

hippocampus

Fig. 13–9. Schematic representation of cholinergic innervation of neocortex and hippocampus from basal forebrain nuclei, as seen from medial surface of the hemisphere. The nuclei of the medial septum and of the diagonal band of Broca contain large cholinergic neurons that innervate the hippocampus. Corresponding neurons in the basal nucleus of Meynert send cholinergic axons to supply the neocortex. Loss of neurons from these basal nuclei may account for the decreased activity of choline acetyltransferase in cortex of AD.

nuclei has been reported in AD, but not in Huntington's disease, another cause of dementia. There are conflicting reports regarding loss of neurons from the basal nucleus in Parkinson's disease, with or without dementia. The disappearance of neurons from these basal forebrain cholinergic nuclei may explain the low choline acetyltransferase activity levels in the cortex of AD brains.

One theory holds that as neurons of the basal nucleus of Meynert begin to deteriorate in their terminal portions, the degenerating neurite terminals form an immature plaque that later attracts amyloid. When the distal processes of these neurons disappear completely, only the end-stage plaque remains. Aging monkeys have cortical plaques with neurites rich in acetylcholinesterase activity. Monkeys older than those have end-stage plaques,

devoid of neurites and acetylcholinesterase activity.

The cholinergic hypothesis for AD was appealing because it offered (1) a schema analogous to the dopaminergic model of Parkinson's disease, and therefore (2) a basis for trials of substitution therapy. However, there have been inconsistencies in the findings from various laboratories in experiments testing the cholinergic hypothesis. Responses of patients with AD to cholinomimetic drugs and other agents to promote cholinergic transmitter function have been spotty and disappointing.

Should the cholinergic system deficiency prove to be important in AD, one would still have to deal with the question of what causes the loss of cholinergic neurons. Is there a critical decline in trophic factors essential for healthy cholinergic neurons? If so, what leads to that decline?

Do cholinergic deficiencies result from the same factors that give rise to plaques or tangles or loss of cortical neurons? Of course, there is the possibility that the cholinergic defects are secondary rather than primary in AD.

Other theories. There is nearly uniform agreement that a genetic factor is present, even though AD is probably multifactorial in origin. The data are still unsatisfactory, but it appears the risk of AD is about fourfold if an individual has a first-degree relative with the disease.

Since aluminum salts can produce neurofibrillary tangles in experimental animals (albeit without the characteristic paired helical filaments) and since there were early reports of increased aluminum content in AD brains, it remains possible that aluminum toxicity may be a factor. Other investigators have not been able to duplicate the finding of a generally increased aluminum content in the cortex compared to age-matched controls, but there may be a selective increase of aluminum content in the nuclei of tangle-bearing neurons. That nuclear increase may only reflect neuronal damage and not its cause, since aluminum accumulates with aging and with various kinds of neuronal dysfunction. Patients with chronic renal disease who develop dialysis dementia with large amounts of aluminum in the brain do not develop the structural changes of AD.

The theory that AD may be caused by an unconventional virus arose because other disorders previously considered to be degenerative, such as kuru and Jakob-Creutzfeldt spongiform encephalopathy, have been shown to be due to transmissible unconventional agents, akin to scrapie in lower animals. The scrapie agent (a proteinaceous infectious particle, or "prion") in certain strains of laboratory mice gives rise to an encephalopathy with amyloid and neuritic plaques identical in all respects to the plaques of AD except

for the absence of PHF in the neurites. There have been many attempts to transmit AD or a spongiform encephalopathy by injection of AD brain into laboratory animals, but these efforts have not been successful, in contrast to their regular success in the transmission of scrapie, kuru, and Jakob-Creutzfeldt disease. Negative evidence on the transmissibility of AD is not impressive, however, when one considers that two chronic brain diseases caused by viruses (subacute sclerosing panencephalitis and progressive multifocal encephalopathy) have not been transmitted to subhuman primates. A link between the virus and cholinergic theories is possible because one of the noncytopathic effects of virus infection is the suppression of "luxury" cellular function (such as cholinergic activity) in normal appearing cells.

An immunologic mechanism has been suggested because of the presence of amyloid in the neuritic plaques and in walls of blood vessels. Furthermore, the age-related incidence of AD parallels age-related changes in immunoregulatory mechanisms. However, the debate on the significance of the amyloid and associated immunoglobulins was cited earlier.

Alzheimer's disease must still be regarded as a disorder of unknown cause whose mechanisms are poorly understood. There is no certain relationship of the clinical phenomena to the histological, ultrastructural, or chemical changes in the brain. These are fertile areas for research, made mandatory by society's needs.

REFLECTIONS

Is Alzheimer's disease an exaggeration of normal aging?

An affirmative answer to this question is suggested by the progressive rise in the incidence of the disorder with each decade from the age of 60 to 90, and by the occurrence of small numbers of plaques and tangles in the cortex of nondemented elderly subjects. The mild loss of neurons from cerebral cortex and basal nucleus of Meynert in healthy aging can be compared with the more marked neuronal loss from those regions in AD. Furthermore, the histological signs of Alzheimer's disease are found almost uniformly in the cortex of patients with Down's syndrome when they pass the age of 35 or 40, accompanied by signs of precocious aging elsewhere in the body.

On the other hand, contrary evidence has been adduced. The incidence of AD appears to decrease after the age of 90. According to the limited evidence available, patients with progeria do not develop dementia or the histological changes of AD. Furthermore, there is no increase of lipofuscinosis in AD brains as compared with age-matched controls. Another histological point is the reported lack of a continuum between the rare neocortical tangle in nondemented elderly and the vast numbers of neocortical tangles in AD. Finally, electroencephalographic and evoked potential studies suggest differing sequential changes in healthy aging as compared with AD.

There are conflicting reports on whether patterns of declining psychometric performance in aging are similar to or different from those found in AD. Suffice it to say that the question posed above cannot be answered at present. The answer may only be forthcoming when the causes of both aging and of AD are understood.

Relationship of clinical manifestations to brain changes

This important issue still awaits investigation. The present state of understanding the mechanisms underlying Alzheimer's disease has been reviewed. Even for the healthy elderly there are no useful quantitative data comparing clinical performance with changes in brain anatomy, physiology, or chemistry. Some speculations have been offered. For instance, it is tempting to relate the more benign syndromes of forgetfulness in the elderly to the small numbers of neuritic plaques and neurofibrillary tangles found in the hippocampuses of most nondemented elderly. One of the most striking features in the clinical neurology of the normal aged is their susceptibility to delirium under metabolic stress. Does that vulnerability result from age-related loss of redundancy in critical neuronal systems such as the numbers of neurons, dendrites, or synapses, or activity levels of certain transmitter or other enzymatic systems?

Relationship between mind and brain

It is reasonable to assume that neuronal connections of increasing complexity underlie some kinds of learning and memory, such as innate or instinctual behavior. Furthermore, it is likely that changes in efficiency of certain synapses result from repeated use of certain neural circuits, lead to enhancement of one or a few possible pathways over others, and give rise to a certain kind of elementary learning and memory. How much more difficult it will be to understand the neurobiology of human memory that involves percepts or experiences, to understand the basis of human perception, thinking, and experiencing—and their recapitulation when people learn or remember. Then what of human integrative behaviors beyond learning and memory? What of conception, imagination, creativity, volition, emotion, judgment, wisdom? What are the mechanisms of changes in those capacities with normal aging and of their deterioration in the syndromes of dementia, such as Alzheimer's disease?

These questions call to mind the words of the artist Georges Braque in another, but related, context: "What matters in art is the part that cannot be explained." The aspects of human brain function that are truly important to behavior are those that we do not understand. Are we far removed from being able to design experiments to pursue the answers? Just as there are many examples of the elucidation of normal physiology and chemistry from study of disease states elsewhere in medical science, perhaps future investigation of the brain disorder in Alzheimer's disease will lead to better understanding of normal brain-mind interrelationships.

GENERAL REFERENCES

Bartus, R. T., R. L. Dean III, B. Beer, and A. S. Lippa. The cholinergic hypothesis of geriatric memory dysfunction. *Science* 217:408–17, 1982.

Buell, S. J. Golgi-Cox and rapid Golgi methods as applied to autopsied human brain tissue: widely disparate results. *J. Neuropath. Exper. Neurol.* 41:500–7, 1982.

Corkin, S., K. L. Davis, J. H. Growdon, E. Usdin, and R. J. Wurtman (eds.). *Alzheimer's Disease: A Report of Progress in Research.* New York, Raven Press, 1982.

Kandel, E. R., and J. H. Schwartz. Molecular biology of learning: Modulation of transmitter release. *Science* 218:433–43, 1982.

Katzman, R., and R. Terry. *The Neurology of Aging.* Philadelphia, Davis, 1983.

Katzman, R. (ed.). *Biological aspects of Alzheimer's disease.* Banbury Report #15. Cold Spring Harbor Laboratory, 1983.

Miller, E. Cognitive assessment of the older adult. In *Handbook of Mental Health and Aging,* J. E. Birren and R. B. Sloane (eds.). Englewood Cliffs, N.J., Prentice-Hall, 1980, pp. 520–36.

Nottebohm, F. A brain for all seasons: cyclical anatomical changes in song control nuclei of the canary brain. *Science* 214:1368–70, 1981.

Prusiner, S. B. Novel proteinaceous particles cause scrapie. *Science* 216:136–144, 1982.

Rogers, J., S. F. Zornetzer, and F. E. Bloom. Senescent pathology of cerebellum: Purkinje neurons and their parallel fiber afferents. *Neurobiol. Aging* 2:15–25, 1981.

Sinex, F. M., and C. R. Merrill (eds.). Alzheimer's disease, Down's syndrome, and aging. *Ann. N.Y. Acad. Sci.* 396:1–192, 1982.

Squire, L. R. The neuropsychology of human memory. *Ann. Rev. Neurosci.* 5:241–73, 1982.

Wells, C. E. (ed.). *Dementia,* 2d ed. Philadelphia, Davis, 1977.

Wisniewski, H. M., G. S. Merz, P. A. Merz, G. Y. Wen, and K. Iqbal. Morphology and biochemistry of neuronal paired helical filaments and amyloid fibers in humans and animals. In *Progress in Neuropathology,* vol. 5, H. M. Zimmerman (ed.). New York, Raven Press, 1983, pp. 139–50.

14.

Demyelinating Diseases

JOHN N. WHITAKER

Demyelinating diseases partially or totally destroy the myelin sheath. Demyelination refers to loss of myelin that has been formed, in contrast to *dysmyelination,* in which the myelin sheath is never formed properly. Dysmyelination is usually the result of metabolic disturbances affecting the synthetic or degradative mechanisms of myelin formation.

Demyelination may affect the central or peripheral nervous system and may appear as a primary or secondary phenomenon. In primary demyelination the myelin unit, i.e., the compact myelin sheath and its supporting glial cell, is damaged selectively or preferentially. This can occur through effects on meylin itself or on the oligodendrocyte in the central nervous system or the Schwann cell in the peripheral nervous system, altering the ability of these two cells to synthesize and maintain myelin. The loss of myelin in secondary demyelination results from neuronal disease processes that lead to a loss of axons and preclude the axoglial interaction required for myelination. A number of neurological disorders in humans may be associated with a selective effect on the central nervous system myelin unit. These

include certain viral infections, nutritional deficiencies and parainfectious reactions. The most common is multiple sclerosis. General clinical and pathological features and the laboratory abnormalities in multiple sclerosis will be described in the sections that follow. Current views on its etiology and pathogenesis will then be considered. Disorders of peripheral nervous system myelin are covered in Chapter 2.

CLINICAL AND PATHOLOGICAL FEATURES OF MULTIPLE SCLEROSIS

In 1868 Jean-Martin Charcot published the first clinical-pathological correlation of multiple sclerosis, emphasizing the multiple areas of central nervous system myelin loss in patients with a combination of neurological deficits. The diagnosis of multiple sclerosis rests on clinical grounds. Adjunctive, but not diagnostic, laboratory tests are available. The major requirements for a diagnosis of multiple sclerosis are multiple lesions within the central nervous system occurring at different times. Any area of the central nervous system may be involved, but certain manifestations are

Table 14–1. Frequency of symptoms and signs in multiple sclerosis

Function affected	At onset (%)	During disease course (%)
Cerebral	4	40
Visual	35	65
Coordination	20	80
Strength	45	90
Sensation	40	90
Genitourinary	10	65

more common at the onset of disease (Table 14–1). The presenting symptoms are likely to be an indication of those lesions that greatly affect function and are noted by patients, rather than a reflection of the sites of preference for the initial myelin damage. The most common deficits are paresis, paresthesias, visual impairment, and incoordination; mental, sexual, and urinary dysfunction are common in later stages of the disease. The extent of neurological deficit, the rate of progression, and the frequency of exacerbations are highly variable from one individual to the next. While some patients experience a debilitating disease, 10%–15% of patients will have a mild course, sometimes referred to as benign multiple sclerosis. Approximately 90% of persons with multiple sclerosis will experience exacerbations and remissions, averaging two every three years, especially during the first five years of the disease. Exacerbations may appear suddenly over a period of minutes to hours, may develop over a period of hours to a week (the most common type), or may arise gradually over a period of many weeks. Remission is usually incomplete, causing the degree of disability to increase with time. In approximately 10% of cases, multiple sclerosis is insidiously progressive without exacerbations or remissions.

Multiple sclerosis typically affects those between 20 and 40 years of age and rarely occurs outside the age span of 10 to 50. There is a female to male predominance of approximately 1.5 to 1. The disease is twice as common in whites as it is in blacks in the United States and more common in these groups than in Orientals. Although the quality of life may markedly diminish because of disability, average life expectancy is at last 85% that of an age-matched control population. The cause of death in 70% of patients with multiple sclerosis is related to a respiratory or urinary tract infection.

The pathological changes (Figs. 14–1, 14–2; Table 14–2 underlying multiple sclerosis involve both segmental demyelination and inflammation in the central nervous system. As expected in primary demyelination, myelin is decreased or lost, and axons are relatively preserved. Cellular elements around blood vessels and infiltrating tissue are present in the acute lesion and consist mainly of lymphocytes and macrophages. Plasma cells are found in abundance around blood vessels or in the parenchyma of the brain. Oligodendrocytes are often, but not always, diminished. Older lesions are associated with hypertrophy and hyperplasia of astrocytes, leading to gliosis and firmness, which form the basis for the term "sclerosis." Chemical alterations in the injured tissue of multiple sclerosis reflect the loss of myelin components, the increase in proteinases and lipases from phagocytic cells, and the increase of IgG from the infiltrating plasma cells.

Myelin plays a critical role in the transmission of nerve impulses by producing saltatory rather than continuous conduction. The loss or reduction of myelin slows or blocks impulse conduction, producing negative effects such as paralysis or decreased vision. Ephaptic conduction from one partially demyelinated nerve fiber to another or ectopic impulse generation in a demyelinated region results in positive effects such as trigeminal neuralgia, dysesthesias, and Lhermitte's sign. The latter consists of paresthesias in the back and extremities when the neck is flexed and is thought to arise from mechanical stim-

A

B

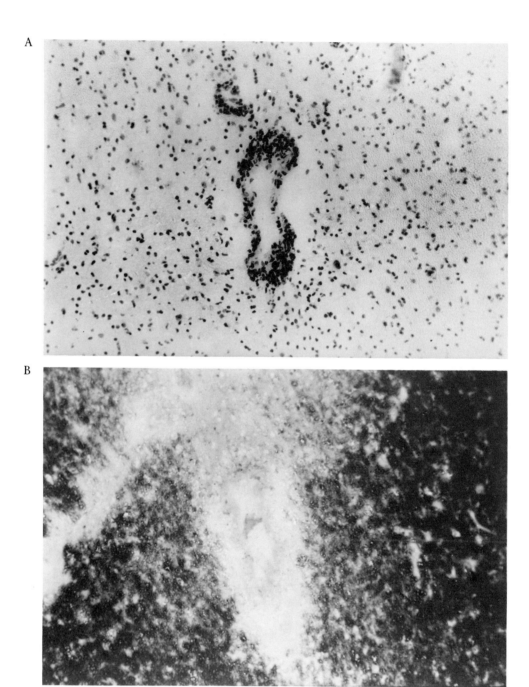

Fig. 14–1. Serial cryostat sections, stained with hematoxylin and eosin (**A**) or Luxol fast blue (a stain for myelin) (**B**) of an acute phase lesion in cerebral white matter obtained postmortem from a patient with multiple sclerosis. The perivascular mononuclear inflammatory cell reaction (**A**) is accompanied by myelin loss (**B**). Normally, the darkly stained myelin (**B**) would extend to the vascular rim. × 265. (From Whitaker, 1978).

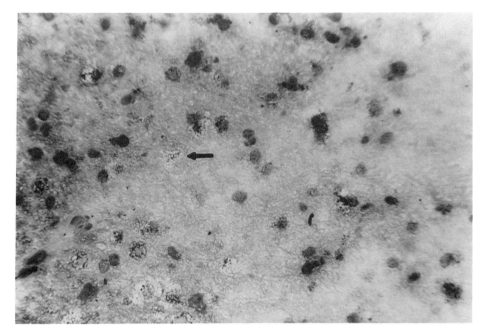

Fig. 14–2. Cryostat section of cerebral white matter stained with Luxol fast blue showing changes of a more chronic lesion of multiple sclerosis. The paleness indicates loss of myelin. Phagocytic cells (arrow) with engulfed myelin are evident. × 665. (From Whitaker, 1978).

Table 14–2. Changes in central nervous system tissue components and composition in multiple sclerosis

Neurons: Selectively or preferentially preserved
Myelin: Diminished or absent
Glia: Oligodendrocytes usually decreased; Astrocytes and microglia increased
Infiltrating cells: Lymphocytes, macrophages, and plasma cells
Chemical changes: Decreased myelin components and markers of oligodendrocytes; increase in astrocytic components; increased proteinase and lipase activity, cholesterol esters, triglycerides, H_2O and IgG

ulation of demyelinated fibers in the posterior columns of the cervical spinal cord. These changes and their basis are described more fully in Chapter 1.

LABORATORY AND DIAGNOSTIC STUDIES

Several special laboratory tests, including evoked potentials, radiographic cranial imaging, and examination of cerebrospinal fluid IgG, may be used to assist in the diagnosis of multiple sclerosis. Although none of these studies are specific for multiple sclerosis, they are often helpful when considered together with the clinical picture.

Evoked potentials are measured following visual, auditory, or somatosensory stimulation. These tests detect loci of slowed nerve conduction velocity and, inferentially, areas of demyelination in the central nervous system that are not apparent clinically. Visually evoked potentials (Fig. 14–3) are elicited by flashing a bright light or showing a shifting checkerboard pattern, which produce an evoked potential detected over the occipital lobes. Since the reduction or loss in the myelin sheath leads to a slowing of the conduction velocity, lesions of the visual pathways in multiple sclerosis may result in increased latencies for visually evoked potentials. Measurements of visually evoked poten-

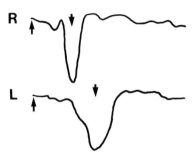

Fig. 14–3. Recording of pattern-shift visually evoked response in a patient with left optic neuritis and multiple sclerosis. The latency between stimulus (↑) and first major positive wave (↓) (positive is downward) recorded at the occiput is normal in the right (R) eye but markedly prolonged in the left (L) eye.

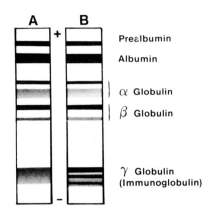

Fig. 14–4. Agarose gel electrophoresis of cerebrospinal fluid proteins from a normal control (A) and a patient with multiple sclerosis (B). Distinct bands are present in the immunoglobulin region in B and are designated as oligoclonal bands.

tials may uncover abnormalities in up to 40% of patients with multiple sclerosis in whom there is no history of optic neuritis or of clinical abnormalities affecting vision. Other evoked potentials may be similarly used. Brainstem auditory evoked responses detect abnormalities in conduction of auditory stimuli through the brainstem, and somatosensory stimuli are used to identify abnormalities in ascending sensory tracts.

Imaging procedures, notably cranial computed tomography, may be useful in the diagnosis of multiple sclerosis and in excluding other causes of the patient's neurological problem. Parenchymal foci and periventricular hypodense areas may be present. Areas of uptake after intravenous injection of contrast material may also be noted in new or active lesions and reflect an alteration of the blood-brain barrier. Initial studies with nuclear magnetic resonance indicate that it is superior to computed tomography in the detection of areas of demyelination.

Cerebrospinal fluid is examined for quantitative and qualitative abnormalities of IgG and for indicators of myelin damage. Conventional cerebrospinal fluid tests of cell number, cell type, protein concentration, and glucose concentration are typically normal or near normal, although there may be a slight mononuclear pleocytosis immediately following an exacerbation. In approximately 70% of patients with multiple sclerosis there is a quantitative increase in cerebrospinal fluid immunoglobulins, primarily in the IgG class. The qualitative abnormality is that of oligoclonal "bands" (Fig. 14–4). These consist of both IgG and free light chains that migrate as discrete bands on agarose gel electrophoresis or isoelectric focusing. The oligoclonal bands are thought to arise from a small number of lymphoid cell clones *in situ* in the central nervous system. Oligoclonal bands are present in cerebrospinal fluid in 80%–90% of patients with multiple sclerosis. The quantity of IgG and its presence or pattern show little relationship to disease activity. Components of the central nervous system myelin sheath may appear in cerebrospinal fluid coincident with demyelination. Myelin basic protein is the most fully studied of these protein markers. Myelin basic protein, or its peptides, enters cerebrospinal fluid at the time of myelin injury, providing an indication of recent myelin damage. Neither basic protein nor oligoclonal bands in cerebrospinal fluid is unique to multiple sclerosis. Myelin basic protein or its fragments may be found in cerebrospinal fluid after any type of acute central nervous system myelin damage. Oligoclonal bands are present in cerebrospinal fluid in disorders such as neurosyphilis or subacute sclerosing panencephalitis, in which a hyperimmune state exists within the central nervous system.

ETIOLOGY AND PATHOGENESIS OF MULTIPLE SCLEROSIS

The etiology and pathogenesis of multiple sclerosis are unknown. Available evidence indicates that a combination of environmental factors and host susceptibility, probably manifested in the immune system, governs its development.

Epidemiology

Approximately 125,000 persons in the United States have multiple sclerosis, but the disease has a very uneven distribution (Fig. 14–5) throughout the world. The area of greatest prevalence (number of cases per unit population at a given time) is in the temperate zones of North America, Europe, South Australia, and New Zealand, where it is 30–80 cases per 100,000 population. Nearer the equator, the prevalence of the disease declines. This pattern does not hold throughout the world, however. The most notable exception is in Japan, where the disease is 5% of that expected at the same latitude in the United States.

The uneven distribution of multiple sclerosis has permitted analysis of the differences in areas of high and low prevalence. In studies of migration of individuals from high to low prevalence regions, it has been shown that the environmental influence is exerted sometimes prior to age 15. This finding has been demonstrated in studies of populations that have immigrated to South Africa and to Israel or have migrated within the United States. Immigration after age 15 to an area of low prevalence results in prevalence statistics that are similar to the region of origin. Movement before age 15 produces prevalence rates of the new area in the immigrant population. These observations need not imply a rigid cutoff of an environmental influence at age 15 and are too limited to be completely conclusive. However, they do indicate changes in susceptibility to a potentially causative effect before puberty, many years before the clinical manifestations of multiple sclerosis appear.

The incidence (number of cases per unit population per unit time) of multiple sclerosis has remained nearly constant in some regions over the last 50 years, but in certain areas there is evidence for an "epidemic" of the disease. In the Faroe Islands, for example, there was no record of the disease from the early 1920s until 1943, but from 1943 to 1960 there were 24 cases in a population of 35,000. These cases of multiple sclerosis appeared in individuals who lived near the encampment sites of British soldiers stationed in the Faroe Islands between the years 1940 and 1945. An influence of the physiological changes at puberty on the latency between exposure and appearance of the disease has been observed in these cases. For adults the time between exposure and appearance of disease was five years, whereas for those who were prepubertal in 1940–5, the disease appeared approximately five years after puberty. The cause of this apparent epidemic is still under study, but an infectious agent must be considered. Less-striking increases of multiple sclerosis also appeared in Iceland following the influx of Canadian and British armed forces there in the early 1940s.

Racial factors, in addition to those of geography, also play a role in the epidemiology of multiple sclerosis. Certain populations, including Orientals, Eskimos, and the Bantus have a very low prevalence of the disease. Despite the differences in prevalence among races, the

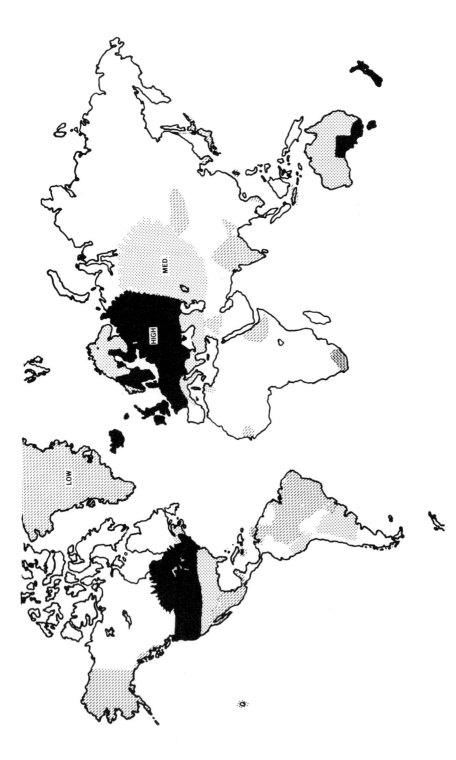

Fig. 14–5. Worldwide geographical distribution of multiple sclerosis demonstrating the uneven prevalence of the disease. High prevalence areas are indicated in black, medium prevalence areas with dots, and low prevalence areas with diagonal marks. Data are unavailable for the regions shown in white. (From J. F. Kurtzke. Geographic distribution of multiple sclerosis: An update with special reference to Europe and the Mediterranean region. *Acta neurol. Scand.* 62:65–80, 1980).

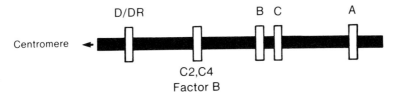

Fig. 14–6. The human major histocompatibility complex on the short arm of the sixth chromosome. The centromere is to the left. Each of the four loci (A, C, B, D/DR) shown is polymorphic. Gene products of the A, C, and B loci show biochemical similarities, are present on the surface membranes of all cells, and are designated as Class I. Different gene products, designated as Class II, are coded for by the D/DR loci and are found predominantly on immunocompetent cells. Cells bearing Class II gene products are involved in presentation of antigen to helper and suppressor cells. The gene locus between the B and D/DR loci is involved in the control of complement factors.

features of the disease and its onset tend to be the same throughout the world. However, optic nerve and spinal cord involvement are relatively more common in the Japanese, and the lesions in these sites tend to be more necrotic.

Host susceptibility

Multiple sclerosis is 12–20 times more common among those with family members who have the disease, indicating a probable genetic effect. Markers of gene products have been studied in an attempt to understand this effect and its role in host susceptibility. The most helpful information has come from analysis of histocompatibility antigens, which in the human are products of a group of gene loci located on the short arm of the sixth chromosome (Fig. 14–6). Each species has a group of such loci, designated as the major histocompatibility complex, controlling the recognition of self and nonself. In the human the antigenic gene products of the major histocompatibility complex are referred to as HLA (histocompatibility leukocyte antigen); in the mouse they are called H-2. The gene products coded for by the loci of the major histocompatibility complex can be detected on the surfaces of cells, commonly peripheral blood lym-

phocytes, and have been used in studying host susceptibility in multiple sclerosis and other diseases.

The major histocompatibility complex in the human consists of four major gene regions (Fig. 14–6), each very polymorphic. Products of the A, C, and B loci are grouped as class I and are present on the surface membrane of all nucleated cells. Products of the D/DR locus are also present on cell surface membranes but are generally restricted to immunocompetent cells. In Caucasian patients with multiple sclerosis, there is a twofold increase in frequency of HLA-B7 and HLA-A3 and a decline in HLA-A12. The usefulness of markers has been enhanced by examining the frequency of the D and DR region antigens, which are more difficult to analyze. The DR2 antigen has a threefold greater frequency in patients with multiple sclerosis than in controls. The major histocompatibility complex, in particular the D/DR locus, influences or controls the immune response, thus raising the prospect that these correlations point to an immunogenetic abnormality in multiple sclerosis. However, the lack of concordance for multiple sclerosis in identical twins and the imperfect correlation of HLA type with the presence of the disease in families with two or more cases indicate that other factors are necessary for the disease to occur. One possibility is an as yet unidentified gene that influences susceptibility or resistance to multiple sclerosis that is near, but not in, the major histocompatibility complex.

Immunological abnormalities

Immunological investigations of patients with multiple sclerosis have revealed abnormalities in peripheral blood, cerebrospinal fluid IgG, and central nervous system tissue. It is still unclear which of these changes might be related to the cause of multiple sclerosis. Before reviewing the immunological investigations conducted on the disease, it is necessary to describe some of the cells of the immune system and their products briefly.

An immune response to a soluble antigen consists of the combined effort of lymphocytes preceded by the action of an accessory cell, typically the macrophage, in processing the antigen. The cells interacting in this initiation of the immune response must be histocompatible, i.e., have the same HLA type. The HLA type would be expected to determine or influence the generated immune response. The lymphocyte population involved in an immune response is very heterogeneous. It consists of different lymphocyte subsets with varied functions and markers, identified by functional assays or monoclonal antibodies. Lymphocytes are derived from a bone marrow stem cell that may develop along two major routes. Some stem cells migrate to the thymus, where they proliferate and acquire membrane markers and the capacity to function in selected ways. Most cells die within the thymus, but some enter the peripheral blood and circulate, while others are eventually deposited in the medullary and paracortical areas of lymph nodes. These cells are referred to as T lymphocytes. They have a receptor for sheep erythrocytes, little surface membrane immunoglobulin, and a membrane marker designated as T_3. T lymphocytes are involved in the events of cellular immunity and participate in the effector functions of cytotoxicity, lymphokine release, and proliferation on exposure to antigen or mitogens. T lymphocytes may also serve an immunoregulatory function in promoting (T helper cells bearing the T_4 antigen) or suppressing (T suppressor cells bearing the T_5 or T8 antigen) an immune response. Other bone marrow stem cells are activated elsewhere (in a site still unknown in mammals) and are modified to become B lymphocytes. These cells have readily detectable surface membrane immunoglobulin (IgM or IgD) but do not have receptors for sheep erythrocytes. The cells circulate or reside in follicles and germinal centers of lymph nodes. They are able to synthesize and secrete antibody in association with a transformation into plasma cells. Approximately 65% of peripheral blood lymphocytes are T cells and 20% B cells; the remainder are called null cells.

Many immunological studies of patients with multiple sclerosis have been undertaken on peripheral blood to analyze cell types, cell products, and serum factors. Studies of blood or serum immunoglobulins, complement, immune complexes, other serum proteins, T- and B-lymphocyte numbers, T-lymphocyte sensitization to antigens, and lymphocyte responses to mitogenic lectins have disclosed no consistent abnormality in multiple sclerosis. However, abnormalities are detected when the regulation of these events, rather than the effector functions of lymphocytes, is studied. These abnormalities consist of diminished suppressor function and usually a decline in suppressor T-lymphocyte (T_5 or T8) numbers during periods of exacerbations. There is also evidence for enhanced B-cell activity and T-helper function. Each of these alterations would bring about a hyperimmune status.

Changes in cerebrospinal fluid

An elevation of cerebrospinal fluid IgG and oligoclonal bands is found frequently in patients with multiple sclerosis, as already mentioned. The origin and features of this IgG and its antibody activity have been of much interest. Protein and immunoglobulin levels in cerebrospinal fluid may change through several different mechanisms. Normally there is a ratio of approximately 1 to 200 between protein in the cerebrospinal fluid and that in the blood. An increase in serum protein and IgG levels would lead to a new equilibrium and an increase of both levels in cerebrospinal fluid. There may also be an increase in transfer of protein from blood to cerebrospinal fluid because of an alteration of the blood-brain barrier. In both situations the ratio of IgG to total protein in the cerebrospinal fluid would be the same as that in blood. In a third situation, and the one that pertains in multiple sclerosis, the relative amount of IgG to total protein in cerebrospinal fluid is increased. Available evidence shows that although there is a slight increase of permeability of the blood-brain barrier in multiple sclerosis, the major explanation for the increase in IgG in cerebrospinal fluid is in situ synthesis by lymphoid tissue within the central nervous system, where as much as 100 mg of IgG may be synthesized daily. The cellular origin of the IgG is thought to be the plasma cells, which have been estimated to be as high as 10^8 in the brain of a patient with the disease. Plasma cells are rarely seen in normal human brain.

The pattern of oligoclonal bands present in the cerebrospinal fluid varies from one patient to another, but changes little during the course of the disease in a given patient with multiple sclerosis. The increased IgG level in cerebrospinal fluid represents both polyclonal and oligoclonal IgG. The nature of the antibody activity in the oligoclonal bands and in the polyclonal response has not been identified. It is known that in cerebrospinal fluid of individuals with multiple sclerosis there is an increase in antibody against certain viruses, particularly rubeola, with evidence that much of the antiviral antibody is produced in the central nervous system. In other diseases such as subacute sclerosing panencephalitis and neurosyphilis, in which oligoclonal bands are commonly found, the oligoclonal bands have antibody activity against the causative infectious agent. However, antibody against viruses, viral components, or neural tissue antigens has rarely been detected in the oligoclonal bands in multiple sclerosis. The general interpretation of the alterations in cerebrospinal fluid immunoglobulin in multiple sclerosis is that they represent either chronic stimulation by unusual or unidentified antigens or that they reflect impaired regulation of immunoglobulin synthesis, so that the resultant antibodies are "nonsense" in their activity. This might occur as a result of the diminished suppressor T lymphocytes present in both blood and cerebrospinal fluid during periods of disease activity. In addition to the mild pleocytosis that may occur during an exacerbation, cells in the cerebrospinal fluid of patients with multiple sclerosis can be demonstrated by flow cytometry to be activated, more so during periods of disease activity. This suggests constant stimulation or lack of suppression with periodic accentuation of this phenomenon.

Changes in brain

Changes in the brain relate to the disease mechanisms and the mechanism for tissue injury. It is still unclear whether an autoimmune attack, a chronic viral infection, or a combination of these two or other factors is involved. An increase in plasma cells and IgG in the lesions of multiple sclerosis has already been discussed. When different lesions from the same brain have been obtained postmortem and individually analyzed, the extracted oligoclonal

Table 14–3. Immunological abnormalities in multiple sclerosis

Accumulation of plasma cells and in situ IgG synthesis in the central nervous system
Increased immunoglobulin levels and antiviral titers and the presence of oligoclonal bands of IgG in the cerebrospinal fluid
Decreased suppressor cell activity and number of suppressor T lymphocytes bearing T5 and T8 markers in peripheral blood during periods of disease activity

bands are not identical in each lesion sampled. This has been interpreted as evidence for different clones responding to different antigens and also as further support for an immunoregulatory defect. Numerous studies of brain specimens, body fluids, and non-neural tissues have provided no definitive evidence for a causative virus infection in multiple sclerosis.

The abnormalities related to the immune system that occur in multiple sclerosis are summarized in Table 14–3. An explanation of how these changes might relate to disease production remains elusive. The most impressive (although inconstant) changes in peripheral blood are those related to the decline in suppressor T lymphocytes at the time of disease activity. The nature of this decline is still unknown, but it could possibly be due to infiltration of the central nervous system by these cells or to changes in their migratory pattern in the body so that they are less represented in the sampled peripheral blood. The decline in suppressor T lymphocytes could also be the result of the loss of their markers, either by destruction of the cell itself, or by "modulation" of the surface antigen by some event leading to both loss of surface marker and suppressor function. Present evidence indicates that the suppressor cells are not sequestered in the central nervous system but that their marker antigen is altered at the time of disease activity. It is unclear how an abnormality of a subset of lymphocytes might

be related to a primary demyelinating disease of the central nervous system.

The possibility of autoimmunity

The possibility that a myelin antigen provokes an autoimmune response has been considered as an etiologic mechanism in multiple sclerosis. There is a component of normal myelin that has the capacity to induce inflammatory demyelination in laboratory animals when injected with complete Freund's adjuvant. The responsible constituent is myelin encephalitogenic or basic protein, a protein with a molecular weight of 18,500 and accounting for 30% of central nervous system myelin proteins. A similar induction of inflammatory demyelination probably produced the acute disseminated encephalomyelitis that developed in a small percentage of humans receiving the Pasteur treatment for rabies, which involved repeated injections of dried rabbit spinal cord. Myelin basic protein with complete Freund's adjuvant can induce a disease characterized by perivascular inflammation and coexistent demyelination in guinea pigs, rabbits, monkeys, and certain strains of rats and mice. The acute variety of experimental allergic encephalomyelitis is similar to acute disseminated encephalomyelitis in humans, but is unlike most cases of multiple sclerosis. By altering the immunization program it is possible to induce a chronic form of experimental allergic encephalomyelitis that does bear many similarities to the disease. In addition, myelin basic protein, or its fragments, enters cerebrospinal fluid at the time of central nervous system myelin damage and antibody in cerebrospinal fluid to myelin basic protein may be concurrently demonstrated. The influence of released antigen or provoked immune response on the perpetuation of demyelinating disease remains a possibility, although neither is specific for multiple sclerosis.

Consideration of pathogenesis of Multiple Sclerosis

It is possible to relate some of the foregoing observations to provide a framework for speculative, but not conclusive, statements about the etiology or pathogenesis of the tissue injury in multiple sclerosis. It has been particularly difficult to determine which events are primary and which are secondary to the disease. There is no evidence that the central nervous system myelin unit of multiple sclerosis patients is intrinsically abnormal, rendering it more susceptible to injury. It is assumed that the initial occurrence involves damage to the central nervous system myelin sheath or to the oligodendrocyte. Although cellular and humoral immunity against both can be detected in multiple sclerosis patients, such immunity is not disease specific. Nor has a virus or viral component been convincingly demonstrated, although antibodies to rubeola and to other viruses are produced within the central nervous system. Whether the initial tissue injury precedes or follows the arrival of infiltrating hematogenous cells or activation of resident cells of the central nervous system is also unknown. Mononuclear cells are evident, especially in a perivascular location in acute lesions, and phagocytosis of myelin is followed by degradation of proteins and lipids. Released myelin components, such as myelin basic protein, can be detected in cerebrospinal fluid and could participate in the stimulation of a humoral or cellular immune response directed at the central nervous system myelin unit. During these events, astrocytes presumably proliferate and invading lymphocytes transform into plasma cells. Although remyelination takes place in the central nervous system of certain mammalian laboratory animals and in the human peripheral nervous system, it is very limited in the human central nervous system.

DISEASE MANAGEMENT

Therapeutic approaches in multiple sclerosis may involve interference with demyelination, enhancement of remyelination, or promotion of the function of demyelinated axons. Most efforts to date have been directed at changing immune function, based on the premise that an immunological attack on myelin of the central nervous system is present. At the present time most therapy is designed to suppress the immune system, but stimulation of the immune system has also been advocated. These contrasting approaches reflect the lack of fundamental knowledge about the etiology and pathogenesis of multiple sclerosis. A variety of immunosuppressive and immunopotentiating substances has been tried, but there is no evidence that any of these alters the overall course of the disease. A randomized trial has shown that adrenocorticotrophic hormone produced slightly more rapid recovery from exacerbations of the disease, but there was no long-term benefit when compared to placebo.

Although the natural history of multiple sclerosis cannot be altered, infections and metabolic disturbances in patients with the disease are frequent and require careful medical management. Any elevation in body temperature may produce a profound worsening that is not caused by the disease itself and that therefore should subisde once the infection or metabolic disturbance is corrected. It is also possible to treat certain of the symptoms that often trouble patients with multiple sclerosis. Flexor spasms may be treated with spasmolytic agents such as baclofen. Urinary bladder dysfunction, a very common and debilitating problem in many patients, should be assessed by urodynamic testing so that therapy can be directed at the cause of the urinary disturbance, i.e., failure to store urine or to empty the bladder. The paroxysmal problems of pain and tonic spasms sometimes respond to anticonvulsants. Symptoms are likely to become worse with fatigue (Chap. 1), so careful planning of daily activities is important. Assistance from physical and occupational therapists is very helpful in enabling patients with the disease to function as effectively as possible despite their disabilities.

SUMMARY

Multiple sclerosis is a primary demyelinating disease of the central nervous system. Both environmental and host factors appear to play a role in its etiology. The environmental effect is exerted years before the appearance of the disease. The genetic effect may be exerted through the immune system. The most consistent immunological abnormalities in multiple sclerosis are a hyperimmune in situ response within the central nervous system and defective immunoregulation. An autoantigenic protein is a component of normal myelin and may also be related. Symptomatic therapy is available, but there is as yet no treatment to alter the natural history of the disease.

GENERAL REFERENCES

Allen, I. V. The pathology of multiple sclerosis. *Neuropath. Appl. Neurobiol.* 7:169–82, 1981.

Eldridge, R., H. McFarland, J. Sever, D. Sadowsky, and H. Krebs. Familial multiple sclerosis: clinical, histocompatibility, and viral serological studies. *Ann. Neurol.* 3:72–80, 1978.

Itoyama, Y., N. H. Sternberger, H. DeF. Webster, R. H. Quarles, S. R. Cohen, and E. P. Richardson. Immunocytochemical observations on the distribution of myelin-associated glycoprotein and myelin basic protein in multiple sclerosis lesions. *Ann. Neurol.* 7:167–77, 1980.

Kurtzke, J. F. Epidemiological contributions to multiple sclerosis: an overview. *Neurology* 30:61–79, 1980.

Mattson, D. H., R. P. Roos, and B. G. W. Arnason. Isoelectric focusing of IgG eluted from multiple sclerosis and subacute sclerosing panencephalitis brains. *Nature* 287:335–7, 1980.

Norton, W. T. Formation, structure, and biochemistry of myelin. In *Basic Neurochemistry*, G. J. Siegel, R. W. Albers, B. W. Agranoff, and R. Katzman (eds.). Boston, Little, Brown 1981, pp. 63–92.

Poser, S., J. Wikstrom, and H. J. Bauer. Clinical data and the identification of special forms of multiple sclerosis in 1271 cases studied with a standardized documentation system. *J. Neurol. Sci.* 40:159–68, 1979.

Reinherz, E. H., H. L. Weiner, S. L. Hauser, J. A. Cohen, J. A. Distaso, and S. F. Schlossman. Loss of suppressor T cells in active multiple sclerosis. *N. Eng. J. Med.* 303:125–9, 1980.

Waksman, B. H. Current trends in multiple sclerosis research. *Immunology Today* 1:87–93, 1981.

Whitaker, J. N. The distribution of myelin basic protein in central nervous system lesions of multiple sclerosis and acute experimental allergic encephalomyelitis. *Ann. Neurol.* 3:291–8, 1978.

Whitaker, J. N. and D. S. Synder. Myelin components in the cerebrospinal fluid in diseases affecting central nervous system myelin. *Clin. Allergy Immunol.* 2:469–82, 1982.

15.

Stroke

WILLIAM J. POWERS and MARCUS E. RAICHLE

Stroke is the third most common cause of death in the United States and has been estimated to cost as much as $7 billion a year in medical expenses and time lost from work. This chapter will consider the way in which the brain responds to disturbances in its normal circulation and the disease processes that cause those disturbances. In order to understand these concepts, the normal circulation and metabolism of the brain are reviewed first.

ANATOMY OF THE CEREBRAL CIRCULATION

Arterial blood flows to the brain by way of three major vascular trees: the right and left internal carotid arteries, which supply the anterior two-thirds of the corresponding hemisphere, and the vertebral-basilar system, which carries blood to the brainstem and the posterior parts of both hemispheres. The internal carotid arteries are formed in the neck by the bifurcation of the common carotid arteries into internal and external branches. The external carotid artery supplies blood to the soft tissues of the neck, eye, face, and scalp. From their origin, the internal carotid arteries

travel upwards and enter the base of the skull through the foramen lacerum. After a serpentine course through the petrous bone, they emerge intracranially to lie on either side of the sella turcica and pituitary gland. Here the arteries make an S-shaped bend (the carotid siphon) and give a major branch to the eye, the ophthalmic artery. Each carotid then divides into two major branches: the anterior cerebral artery and the middle cerebral artery (Fig. 15–1). The anterior cerebral artery runs medially and then superiorly, supplying the undersurface of the frontal lobe and the cortical gray matter in the interhemispheric fissure. The representation of the contralateral lower extremity in the primary motor and sensory cortex are included in the vascular territory of this artery (Fig. 15–2).

The middle cerebral artery courses laterally from the bifurcation and immediately gives rise to a series of small penetrating branches called the lenticulostriate arteries (Fig. 15–1). These supply the deep gray and white matter structures of the hemisphere, including the basal ganglia and the fiber tracts descending from the cortex to form the internal capsule. The middle

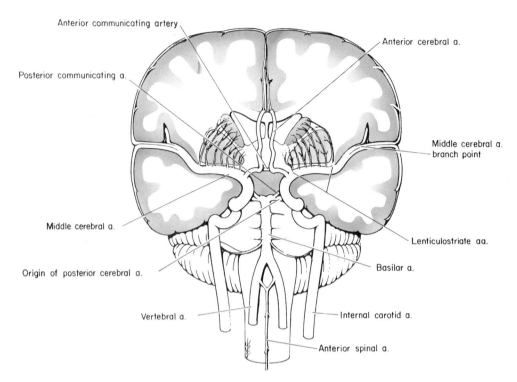

Anterior communicating artery

Posterior communicating a.

Middle cerebral a.

Origin of posterior cerebral a.

Vertebral a.

Anterior cerebral a.

Middle cerebral a.
branch point

Lenticulostriate aa.

Basilar a.

Internal carotid a.

Anterior spinal a.

Fig. 15–1. Coronal section through the front of the brain with the anterior portions of the frontal and temporal lobes removed. The major vessels of the posterior circulation (vertebrals and basilar arteries) and anterior circulation (internal carotid, middle and anterior cerebral arteries) can be seen. Note that these two circulations are potentially one circulation due to the interconnections of the vessels at the base of the brain, called the Circle of Willis (see also Fig. 15–2). Note also the vessels coming off the proximal third of the middle cerebral artery. These lenticulostriate vessels are often damaged by hypertension causing infarction or hemorrhage into the caudate, putamen, and internal capsule.

cerebral artery then runs farther laterally into the Sylvian fissure, where it divides into several major branches that carry blood to the lateral surface of the frontal, parietal, and temporal lobes (Fig. 15–3). Thus, the middle cerebral artery supplies the primary motor and sensory cortex (except for the leg area), the speech areas in the dominant hemisphere, and the deep hemispheric white matter. The latter includes the motor and sensory fibers from all cortical areas as well as the visual fibers running from the geniculate bodies to the occipital cortex.

The vertebral arteries arise from the subclavian arteries at the base of the neck and run upward through bony foramina in the cervical vertebrae to enter the skull through the foramen magnum. Branches from the intracranial vertebral arteries supply the upper cervical spinal cord, the medulla, and the inferior cerebellum. The two vertebral arteries join at the level of the ponto-medullary junction and form the basilar artery, which lies on the ventral surface of the brainstem, supplying blood to the pons, cerebellum, and midbrain (Fig. 15–1). At the level of the midbrain, just

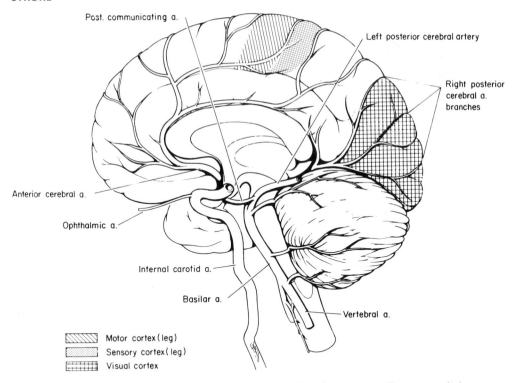

Post. communicating a.

Left posterior cerebral artery

Right posterior cerebral a. branches

Anterior cerebral a.

Ophthalmic a.

Internal carotid a.

Basilar a.

Vertebral a.

Motor cortex (leg)
Sensory cortex (leg)
Visual cortex

Fig. 15–2. Medial aspect of the hemisphere after the corpus callosum, medial thalamus, and midbrain have been sectioned to remove the other hemisphere. The anterior cerebral artery runs from the internal carotid to the posterior third of the corpus callosum. The posterior cerebral artery runs from the top of the basilar artery to the occipital cortex and also supplies the posterior third of the corpus callosum. Note the small posterior communicating artery that joins the posterior cerebral (posterior circulation) to the internal carotid (anterior circulation). Note also the circumferential branches of the basilar artery that supply the lateral aspects of the brainstem and cerebellum.

above the tentorium cerebelli, the basilar artery bifurcates into the two posterior cerebral arteries. After giving off small branches to the medial temporal lobes and thalami, each posterior cerebral artery sweeps backward to supply the occipital lobes (Fig. 15–2). Thus, the vertebrobasilar system supplies the entire brainstem (including the cranial nerve nuclei and motor and sensory tracts bilaterally), both thalami, the medial surfaces of the temporal lobes, and the primary and associative visual cortex in the occipital lobes (Fig. 15–2).

If the flow through any of these major vascular trees is compromised, the area of

brain deprived of blood must be able to be supplied via alternate pathways or suffer permanent damage. Three major potential collateral pathways are available. The most important of these is the Circle of Willis (Fig. 15–1), formed by the posterior communicating arteries (which connect the posterior cerebral and internal carotid arteries) and by the anterior communicating artery (which connects the anterior cerebral arteries). These communicating arteries allow blood to circulate between the three major vascular trees at the base of the brain. Thus, the circle of Willis provides a potential route for blood to bypass a stenosis or obstruction occur-

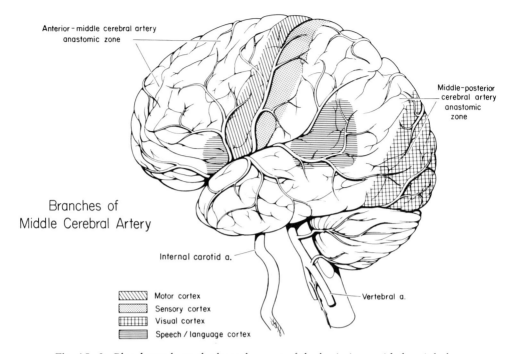

Branches of
Middle Cerebral Artery

Anterior-middle cerebral artery
anastomic zone

Middle-posterior
cerebral artery
anastomic
zone

Internal carotid a.

Vertebral a.

▨ Motor cortex
▦ Sensory cortex
▥ Visual cortex
▤ Speech / language cortex

Fig. 15–3. Blood supply to the lateral aspect of the brain is provided mainly by the middle cerebral artery. Note the anastomotic zones ("watershed areas") between the middle cerebral and anterior cerebral arteries anteriorly and superiorly, and between the middle and posterior cerebral arteries posteriorly.

ring in the neck. However, one or more of these communicating arteries may be absent or nonfunctional in as much as one-third of the population. An anastomosis between the extracranial and the intracranial circulations forms another major collateral pathway. Branches of the external carotid arteries supplying the orbit anastomose with branches of the ophthalmic artery, and branches of the external carotid artery supplying the muscles of the scalp posteriorly anastomose with branches of the vertebral artery. These channels can enlarge to provide a significant amount of blood flow to the brain, especially in situations where flow in the cerebral vessels decreases gradually. The third available collateral pathway consists of end-to-end arterial anastomoses of the superficial cortical branches of the anterior, middle, and posterior cerebral arter-

ies where their vascular territories abut, the so-called watershed or border zone areas (Fig. 15–3). The effectiveness of all of these collateral pathways is variable and, to a degree, will determine the amount of damage to the brain that will result when blood flow in a major vessel is decreased.

The venous drainage of the brain can be separated into a superficial and a deep system (Fig. 15–4). The surface of the hemispheres are drained by superficial veins flowing into the superior sagittal sinus. The underside of the brain and deep structures are drained by a series of veins that eventually unite to form the straight sinus. This vessel joins the superior sagittal sinus at the confluence of sinuses or the torcular Herophili. Flow from the torcular divides into the right and left lateral sinuses, proceeding through the jugular foramina in the base of the skull to form the internal

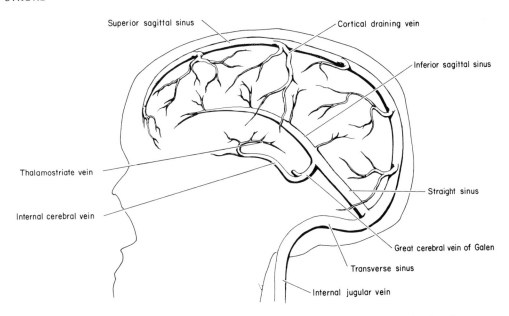

Fig. 15–4. Venous drainage from the brain proceeds through a superficial and a deep system. The hemispheres drain superiorly into the superior sagittal sinus. Deep aspects of the hemisphere and the thalamus drain into the straight sinus. These join to form the two lateral, then two sigmoid sinuses, which ultimately form the internal jugular veins.

jugular veins in the neck. Collateral pathways exist both within and between the superficial and deep systems.

PHYSIOLOGY OF THE CEREBRAL CIRCULATION

The normal adult brain receives 20% of cardiac output, resulting in an average cerebral blood flow of 750 ml per minute, or 50 ml per 100 g brain per minute. Further analysis of cerebral blood flow data reveals a fast-flow component of approximately 70–80 ml per 100 g per minute and a slow component of 20–30 ml per 100 g per minute. The former has been related to flow through gray matter and the latter to flow through white matter.

Factors affecting cerebral blood flow

Blood Pressure. In a normal adult human, cerebral blood flow is kept very constant over a wide range of perfusion pressures. This phenomenon is known as *autoregulation.* When systemic blood pressure falls cerebral vessels automatically dilate, keeping blood flow constant. Conversely, with high systemic pressure cerebral blood vessels constrict. Perfusion pressure in the brain represents the difference between the mean arterial blood pressure and the intracranial pressure plus the venous pressure. Under normal circumstances, the intracranial pressure and the venous pressure are relatively low compared to arterial blood pressure, and the mean arterial blood pressure is viewed as the effective perfusion pressure. Autoregulation usually fails when the mean arterial blood pressure falls below 60 mm Hg. At this point cerebral arteries are dilated maximally. The exact mechanism by which cerebral vessels dilate when perfusion pressure falls and constrict when perfusion pressure rises is complicated. Neurogenic, myogenic, and metabolic factors all play a role. Autoregulation is constantly changing and is of major importance for maintaining metabolic and physiologic homeostasis. Not only does it protect the brain from changes in perfusion pressure due to changes in body posture, but it also protects against narrowing or occlusion of major vessels in the neck, increased intracranial pressure, and decreased cardiac output. Of note, autoregulation is lost in areas of acute ischemia, necessitating meticulous control of blood pressure in patients with stroke to avoid further injury to the brain.

Carbon Dioxide. Carbon dioxide is a potent vasodilator of cerebral blood vessels. A 1 mm Hg change in the partial pressure of arterial carbon dioxide produces a 2% change in the cerebral blood flow. This provides a link between brain metabolism and blood flow, since the end product of oxidative metabolism is carbon dioxide. The action of carbon dioxide on the cerebral vessels, however, appears to be mediated by changes induced in the perivascular concentration of hydrogen ions rather than by a direct action of carbon dioxide on the vascular wall. Carbon dioxide is hydrated by carbonic anhydrase to form carbonic acid, which provides the hydrogen ion. In addition, the local accumulation of such acidic metabolic end products as lactate and pyruvate lowers the perivascular pH to produce vascular dilation and increase flow. As a result, local increases in the functional activity of the brain are associated with local increases in cerebral blood flow.

Oxygen. Although essential for the functioning and survival of the brain, oxygen has only a modest effect on cerebral circulation compared to carbon dioxide. Arterial oxygen tensions greater than 50 mm Hg have no measurable effect on cerebral circulation. Tensions below this level appear to have a vasodilator action. When arterial oxygen tension remains above 50 mm Hg, the nervous system is able to

maintain a constant supply of oxygen by adjusting the amount of oxygen extracted from the blood to changes in cerebral blood flow. As hypoxemia becomes severe there is an acceleration of anaerobic glycolysis in brain. Lactic acid accumulates and the subsequent pH shift causes vasodilation and increase in flow.

Glucose. This primary substrate for brain metabolism has no effect on cerebral blood flow. A blood glucose level low enough to produce deep coma is not associated with any change in cerebral blood flow.

Autonomic Nervous System. Nerve fibers, both adrenergic and cholinergic, supply cerebral blood vessels. A wide variety of physiological and anatomical studies of this system have, to date, produced conflicting results, and its role in the regulation of cerebral blood flow remains an enigma. Recent studies indicate that sympathetic nerve fibers to cerebral blood vessels can serve a protective function. Sudden increases in systemic arterial blood pressure can produce disruption of the blood-brain barrier in animals in whom the sympathetic nerves to cerebral blood vessels have been removed.

Blood Viscosity. Marked increases in blood viscosity may decrease cerebral blood flow. Observations on some patients with polycythemia vera, which inceases viscosity, have found a decrease in cerebral blood flow. However, this observation has not been confirmed experimentally even though a variety of means has been employed to change blood viscosity. Changes in blood flow and symptoms of cerebral ischemia in patients with polycythemia may well be related to changes in oxygen delivery rather than blood viscosity.

Temperature. Changes in temperature do not affect cerebral blood flow when body temperature remains in the range of 35° to 40°C. Below 35°C, cerebral blood flow has been shown to decrease 7% per degree change in temperature; between 40° and 42°C, it increases 30%–50%. These changes in cerebral blood flow are probably related to alterations in metabolism as a consequence of changing temperature.

Under normal circumstances, the cerebral blood flow is sufficient for the brain's metabolic needs. Sudden increases in metabolic requirements, such as those that occur with seizures, are met by increases in cerebral blood flow. Conversely, when cerebral blood flow is decreased, the brain merely extracts more oxygen and glucose per unit volume of blood. The brain's metabolic rate will thus continue to be normal with decreasing blood flow, until so much oxygen has been extracted that the cerebral venous oxygen tension falls to about 20 mm Hg. To reach this value, the cerebral blood flow must fall to less than 50% of the normal value. At this point, the oxygen tension in the brain tissue remote from capillaries falls to levels that will no longer maintain metabolism. This 50% margin of safety is obviously reduced when insufficient oxygen reaches the blood, e.g., under conditions of high altitude, alveolar hypoventilation, pulmonary disease, or when the oxygen-carrying capacity of blood is reduced by anemia, methemoglobinemia, or carbon monoxide poisoning.

PATHOPHYSIOLOGY OF CEREBRAL VASCULAR DISEASE

Damage to the brain as a result of cerebral vascular disease can be divided into two major categories: (i) insufficient blood supply to meet the metabolic needs, i.e., ischemia or infarction, and (ii) hemorrhage. Although there are many causes for each of these, the mechanism of injury to the tissue in each case is very similar.

Ischemia/infarction

As described in the preceding sections, four factors protect the CNS against focal or generalized reduction in substrate supply: (i) anastomoses within the arterial tree, primarily at the circle of Willis; (ii) autoregulation of blood flow in response to changes in perfusion pressure; (iii) increased cerebral blood flow; and (iv) increased extraction of glucose and oxygen from the perfusing blood. At times of generalized circulatory crises, these mechanisms are supplemented by systemic adjustments in blood flow that redistribute blood to the CNS from other regions of the body. Despite this physiological insurance, cerebral blood flow and arterial concentrations of oxygen and glucose fail to meet tissue metabolic needs under a variety of circumstances. The general consequences of this failure are discussed in this section.

The consequences of nutritional deprivation of the CNS, whether the result of interference with the supply of nutrients (hypoxia or hypoglycemia) or their delivery (ischemia), are similar in many respects. When neural tissue is deprived of oxygen or glucose the functional and structural changes that can occur depend on the duration of the insult. When hypoxia or ischemia persists for less than a minute, as might occur with vasodepressor syncope, postural hypotension, or decreased cardiac output (Stokes-Adams attack), clinical signs of impaired function (loss of consciousness, generalized convulsions, pupillary dilation, and loss of EEG activity) may be transient. When oxygen deprivation lasts longer, neurons in the affected area ultimately undergo necrosis; pyramidal cells of the neocortex, the hippocampus, and the Purkinje cells of the cerebellum are most sensitive. Often these changes are multifocal, relatively small, widely separated, and recognized only by microscopy. If oxygen deprivation is more severe or prolonged, the cerebral cortex may appear narrowed and show microscopic evidence of pseudolaminar necrosis. In this state there is relative preservation of the superficial and deep cortical

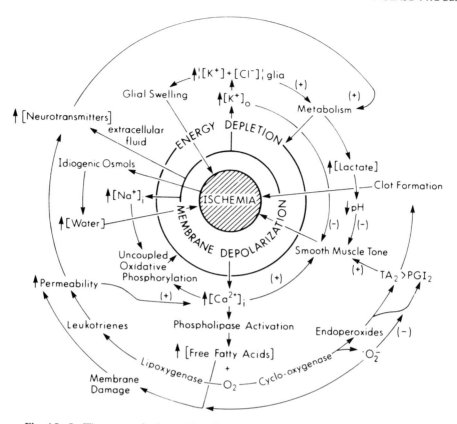

Fig. 15–5. Tissue metabolic and biochemical events produced in brain tissue by ischemia. The temporal sequence of primary events is depicted in a radial fashion beginning at the center of the figure. Interrelationships are depicted circumferentially. Those involving stimulation are indicated by $(+)$ and those resulting from inhibition by $(-)$. TA_2, thromboxane A_2; PGI_2, prostacyclin; O_2^-, the superoxide anion radical.

layers with necrosis of middle layers. White matter may show demyelination or necrosis. If still more severe or prolonged hypoxia occurs, a relatively large area of gray and white matter will undergo complete necrosis (infarction). When cardiac arrest results in diffuse brain ischemia for longer than 4 minutes neurological damage invariably occurs. Patients who eventually awake are often demented, or show multifocal deficits, some with seizures. Others never truly regain consciousness, but remain in a persistent vegetative state with only brainstem function.

Many factors contribute to irreversible ischemic cell damage. Identification of these cytotoxic factors is crucial to developing a rational approach to the protection of brain threatened by ischemia. What emerges from a review of the literature is a complex picture of interacting and cascading events that tend to reinforce the initial ischemic insult and initiate biochemical reactions that ultimately destroy vital cellular elements (Fig. 15–5). Briefly summarized, these events are as follows: Interruption of cerebral blood flow results in loss of consciousness within 10 seconds and cessation of spontaneous and evoked electrical activity within 20 seconds. Within several minutes after the loss of electrical activity there are major disruptions of normal tissue ion homeostasis. Ion-sensitive microelectrodes placed in the extracellular fluid space of the brain record a marked increase in potassium concentration and a fall in sodium and calcium concentrations. The movement of sodium and calcium into the cell plus the release of calcium from mitochondria and endoplasmic reticulum results in a substantial rise in both the intracellular sodium and free calcium concentrations. Two important biochemical events occur as a result of anaerobic metabolism of glucose in ischemic brain tissue. First, energy stores of the tissue (i.e., phosphocreatine and adenylate energy charge) are depleted. Second, lactic acid is produced in excessive amounts and accumulates in the tissue, leading to cellular acidosis. Finally, alterations in the blood-brain barrier also occur. With the exception of the loss of consciousness and electrical activity, all these events are thought to have important implications for cell survival.

Several specific features should be emphasized because of the important implication they may ultimately have in the management of patients. First, a disturbance in calcium homeostasis within the ischemic cell may be a critical feature in producing ultimate death of the cell, although the exact biochemical and metabolic events initiated by calcium remain to be determined. Second, cellular acidosis due to accumulation of lactate within ischemic tissue appears to have a deleterious effect. Excessive accumulation of lactate may, in fact, contribute directly to irreversible cell damage. This fact may have important implications for the management of patients. Thus, in the adult, elevated blood glucose levels preceding infarction may well predispose to a worse outcome because higher tissue glucose levels lead to a greater accumulation of lactate when the brain must resort to anaerobic glycolysis. On the other hand, anoxemic infants may benefit from administration of glucose because of their increased capacity to clear metabolically produced lactate from the tissue. Third, a variety of factors initiated by ischemia appears, in turn, to contribute to further tissue damage. These include the rise in extracellular potassium concentration, which paradoxically stimulates metabolism while further impeding substrate delivery by causing cell swelling; the release of neurotransmitters capable of stimulating metabolism; and the release of a variety of vasoactive substances capable of disrupting blood flow in relation to the metabolic needs of the tissue.

Hemorrhage

The effect of intracranial hemorrhage on the brain is due to two very disparate mechanisms. The first is simply the action of blood as a mass. When an artery ruptures intracranially, a volume of blood under pressure is suddenly introduced into an enclosed, poorly distensible space. This leads to a sudden rise in intracranial pressure that may transiently impede all arterial inflow. If the bleeding occurs into the substance of the brain rather than solely into the subarachnoid space, the mass of blood will destroy cerebral tissue and produce a localized neurological deficit. This intracerebral blood clot also acts as a mass lesion and, if large enough, can cause transtentorial or tonsillar herniation and death. Blood under high pressure may enter into the ventricular system directly, leading to coma and death within minutes to hours. The fatal result of blood entering the ventricular system is thought to be due to a mechanical insult transmitted to the brainstem rather than the kind of irritative effect seen in subarachnoid hemorrhage. Two observations support this view. First, the sudden injection of saline into the lateral ventricles of dogs creates acute pressure gradients between the anterior and posterior fossa, which produce rapid medullary failure, whereas similar injections over the surface of the hemisphere have no such effect. Second, blood experimentally introduced into the ventricular system fails to elicit the prominent chemical meningitis seen with similar injections into the subarachnoid space.

The second effect of intracranial bleeding is due to the irritative effect of the blood itself. Bleeding into the subarachnoid space causes a sterile inflammation of the meninges accompanied by varying degrees of headache, fever, and stiff neck together with pleocytosis, high protein and low glucose concentrations in the cerebrospinal fluid. Cerebral arterial spasm is a less common, but more serious, complication of subarachnoid hemorrhage. Spasm most commonly occurs following rupture of saccular (berry) aneurysms, and rarely after hemorrhage caused by head trauma or arteriovenous malformations. After a delay of several hours or a few days, the larger cerebral arteries may go into spasm that can persist for several weeks. This spasm can be severe enough to cause large cerebral infarctions. The pathophysiologic mechanism is uncertain, but most likely involves vasoconstrictive substances generated by the extravasated blood. Serotonin, prostaglandins, angiotensin, and histamine have all been proposed as etiologic agents.

DISEASES CAUSING STROKE

Ischemia/infarction

Cerebral infarction is the most common type of stroke, comprising 80%–90% of most series. The specific causes of arterial ischemia and infarction can be divided into two general categories: those that cause global ischemia (a decrease in blood flow to the entire brain) and those that cause focal ischemia (a decrease in blood flow to a specific area within the brain).

Global ischemia or infarction is caused by diseases that decrease the systemic blood pressure either by lowering cardiac output or by decreasing systemic vascular resistance (Table 15–1). These are rare causes

Table 15–1. Causes of global cerebral ischemia

Decreased cardiac output
  Cardiac arrest
  Cardiac arrhythmias
  Valvular heart disease
  Myocardial failure
  Pulmonary embolism
  Vasovagal syncope
  Hypovolemic shock

Decreased peripheral vascular resistance
  Autonomic insufficiency (including drugs)
  Vasovagal syncope
  Septic shock

---

of stroke. Even in people with stenosis of the internal carotid arteries, a decrease in systemic blood pressure will usually cause loss of consciousness rather than focal cerebral infarction. There are occasional well-documented cases, however, in which a decrease in blood pressure causes persistent neurological deficits in the territory supplied by a stenotic artery. More commonly, a period of hypotension will cause infarction in the watershed or border zone areas between the major vascular territories. If the ischemia is moderate, focal infarction of these areas may result. If the ischemia is severe and prolonged, infarction of the entire brain can occur.

The most common cause of focal cerebral ischemia and infarction is atherosclerosis (Table 15–2). It causes 60%–70% of all strokes and over three-quarters of cerebral infarctions. The prevalence of atherosclerosis of the major cerebral vascular trees increases with age, occurring earlier in life in men than in women. It has a predilection for certain sites. In the carotid circulation, the most common site is the first few centimeters of the internal carotid artery in the neck. The next most common site is the carotid siphon. In the vertebrobasilar circulation, atherosclerosis most commonly occurs at the origin of the vertebral arteries in the neck, in the distal intracranial portion of the vertebral arteries, and in the basilar artery. Ather-

Table 15–2. Causes of focal cerebral ischemia

Cervical-cerebral vascular disease

Atherosclerosis	Arterial hyalinosis
Fibromuscular dysplasia	Arterial dissection
Vascular trauma	Migraine
Vasospasm	Meningitis: syphilitic, tuberculous, fungal, bacterial
Vasculitis: giant cell (temporal) arteritis, granu-	Connective tissue diseases: Ehlers-Danlos, pseu-
lomatous angiitis, polyarteritis, systemic lu-	doxanthoma elasticum
pus erythematosis	Metabolic diseases: homocystinuria, Fabry's dis-
	ease

Systemic embolism

Valvular heart disease: cogenital, rheumatic, mitral valve prolapse, prosthetic, infective endocarditis, non-
bacterial thrombotic (marantic) endocarditis
Cardiac thrombus: myocardial infarction, atrial fibrillation, ventricular aneurysm, cardiomyopathy
Paradoxical
Tumor embolism
Fat embolism
Air embolism

Hematologic disorders

Oral contraceptives, pregnancy, puerperium
Thrombocytosis
Hyperviscosity
Sickle cell disease
Thrombotic thrombocytopenic purpura
Paroxysmal nocturnal hemoglobinuria
Inflammatory bowel disease

---

osclerosis distal to the circle of Willis is uncommon, but does occur, particularly in the stem of the middle cerebral artery.

Many pathological and radiographic studies have shown an association between atherosclerosis of the internal carotid artery and infarction in the territory of the middle cerebral artery or atherosclerosis of the vertebrobasilar system and infarction in the brainstem or occipital lobes. Atherosclerosis can cause infarction either by producing sufficient stenosis to cause a decrease in blood flow or by serving as a source for emboli that are carried distally until they cause occlusion of smaller intracranial vessels. Since the cross-sectional area of a vessel must be decreased to a few square millimeters before flow is diminished, decrease in flow is a viable explanation only in those cases with severe stenosis or total occlusion. Such severe disease is unusual. A more common finding in people with recent hemispheric strokes is slight to moderate stenosis or an ulcerated plaque in the carotid artery. This is sometimes associated with occlusion of one or more small intracerebral arteries, suggesting emboli. Several fortuitous observations of retinal and cortical arteries have disclosed emboli that are composed of either platelet-fibrin thrombi or atheromatous debris. Thus, the major cause of atherosclerotic ischemia and infarction in the carotid circulation appears to be emboli, predominantly composed of platelets, which originate from atherosclerotic plaques. The vertebrobasilar circulation is somewhat different. Since small branches of these arteries run directly to the brain substance, the atherothrombotic process of the major vessels can cause occlusion at the origin of these branches as well as embolization.

The association between atherosclerosis and cerebral infarction, while common, is not invariable. There are many people with severe atherosclerosis of the carotid and vertebrobasilar arteries who never develop cerebral ischemia or infarction. Those factors that determine when atherosclerotic plaques will produce cerebral ischemia remain poorly understood.

Several theories have been advanced to explain the evolution of these plaques from asymptomatic to symptomatic lesions. Atherosclerosis decreases the capacity of arterial walls to synthesize prostacyclin, a prostanoid with a potent, antiaggregatory action on platelets. When the synthesis of prostacyclin is sufficiently inhibited, the plaque may become thrombogenic. Others have proposed that sudden hemorrhage into the plaque is linked to the occurrence of symptoms, either by exposing the thrombogenic internal contents of the plaque or by causing a sudden decrease in the luminal size with a corresponding drop in flow. Similarly, disease progression may result in a change from a predominately smooth, fibrous lesion to a friable, ulcerated, thrombogenic one. The amount of atherosclerosis elsewhere may also be an important determinant. Stenosis in other cerebral vessels may prevent adequate collateral circulation to an area of the brain rendered ischemic by low flow or emboli, and thus contribute to the occurrence of symptoms.

Other causes of cerebral ischemia and infarction are listed in Table 15–2. Although the etiologies vary widely, the end result to the cerebral tissue is the same: lack of an adequate blood supply to meet the metabolic needs. These other causes may be divided into three general groups: those due to primary disease of the cerebral blood vessels, those due to emboli to the brain from other sources, and those due to disorders of the blood itself. After atherosclerosis, the second most common cause of cerebral infarction due to primary arterial disease is arterial hyalinosis. This is a degenerative disease of small arteries within the brain caused by chronic hypertension. It results in small infarcts called lacunae, which most commonly occur deep within the hemispheres or brainstem. Among the many causes of cerebral emboli, those arising in the heart are of the most clinical importance, comprising 10%–15% of all cerebral infarcts. Primary diseases of the blood are rare causes of stroke and produce cerebral ischemia by causing intravascular thrombosis or decreases in blood flow due to increased viscosity.

Table 15–3. Causes of cerebral venous infarction

Infective
  Chronic otitis media
  Orbital cellulitis
  Meningitis

Noninfective
  Pregnancy, puerperium, oral contraceptives
  Dehydration
  Trauma
  Neurosurgery
  Tumor invasion
  Nonmetastatic effect of cancer
  Inflammatory bowel disease
  Sickle cell anemia
  Paroxysmal nocturnal hemoglobinuria
  Polycythemia

Obstruction of the cerebral venous drainage can also produce infarction. The resultant rise in venous pressure leads to a decrease in perfusion pressure, thus causing tissue ischemia. Causes of cerebral venous infarction are commonly divided into infective and noninfective etiologies (Table 15–3). Infection of the middle ear and mastoid region can spread through the bone to the adjacent lateral sinus or internal jugular vein producing thrombosis. This complication of ear infection is becoming less common as the incidence of chronic otitis declines. Abnormalities of blood clotting now account for the majority of cases of cerebral venous thrombosis. The most common of these is produced by the changes that accompany pregnancy, the puerperium, and use of oral contraceptives.

Hemorrhage

Intracranial hemorrhage due to cerebral vascular disease is much less common than cerebral infarction, comprising only 10%–20% of all strokes. Of these, the vast ma-

Table 15–4. Causes of cerebral hemorrhage

Primary intracerebral (hypertensive) hemorrhage
Saccular (berry) aneurysms
Arteriovenous malformations
Infective (mycotic) aneurysms
Vasculitis
Tumor with hemorrhage
Hematologic disorders

jority are due to primary intracerebral hemorrhages, ruptured saccular (berry) aneurysms, and arteriovenous malformations (Table 15–4).

Primary intracerebral hemorrhage accounts for approximately 10% of all strokes. Its pathogenesis is closely linked to that of hypertension. Up to 90% of patients who suffer a primary intracerebral hemorrhage have a past history of high blood pressure. Primary intracerebral hemorrhage has a predilection for certain areas of brain: the basal ganglia, thalamus, cerebellum, and pons being the most commonly affected in that order. The most common associated pathological finding is tiny (up to 2 mm) aneurysms arising from small penetrating arteries in these regions. Rupture of these Charcot-Bouchard aneurysms is the most likely cause of primary intracerebral hemorrhage, although rupture of arterial vessels weakened by hyalinosis may also play a role.

Saccular (berry) aneurysms cause about 10% of all strokes, but are the most common cause of nontraumatic hemorrhage into the subarachnoid space. These are larger than Charcot-Bouchard arterial aneurysms, ranging from several millimeters to several centimeters in size, and occur primarily at the branch points of large vessels at the base of the brain. The most common locations are the anterior communicating artery, the posterior communicating artery, and the branching point of the middle cerebral artery. These aneurysms are sac-like dilatations caused by a defect in the media and internal elastic lamina of the arterial wall. Whether these defects in the wall are congenital or ac-

quired is not certain. When they rupture, bleeding occurs either into the subarachnoid space or into the substance of the brain itself.

Arteriovenous malformations are rarer than saccular aneurysms, accounting for only 5% of subarachnoid hemorrhages, but are the most common cause of nontraumatic subarachnoid hemorrhage before the age of 20. These malformations are congenital, developmental anomalies in which the normal capillary bed between arterial and venous circulations fails to form in one part of the brain. Instead, there is a mass of large, thin-walled vessels carrying arterialized blood under high pressure. These vessels can rupture, causing either subarachnoid or intracerebral hemorrhage. Arteriovenous malformations may also cause seizures, headache, and transient episodes of neurological dysfunction similar to those seen with cerebral ischemia. These latter symptoms have been explained on the basis of a shunting phenomenon, with the flow through the malformation "stealing" blood from adjacent areas of the brain. Arteriovenous malformations may occur anywhere within the brain, but are most common in the frontal and parietal lobes.

CLINICAL FEATURES OF STROKE

The hallmarks of the clinical presentation of stroke of any kind are the sudden onset of a neurological deficit. Other entities such as hypoglycemia, tumor, subdural hematoma, and epilepsy may mimic the clinical presentation of stroke and should always be considered.

The onset of stroke is usually abrupt, with the maximum neurological deficit occurring within a few minutes or at the most, half an hour. Further progression may occur, but also tends to happen in an abrupt stepwise manner rather than as a slow, steady decline. The neurological dysfunction caused by stroke is most often focal, reflecting the involvement of discrete regions of the brain. The major exception to this is the rupture of saccular aneurysms into the subarachnoid space. Rupture of a saccular aneurysm usually produces severe headache, confusion, and lethargy, sometimes with loss of consciousness without evidence of focal brain dysfunction.

The clinical manifestations of cerebral hemorrhage or infarction depend on several factors. More important than the size of the lesion is its location. Lesions less than a cubic centimeter in size that occur in strategic areas such as the internal capsule or brainstem can cause total paralysis or even death. A much larger lesion occurring in another part of the brain, such as the frontal lobe, may produce virtually no symptoms. However, both large infarcts with significant edema and large hemorrhages can cause herniation and death regardless of their location. The actual size of the cerebral infarction will be determined to a great extent by the adequacy of collateral circulation. Since this is highly variable, internal carotid artery occlusion may produce no infarction at all, or cause infarction of the entire anterior two-thirds of the hemisphere.

Determining which part of the brain is affected by a stroke is very important. Since radiologic investigations may be normal or fail to distinguish between new and old lesions, localization based on the clinical neurological findings is crucial. Ischemia or infarction in the carotid circulation produces motor or sensory deficits on the opposite side of the body. Involvement of the dominant (left) hemisphere often produces abnormalities in language function (aphasia). If the lesion involves the deep white matter, it will cause dysfunction of the face, arm, and leg and may also produce visual field defects. More superficial lesions involving the territory supplied by the middle cerebral artery will spare the leg since the cell bodies in the interhemispheric fissure (supplied by the anterior cerebral artery), as well as the descending

fibers through the internal capsule, will not be involved. Ischemia of the eye, causing transient monocular blindness (amaurosis fugax), can be produced by decreased flow through the ophthalmic artery and is characteristic of carotid artery disease. Ischemia in the vertebrobasilar system characteristically produces signs of brainstem dysfunction with cranial nerve dysfunction and motor or sensory deficits on the opposite side of the body or bilaterally. Visual symptoms may occur with atherosclerosis in the vertebrobasilar system due to low flow through posterior cerebral arteries to the occipital lobes. Cerebellar involvement may produce ataxia. Smaller brainstem strokes can produce unilateral motor or sensory deficits. Thus, unilateral motor or sensory deficits and visual field defects can occur with either carotid or vertebrobasilar lesions. By themselves, they do not provide enough evidence for accurate clinical localization, but neighborhood signs are usually helpful.

The clinical differentiation between cerebral hemorrhage and infarction is much less reliable than the localization of these processes. Although the sudden increase in intracranial pressure that accompanies hemorrhage tends to produce headache, vomiting, and an immediate decrease in the level of consciousness, all of these signs may also be seen with infarction, particularly when it occurs in the vertebrobasilar system. The only accurate way to differentiate hemorrhage from infarction is by CT scan and lumbar puncture.

The temporal course of stroke is somewhat variable. In general, cerebral hemorrhages produce deficits that are maximal immediately and remain stable for the next several days unless herniation, vasospasm, or recurrent bleeding occurs. The course of ischemic deficits is more unpredictable. They may resolve completely, leaving no defect, remain stable, or worsen. If complete clinical resolution occurs within 24 hours, the event is called a transient ischemic attack (TIA). Patients whose ischemic neurological deficit lasts longer than 24 hours are said to have a completed stroke. Some will recover completely and are said to have had a reversible ischemic neurological deficit (RIND). Some patients develop only mild deficits, such as weakness of an extremity rather than complete paralysis, which is called a partial stable stroke or partial completed stroke. Such terms are really misnomers since one-fourth of these patients will become worse in the ensuing week. The mechanism for this progression (stroke in evolution or progressing stroke) is unknown but may involve recurrent embolization, progressive vascular occlusion, thrombus popagating in an already occluded vessel or the ongoing cascade of biochemical events that occur in ischemic tissue.

Functional neurological deficits produced by completed ischemic strokes tend to recover with time. This recovery occurs primarily within the first few months following the stroke. Approximately, one-third of survivors will show major improvement and two-thirds will eventually be capable of functioning independently. The mechanisms responsible for this recovery are poorly understood. The various theories that have been advanced to describe these phenomena can be broadly divided into two groups. The first has to do with alterations in cerebral blood flow and the second to changes occurring within the brain itself. Transient ischemic attacks are most often ascribed to small platelet emboli that occlude a vessel only transiently and then undergo dissolution. The resultant ischemia produces neuronal dysfunction but is not severe enough to cause permanent damage. Thus, when flow is reestablished, function returns. This theory is supported by findings at cerebral arteriography in patients with completed stroke. Embolic occlusions of cerebral vessels are most commonly seen on arteriograms within the first few days and disappear with time. Circulation to an is-

chemic area may also be reestablished by an increase of flow through collateral vessels. This increase may not occur immediately but may develop only over a period of hours or days, perhaps explaining the improvements seen in patients with RIND or completed stroke. Whether or not patients with completed stroke have ischemic regions of brain that will recover function following an increase in blood flow is currently the focus of much research and debate. Neurological recovery may also occur if another part of the brain can assume the functions of the damaged portions. This phenomenon has been documented best in a small group of people who developed aphasia due to infarction of the left cerebral hemisphere, recovered, and then once again became aphasic when a second infarction occurred in the right hemisphere. Although each of these explanations is logical and attractive, the actual mechanisms underlying recovery from stroke remain unknown.

The mortality rate in the early stages of completed stroke depends greatly on the type of cerebral vascular lesion. Approximately 25%–30% of people with cerebral infarction will die during the first 30 days, primarily from either brain herniation or pneumonia. The prognosis for primary intracerebral hemorrhage is much worse. Most series report early mortality rates of 70%–80%. However, these figures antedate the widespread use of CT scanning and probably fail to include smaller hemorrhages with better prognosis. Patients with ruptured saccular aneurysms fare little better. Approximately 20% will die immediately, and another 50% within the next 30 days, primarily due to rebleeding and vasospasm. The prognosis for subarachnoid hemorrhage due to arteriovenous malformation is better, with 80% surviving at the end of the first month.

The long-term prognosis for patients with symptomatic cerebrovascular disease is poor. Of patients with TIAs, 25%–35% will go on to have a stroke within five years;

one-half of these strokes will occur within the first year and one-quarter within the first month. Patients with RIND have a risk of subsequent stroke similar to that for patients with TIA. Patients with a completed cerebral infarction who survive the initial event have approximately a 50% five-year mortality rate. The most common causes of death are heart disease and recurrent stroke. Less information is available about the long-term prognosis in primary cerebral hemorrhage because there are fewer survivors. However, the long-term morbidity and mortality appears to be similar to that for cerebral infarction. Patients who survive rupture of a saccular aneurysm will rebleed at a rate of 3%–4% per year, and two-thirds of these rebleeds will be fatal. Of those who do survive, three-quarters are able to work and only 5%–10% require nursing care. The prognosis for arteriovenous malformation is slightly better, with 85% able to work and less than 5% incapacitated.

CONCLUSIONS

Our understanding of the pathophysiology of stroke is steadily increasing, but the rapidity and complexity of the events that occur with infarction or hemorrhage have made progress in the treatment of acute stroke disappointingly slow. Much more promising results have been obtained when measures have been directed toward preventing stroke. Treatment of chronic hypertension, antithrombotic drug therapy, and carotid artery surgery have all been successful in reducing the occurrence of stroke in patients at high risk.

GENERAL REFERENCES

Jones, H. R., and C. H. Millikan. Temporal profile (clinical course) of acute carotid system cerebral infarction. *Stroke* 7:64–71, 1976.

Jones, H. R., C. H. Millikan, and B. A. Sandok. Temporal profile (clinical course) of acute vertebrobasilar system cerebral infarction. *Stroke* 11:173–7, 1980.

Kontos, H. A. Regulation of the cerebral circulation. *Ann. Rev. Physiol.* 43:397–407, 1981.

Mohr, J. P., L. R. Caplan, J. W. Melski et al. The Harvard Cooperative Stroke Registry: A prospective registry. *Neurology* 28:754–62, 1978.

Raichle, M. E. Pathophysiology of brain ischemia. *Ann. Neurol.* 13:2–10, 1983.

Ross Russell, R. W. (ed.). *Vascular Disease of the Central Nervous System.* New York, Churchill Livingstone, 1983.

Siesjo, B. K. *Brain Energy Metabolism.* New York, Wiley, 1978.

16.

Metabolic Encephalopathy

JOHN C. MORRIS and JAMES A. FERRENDELLI

Normal neuronal activity in the central nervous system relies on the maintenance of an extracellular environment that provides a constant source of essential fuel substrates, is controlled with respect to osmotic, acid–base, and ionic balances, and is safeguarded from potential toxins. In health, these conditions are fully met in brain by the properties of the cerebral circulatory system and the blood-brain barrier (see Chap. 15, 17). However, illnesses that are nonneurologic in origin may nonetheless considerably upset the CNS milieu by affecting, through various means, either the biochemical composition or the intrinsic supply of blood: critical nutrients may be depleted (e.g., hypoxia); homeostatic processes may be overwhelmed (e.g., hypernatremia); endogenous (e.g., uremia) or exogenous (e.g., ethanol ingestion) neurotoxins may be introduced; or cerebral perfusion may be compromised (e.g., cardiac arrest). These changes eventually cause disturbances in neuronal metabolic activity and result in significant neurologic abnormalities. The cerebral impairment, or encephalopathy, produced in this manner is not only an important and frequent sign of underlying

systemic disease, but in some instances may be the primary or sole manifestation of the basic disorder (e.g., hypoglycemic encephalopathy). Despite the diversity of potentially responsible systemic illnesses and intoxications, the fundamental pathogenetic mechanism in all such encephalopathies is a disruption of cerebral metabolic processes. Therefore, the many important neurologic disorders caused by this dysfunction are commonly referred to as the metabolic or toxic-metabolic encephalopathies.

Cerebral metabolic function may be considered at three distinct yet interrelated levels: (i) the subcellular biochemical processes; (ii) the physiological activity of the entire cell; and (iii) the behavior of neuronal systems, ranging from discrete groups to the whole brain. While a wide variety of systemic illnesses and intoxications seemingly cause their neurologic manifestations by disrupting neuronal biochemical mechanisms, the knowledge of the exact molecular disturbances is generally incomplete and much is inferred from the physiological and systems abnormalities. For example, since in most instances neurologic function is completely restored when the underlying disorder is promptly corrected, and because histopathological evidence of fixed neuronal injury is usually absent, the subcellular metabolic lesions responsible for these encephalopathies appear to be fully reversible. Also, because the clinical findings in these disorders almost always indicate bilateral and diffuse cerebral impairment, the biochemical insult presumably affects the entire brain. Differences in sensitivity to the same metabolic derangement may exist among distinct neuronal populations, a phenomenon called selective vulnerability. For example, in Wernicke's disease, the susceptibility to a thiamine deficiency appears restricted to the gray matter in the walls of the third ventricle and specific brainstem regions. Furthermore, focal neurologic deficits (usually nonfixed) are occasionally expressed in the metabolic encephalopathies, albeit perhaps most likely when there is preexisting subclinical cerebral damage.

In general, however, the neurologic syndromes produced by systemic metabolic disorders are characterized by symptoms and signs of diffuse cerebral dysfunction. These tend to appear in an order that mirrors the sensitivity of various regions of the brain to the metabolic insult and initially consist of cortical abnormalities with brainstem involvement occurring later. While frequently found in combination, these manifestations are considered in the following section under four separate headings: (i) altered levels of consciousness; (ii) pupillary and oculomotor dysfunction; (iii) abnormal motor responses; and (iv) disturbances of respiratory control.

CLINICAL MANIFESTATIONS OF THE METABOLIC ENCEPHALOPATHIES
(Table 16–1)

Altered states of consciousness

Consciousness entails not only the total content of thought processes, or cogni-

Table 16–1. Neurologic manifestations of metabolic encephalopathies

---

Altered levels of consciousness
  Clouding of consciousness
  Acute confusional state
  Delirium
  Stupor
  Coma

Oculomotor responses
  Pupillary light reflex: preserved
  Corneal, oculocephalic, and oculovestibular reflexes: generally intact

Motor abnormalities
  Nonspecific
    Paratonia
    Decorticate rigidity
    Decerebrate rigidity
    Flaccidity
  Specific
    Action tremor
    Asterixis
    Myoclonus
    Seizures

Ventilatory disturbances
  Cheyne-Stokes respirations
  Ataxic breathing
  Hyperventilation (Kussmaul breathing)
  Hypoventilation

---

tion, but also the condition of alertness or arousal. Cognitive ability depends in large part on normal activity of the cerebral cortex, whereas alertness and arousal are governed by the activity of the brainstem reticular activating system (see Chap. 10). Perhaps only one normally functioning cerebral hemisphere is required to maintain cognition in the alert state, but consciousness.is not possible without arousal, no matter what the circumstances of the cerebral cortex. Thus, impaired consciousness results from either bilateral hemispheric dysfunction or depression of the reticular activating system, or both. As the cortex is generally more susceptible to metabolic derangements than is the deep gray matter, cognitive disturbances are frequently the initial and possibly the sole manifestation of early or mild metabolic disorders. As the encephalopathic abnormalities progress, the deeper neuronal populations of the brainstem activating structures are affected and the ability to maintain arousal deteriorates and eventually is lost. Within this spectrum, from minor disruption of normal thought processes to inability to arouse the patient, several stages of altered consciousness may be recognized. The first, clouding of consciousness, is expressed by minimal cognitive dysfunction that may be so slight as to escape detection on examination unless carefully compared to the patient's normal intellectual ability and range. Increasingly overt derangements of attentiveness, concentration, orientation, and sensory interpretation are manifested as an acute confusional state. When agitation, hallucinations, and feelings of dread are superimposed in this setting, the clinical picture is called delirium. As the encephalopathy worsens, drowsiness or obtundation becomes apparent and eventually merges into stupor, in which the patient appears to be asleep and is provoked to respond to the environment only by vigorous stimulation. Finally, coma occurs—a deep, sleeplike state—and the patient lacks any organized response to external stimuli. Although a basically stepwise rostral-caudal deterioration through each level of consciousness may be observed with subacute metabolic illnesses, the sudden and dramatic appearance of stupor or coma can be produced by severe disorders, especially those with a rapid course. Therefore, the level of consciousness can serve as a valuable indicator of the severity, rate of progression, and duration of the underlying disease.

Pupillary and oculomotor dysfunction

The response of the pupils to an appropriate light stimulus often provides a reliable means of identifying metabolic encephalopathy from other conditions that alter consciousness. In several specific disorders pupillary reflexes may actually suggest the diagnosis (e.g., opiate intoxication, discussed below). A basic rule is that in metabolic encephalopathy the pupillary light reflexes remain preserved. This rule

generally holds because structural or mass lesions of the brain severe enough to compress the deep reticular activating system and cause changes in consciousness commonly abolish part or all of the pupillary light reflex arc via compressive effects on the third nerve or midbrain (see Chap. 10). However, the absence of the pupillary light reflex does not preclude a metabolic disturbance as the cause. The pupils may be midposition or dilated and fixed to light in instances of severe anoxia, hypothermia, and poisoning with anticholinergic agents or glutethimide.

Again, in contrast to coma from structural cerebral lesions, disturbances of oculomotor function are uncommon in metabolic cerebral depressions, although random or roving conjugate eye movements may be observed. The corneal reflex arc and the oculocephalic responses (doll's eyes) are customarily retained until the patient is deeply comatose, at which point oculovestibular reflexes (cold-water calorics) often still may be elicited (see Chap. 8). Eventually even these responses may be lost in advanced metabolic coma, but the pupillary light reflexes usually remain.

The preservation of the brainstem-mediated corneal, oculocephalic, oculovestibular, and especially pupillary reflexes in comatose patients highlights the relative resistance of these reactions to metabolic depression and provides a useful clinical point of differentiation from structural causes of stupor or coma.

Abnormal motor responses

Several metabolic disorders are associated with specific disturbances in motor function. When present, these motor abnormalities are of great value in the differential diagnosis of an encephalopathic patient. An action tremor commonly occurs in the alcohol and drug withdrawal syndrome. Asterixis, an asynchronous abrupt downward jerking of the hands at the wrists when the arms are outstretched, is frequently encountered in hepatic encephalopathy and is known as "liver flap." However, asterixis may be a manifestation of chronic pulmonary insufficiency and uremic encephalopathy as well. Uremia and anoxia are more commonly associated with multifocal myoclonus. This abnormality consists of arrhythmic, fleeting contractions of muscles or parts of muscles that are often of sufficient force to displace the limb. When permanent cortical damage results from metabolic insult, myoclonic twitching may persist long after the systemic disorder has been corrected. Focal and generalized seizures are most frequently found in anoxic, uremic, and hypoglycemic encephalopathy.

In addition to these characteristic changes in the motor system by different causes of metabolic encephalopathy there are often diffuse or nonspecific changes. Muscle tone is usually increased, exhibited as paratonia, which is defined as fluctuating resistance to passive movement of a limb in all directions. As metabolic encephalopathy worsens patients may exhibit abnormal posturing in response to stimuli, usually rigid extension of arms and legs (decerebrate posturing, see Chap. 10). These postures are more common with structural lesions compressing the brainstem, but have been seen in cases of hepatic encephalopathies, hypoglycemia, or advanced anoxia.

Disturbances of respiratory control

There are two components to the cerebral control of respiration: a cortical-corticospinal tract-spinal respiratory motor neuron system that governs voluntary breathing; and brainstem nuclei that regulate automatic breathing. The major automatic respiratory nucleus is located in the medulla, in the region of the obex, and is made up of a dorsal respiratory group that processes information from glossopharyngeal and vagal afferents and a ventral respiratory group that rhythmically drives the respiratory musculature via vagal and reticulospinal pathways. This brainstem center is also influenced by both peripheral and medullary chemoreceptors that stimulate the respiratory nuclei in conditions of hypoxia, hypercapnea, or acidemia. Metabolic encephalopathies commonly disrupt control of ventilatory function at all levels of organization.

Bilateral hemispheric dysfunction, combined with an heightened sensitivity of brainstem respiratory centers to arterial carbon dioxide tension ($PaCO_2$), produces Cheyne-Stokes respiration. In this disorder an initial hyperventilation is caused by an excessive sensitivity of the medulla to CO_2. Carbon dioxide is blown off until blood carbon dioxide concentration falls below the stimulatory threshold. An apneic state follows until $PaCO_2$ rises to finally reactivate the brainstem centers. Thus, an irregular cycle of hyperventilation followed by a transient apneic phase is created. Damage to brainstem respiratory centers causes both an abnormality of basic respiratory rhythm and a hyposensitivity to chemoreceptor stimulation. This results in ataxic breathing with slow, shallow, irregular respirations that are not increased by either hypoxia or hypercapnea. As the medullary respiratory center is especially sensitive to chemical depression, sedative (particularly opioid) intoxications often result in selective and severe ventilatory depression at relatively early stages of encephalopathy. Conversely, several disorders (e.g., salicylate poisoning; hepatic encephalopathy) directly stimulate the respiratory nuclei to produce hyperventilation and primary respiratory alkalosis.

Ventilatory abnormalities accompanying many metabolic disorders frequently stem not only from interference with cerebral respiratory control mechanisms, but also from coexisting systemic acid–base disturbances. The perpiheral chemoreceptors (carotid bodies) are sensitive to the hydrogen ion concentration (pH) of the blood and stimulate ventilation in conditions of acidemia to increase pulmonary carbon dioxide excretion and return the pH toward normal. This compensatory hyperventilation, or Kussmaul breathing, is a hallmark of the metabolic acidoses, particularly diabetic ketoacidosis and uremia. Metabolic alkalosis occurs secondary to either excessive gastrointestinal or renal acid loss or to ingestion of large quantities of alkali. The alkalosis provokes a compensatory hypoventilation, retention of carbon dioxide, and subsequent lowering of the blood pH.

In summary, altered respiration is almost invariably observed in the metabolic encephalopathies. The Cheyne-Stokes pattern suggests bilateral cerebral hemispheric dysfunction (impaired voluntary control), while ataxic breathing indicates damage to the medullary respiratory centers (impaired automatic control). If hypoxia secondary to pulmonary disease is excluded, hyperventilation represents either direct stimulation of brainstem (e.g., hepatic encephalopathy), or a compensatory response to metabolic acidosis (e.g., uremia). In the absence of severe pulmonary or neuromuscular disease, hypoventilation results from either direct depression of respiratory nuclei (e.g., narcotic poisoning) or from a compensatory reaction to metabolic alkalosis (e.g., alkali ingestion). While combinations of these various alterations do occur (e.g., salicylism produces both a primary respiratory alkalosis and a metabolic acidosis), arterial blood gas determinations combined with assessment of the serum chemistries usually permit the diagnosis of the major component of the ventilatory abnormality.

BASIC ASPECTS OF CEREBRAL METABOLISM

The brain is one of the most metabolically active organs in the body. Neuronal sub-

cellular functions, including anabolic and catabolic processes, active transport of molecules and ions, maintenance of membrane potentials, and transmission of nervous information, proceed at a rate that necessitates a high level of energy utilization—indeed, the highest level of all body tissue. These energy requirements are met by the hydrolysis of high-energy phosphate bonds that are contained in certain molecules, particularly adenosine triphosphate (ATP). In physiologic states, neuronal ATP production, and therefore cerebral energy supply, depends on mitochondrial oxidative phosphorylation that is fueled almost exclusively by the metabolism of glucose.

Oxygen Utilization and Glucose Metabolism

Glucose is rapidly metabolized in nervous tissue, first through the pathway of glycolysis and then through the citric acid cycle (Fig. 16–1). In the cytosol, the anaerobic glycolytic reactions convert each molecule of glucose to pyruvate, generating two molecules of ATP. This level of energy production is inadequate to maintain neuronal activity. Under aerobic conditions, pyruvate enters the mitochondria to undergo oxidation in the citric acid cycle to carbon dioxide and water, with the further generation of 36 molecules of ATP by concomitant oxidative phosphorylation. It is this latter pathway that fulfills cerebral energy requirements and thus underscores the essential role of oxygen in neuronal glucose metabolism and energy production. Metabolites of glucose in the citric acid cycle may also serve as biosynthetic precursors of neurotransmitters, acetyl-CoA for acetylcholine, and amino acids aspartate, glutamate, and GABA. Although neurons do possess small amounts of glycogen as a stored form of glucose and have a limited capacity to utilize other substrates, notably keto acids, neither of these substrates is capable of

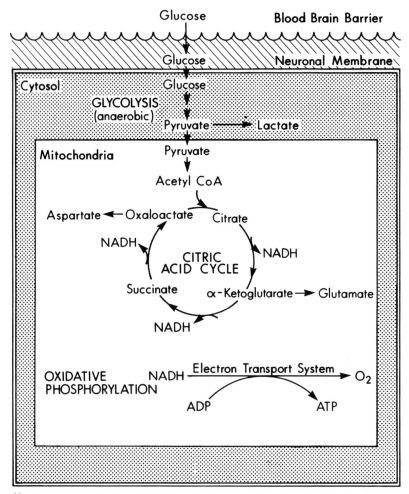

Key:
    Acetyl CoA: acetyl coenzyme A
    NADH: nicotinamide adenine dinucleotide
    O_2: oxygen
    ADP: adenosine diphosphate
    ATP: adenosine triphosphate

Fig. 16–1. Central nervous system glucose metabolism. Glucose is the only major substrate for brain energy metabolism. It crosses the blood-brain barrier by a stereospecific carrier (facilitated diffusion) and is phosphorylated by hexokinase in the cytosol. Small amounts of glucose-6-phosphate are metabolized to glycogen or through the pentose pathway, but most is metabolized by glycolysis to pyruvate. Eighty-five percent of pyruvate is metabolized in mitochondria by oxidative decarboxylation to yield CO_2 and H_2O as products. Fifteen percent is metabolized to lactate. In addition to providing energy, glucose also provides the carbon skeleton for several neurotransmitters, i.e., acetylcholine, glutamate, aspartate, and GABA.

meeting ordinary cellular energy needs for any significant length of time. Therefore, normal neuronal biochemical processes are exquisitely reliant on a generous and constant supply of both oxygen and glucose.

Cerebral blood flow

The circulatory system of the brain allows for the supply of these and other nutrients, and it removes the toxic products generated by metabolic processes. Although the brain comprises only 2% of the body weight, the cerebral blood flow represents almost 20% of the total cardiac output and is dependent on both the systemic arterial pressure and the resistance of cerebral vessels. The diameter of the vascular lumen is altered in response to the carbon dioxide tension and oxygen concentration (PO_2) of the arterial blood. Cerebral vascular resistance is thus subject to dynamic autoregulation and in this manner continually modifies perfusion rate to conform to cerebral metabolic demands. Both regional and global circulatory adjustments transpire and are based on the localization and extent of the underlying cerebral metabolic activity. The ability of these autoregulatory mechanisms to maintain cerebral blood flow may be compromised, however, by a fall in mean systemic arterial pressure below a certain critical level (approximately 60 mm Hg), or by pathologic conditions such as atherosclerosis that directly damage the cerebral vessels.

The neuronal deprivation of essential fuel substances, due either to a primary nutrient deficiency (e.g., hypoxia) or to a disruption of the delivery system (e.g., cardiac arrest), ultimately results in a fall of cerebral ATP levels. When the deprivation persists beyond a certain duration, then energy supply is exhausted at the cost of irreversible neuronal injury and tissue necrosis ensues. The immediate restoration of cerebral energy supply is manda-tory to prevent permanent neuronal damage in those metabolic encephalopathies that impair ATP biosynthesis (e.g., hypoxic-ischemic insults).

Neurotransmission

While severe alterations in brain energy metabolism may occur in hypoxic-ischemic disorders, most metabolic encephalopathies are characterized by normal brain energy metabolism. In these conditions (e.g., hypoglycemia, hepatic failure, uremia) recent animal experiments suggest alterations in ion balance, membrane charge, or neurotransmission.

Neurons maintain concentration gradients of sodium (Na^+) and potassium (K^+) ions across the cell membrane by means of an ATP-dependent $Na^+ - K^+$ pump, for which ATPase is a necessary enzyme. The activities of this membrane-bound system, which consumes 40% of brain energy production, are such that Na^+ is actively extruded from the cell while K^+ is sequestered as the major intracellular cation. The net effect of these ionic fluxes is to create a voltage potential (average: 60–70 mV) across the neuronal membrane with the cell interior negatively charged relative to the extracellular environment. Potentiation of the negative charge causes hyperpolarization of the neuron, while a decrease causes depolarization. A change in the resting membrane potential, produced by alterations in the permeability of the membrane to Na^+, K^+, and chloride (Cl^-) ions, is the foundation for neuronal communication. A reduction in the potential to a threshold level of about −45 mV triggers a large, self-sustaining, all or none depolarizing signal—the action potential—that is propagated down the neuronal axon into its terminal. The arrival of the action potential triggers influx of calcium into the terminal, which facilitates release of neurotransmitters into the synaptic cleft. Neurotransmitters diffuse across the cleft and bind at a stereo-specific receptor site on the postsynaptic membrane.

Receptor activation causes changes in postsynaptic membrane ionic permeability, resulting in depolarization or hyperpolarization of the neuron. Inhibitory postsynaptic potentials hyperpolarize the cell by opening Cl^- channels in the membrane, while excitatory postsynaptic potentials cause neuronal depolarization, primarily by opening Na^+ channels. Furthermore, certain receptor sites are linked to membrane-bound adenyl cyclase and thus permit specific neurotransmitter regulation of postsynaptic cyclic $3',5'$-adenosine monophosphate (cAMP) levels. Because cAMP in turn governs the activity of important intracellular protein kinases, neurotransmitter influence on this "second messenger" system has profound implications for overall cellular function. Neurotransmitter actions are terminated by various mechanisms including degradation by specific extracellular enzymes, uptake by glia, reuptake into the presynaptic terminal, and simple diffusion from the receptor site.

Neurotransmitter substance is manufactured intraneuronally and then stored at the presynaptic terminal in small membranous sacs, or vesicles. The release of neurotransmitter is accomplished by exocytosis, which in turn is dependent on the activation of a mechanism that promotes the fusion of the vesicle with the cell membrane. The essential step in this process is initiated by the depolarizing action potential, for as it reaches the presynaptic terminal it causes the membrane calcium channels to open. The subsequent entry of Ca^{2+} into the terminal down its concentration gradient promotes the fusion of the vesicles with the neuronal membrane and thus is directly responsible for neurotransmitter release. The basic steps comprising neurotransmission are depicted in Figure 16–2.

A number of chemical substances have been identified as neurotransmitters, including the biogenic amines (e.g., norepinephrine, dopamine) and acetylcholine. Of importance in understanding the pathophysiology of metabolic encephalopathies are molecules that are usually found as intermediates in biochemical processes but that are partially compartmentalized for transmitter functions. Two amino acids, glutamate and aspartate, with excitatory properties; two amino acids, gamma-aminobutyric acid (GABA) and glycine, with inhibitiory properties; and a purine nucleoside, adenosine (also inhibitory), may all perform in this regard. Each element of neurotransmitter function, including biosynthesis, storage in synaptic vesicles, release from the presynaptic terminal, interaction with the postsynaptic receptor, and termination of effect, may be influenced (either separately or in combination) by the metabolic encephalopathies. As an example, GABA is generated by the decarboxylation of glutamate, which in turn is derived from alpha-ketoglutarate, a constituent of the citric acid cycle that under normal circumstances is fueled by glucose metabolism. Hypoglycemic conditions cause a decrease in the precursors required for the biosynthesis of these amino acids, and their reduced concentrations and subsequent diminished transmitter activity are probably responsible for some of the neurologic manifestations of hypoglycemia.

PATHOPHYSIOLOGY OF SPECIFIC METABOLIC ENCEPHALOPATHIES

Although the metabolic encephalopathies form a sizable, heterogeneous group of dieseases, they nevertheless all share similar clinical features since they all eventually disrupt neuronal metabolism and/or neurotransmission. However, the specific mechanisms by which these diverse disorders produce their neurologic disturbances are nonuniform, and thus differences do exist. The distinctions in clinical

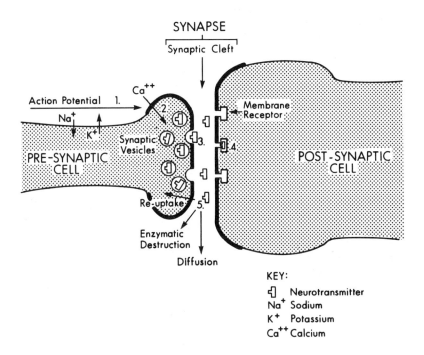

Fig. 16–2. Neurotransmission. (1) The action potential arrives at the axon terminal, opening membrane calcium channels. (2) Calcium ions flow into the terminal and promote fusion of synaptic vesicles with the membrane. (3) The vesicles release neurotransmitter into the synaptic cleft by exocytosis. (4) The released neurotransmitter reversibly binds with specific postsynaptic membrane receptors. (5) Neurotransmitter binding is terminated by reuptake into the presynaptic cell, simple diffusion, or enzymatic destruction.

features, pathophysiologic mechanisms, and neuropathological changes (when present) are partly known for each of the major metabolic disorders. Table 16–2 lists many of the commonly encountered metabolic encephalopathies and classifies them according to their basic manner of metabolic derangement.

Fuel deprivation

Oxygen Deficiency (hypoxic-ischemic encephalopathy). There are two major conditions that are responsible for a diffuse impairment of cerebral oxygen supply. The first is hypoxia, or decreased arterial oxygen tension (decreased PO_2), which results from either a reduction in alveolar oxygen pressure (e.g., high-altitude situations) or from insufficient pulmonary gas exchange (e.g., pneumonia). The second is ischemia, or the cessation of blood flow, which stems from circulatory collapse (e.g., shock) or diminished cardiac output (e.g., cardiac arrest). Ischemia is generally a more serious cerebral insult than hypoxia because the supply of glucose and removal of toxic waste are also compromised. Both conditions yield similar clinical, neurochemical, and histologic lesions that primarily de-

Table 16–2. Classification of the acquired metabolic encephalopathies

---

I. Fuel deprivation
  A. Oxygen
    1. Hypoxia
      a. Decreased atmospheric O_2 tension (e.g., high altitude)
      b. Primary hypoventilation (e.g., opioid intoxication)
      c. Pulmonary disease
      d. Decreased O_2 transport (e.g., carbon monoxide poisoning)
    2. Ischemia
      a. Decreased peripheral vasomotor tone (e.g., shock)
      b. Decreased cardiac output
        1) Rhythm disturbances
        2) Pump disturbances (e.g., myocardial infarction)
  B. Glucose (hypoglycemia)
    1. Hyperinsulinemia (e.g., excessive administration)
    2. Decreased gluconeogenesis (e.g., alcoholic liver disease)

II. Endogenous neurotoxins
  A. Renal failure
    1. Uremia
    2. Dialytic complications
      a. Dialysis dysequilibrium syndrome
      b. Progressive dialysis encephalopathy
  B. Hyperammonemia
    1. Hepatic failure
    2. Portal-systemic shunts
  C. Endocrine dysfunction
    1. Adrenal
      a. Cushing's syndrome
      b. Addison's disease
    2. Thyroid
      a. Thyrotoxicosis
      b. Myxedema

III. Acid–base, water, and ionic imbalances
  A. Acid–base
    1. CO_2 narcosis (pulmonary insufficiency)
    2. Complications of the treatment of acidosis
  B. Water
    1. Hypo-osmolar states (hyponatremia) (e.g., diuretic therapy)
    2. Hyperosmolar states
      a. Hypernatremia (e.g. diabetes insipidus)
      b. Hyperglycemia
        1) Diabetic ketoacidosis
        2) Nonketotic hyperglycemic hyperosmolar coma
  C. Ions
    1. Hypocalcemia (tetany)
    2. Hypercalcemia

IV. Exogenous neurotoxins
  A. Sedative-depressants
    1. Alcohol
      a. Intoxication
      b. Withdrawal syndrome
      c. Wernicke-Korsakoff disease (thiamine deficiency)
    2. Barbiturates
    3. Benzodiazepines
    4. Opioids
  B. Psychoactive drugs
  C. Other drugs
    1. Anticholinergics
    2. Salicylates

pend on the intensity and duration of cerebral oxygen lack.

The chief clinical feature of abrupt cerebral anoxia is loss of consciousness within several seconds. With lesser degrees of hypoxia, a mild clouding of consciousness or an acute confusional state is observed. These minor symptoms are completely reversible. Irreversible neuronal changes may begin after only 2–4 minutes of anoxia, occurring first in the regions of greatest vulnerability (parietooccipital cortex, hippocampus, cerebellar cortex), but eventually extending to the entire neuraxis in a rostral-caudal fashion. The neurologic picture is contingent on the point at which effective cardiorespiratory function is restored. With relatively limited anoxic damage, consciousness may be regained fairly rapidly with neurologic deficits restricted to mild encephalopathy. Long periods of cerebral oxygen deprivation create more serious sequelae, including myoclonic and generalized seizures (often most prominent immediately following resumption of cerebral perfusion), cortical blindness, extrapyramidal disorders, cerebellar ataxia, and memory disorders. With prolonged anoxia, coma may persist for several days and flaccidity mixed with intermittent decerebrate posturing may be present. If brainstem function is preserved (intact pupillary and oculomotor reflexes), the patient will usually recover to some degree but with severe cerebral impairment. If pupillary reflexes are persistently abolished (pupils remain dilated and fixed to light) in anoxic coma, the probability of brain death with an isoelectric EEG and fatal outcome is great.

It has been established that hypoxia alone is sufficient to destroy nerve cells, although mechanisms of the selective susceptibility of certain neurons (e.g., hippocampal pyramidal neurons) to this insult are not known. However, the immediate neuronal depression (reflected by the rapid loss of consciousness) that attends severe hypoxic-ischemic insults is not associated with a concomitant immediate decrease in cerebral energy levels, as might be expected when the supply of O_2 necessary for mitochondrial ATP production is interrupted. Rather, the initial reduction of cellular activity appears related to a slowing of metabolic processes that conserve ATP. The purine nucleoside adenosine, which possesses significant neuroinhibitory properties, is known to be released in large quantities by neurons subjected to hypoxic-ischemic stress and may be involved in this endogenous neuronal depression. After 2 minutes of continued O_2 deprivation, however, even the diminished rate of metabolic activity cannot prevent exhaustion of neuronal ATP stores, and energy-dependent biochemical processes are eventually halted. Failure of the ATP-requiring Na^+–K^+ pump results in the unopposed influx of Na^+ and Ca^{2+} into the cell, loss of the resting membrane potential, and ultimately neuronal edema and death. Recently, cellular acidosis resulting from the accumulation of lactic acid produced by augmented anaerobic metabolism has been implicated as an important mechanism of neuronal destruction in this setting.

The neuropathologic features of hypoxic-ischemic metabolic encephalopathy correlate with the severity of the cerebral injury. Neurons subjected to brief periods of hypoxia appear histologically normal. With prolongation of hypoxia, the first evidence of neuronal damage appears at the electron microscopic level as a swelling of the mitochondria. Light microscopic findings are manifested several hours later and consist of shrunken neurons with pyknotic nuclei and eosinophilic cytoplasm, representing the ischemic cell change. The changes are first apparent in the hippocampus, parieto-occipital cortex, and cerebellum. The necrotic neurons eventually disappear and impart a pseudolaminar appearance to the cerebral cortex and a characteristic loss of pyramidal neurons in Ammon's horn of the hippocampus (hippocampal sclerosis). With profound anoxia, total destruction of all nervous tissue elements may result and produce the clinical picture of brain death.

Glucose Deficiency (hypoglycemic encephalopathy). The brain requires 100–120 g of glucose per day to meet chemical energy needs. Following excessive administration of insulin or, less commonly, with a failure of gluconeogenesis in patients with hepatic disease (e.g., chronic alcoholics), the brain becomes deprived of its primary substrate. An encephalopathic process is created in which the primary alteration is a reversible depression of neuronal metabolic activity. Only after protracted glucose deprivation do lethal cellular changes occur.

Clinically, alterations of consciousness (confusion or delirium) develop insidiously over several minutes to an hour as the blood glucose level falls below 40 mg per 100 ml (normal range, 60–110 mg per 100 ml). As the deprivation worsens, stupor intervenes and one or more convulsions may occur; rarely, seizures may be the initial manifestation of hypoglycemia. Infrequently, focal neurologic deficits may imitate a stroke, but these signs are transient and often shifting in nature. With profound reduction of the blood glucose content to 10 mg per 100 ml or below, deep coma ensues occasionally with evidence of brainstem dysfunction, such as decerebrate posturing. Pupillary reflexes remain intact. Electroencephalographic studies reveal progressive slowing concomitant with falling glucose levels. With prompt correction of hypoglycemia, full neurologic recovery without sequelae is the rule. However, with intense or prolonged glucose deprivation or following repeated hypoglycemic episodes, irreparable cerebral damage can occur.

The deficient provision of glucose to the brain is directly responsible for these neurologic abnormalities, but by mechanisms that are not dependent on a fall in cerebral energy levels. Indeed, despite the customary nearly exclusive use of glucose as the substrate for neuronal ATP production, cerebral high-energy phosphate compounds are maintained at normal levels during hypoglycemic conditions. In part, the substitution of non-glucose-derived substrates, especially keto acids, in the citric acid cycle accounts for the conservation of energy. More importantly, the cerebral metabolic rate (as measured by oxygen consumption and energy utilization) becomes markedly depressed during hypoglycemia. The exact mechanisms by which neuronal depression is achieved are not known, but may relate to impaired biochemical processes that depend on non-energy-related aspects of glucose metabolism. In particular, glucose deprivation produces marked alterations in the concentrations of important neurotransmitters that are also intimately linked to glucose metabolism by the citric acid cycle. These perturbations may ultimately be found responsible for many of the biochemical, physiologic, and clinical abnormalities of hypoglycemia. For example, reduced GABA levels in hypoglycemic conditions may lead to impaired inhibitory neurotransmission with a subsequent increase in spontaneous neuronal firing culminating in clinical seizures. Furthermore, by reducing levels of glutamine (which is derived from glutamate), hypoglycemia may interfere with cerebral metabolism of nitrogenous catabolic byproducts and thus permit the accumulation of toxic levels of ammonia. The more gradual onset and course of neurologic dysfunction in hypoglycemia, as compared to hypoxic-ischemic encephalopathy, as well as the greater potential for neuronal recovery with similar durations of substrate deprivation, indicate that the brain may tolerate glucose lack for longer periods than it does oxygen deficiency.

Lasting cerebral injury can occur, however, in severe and protracted hypoglycemic encephalopathy, and the neuropathological changes remarkably resemble those of hypoxic-ischemic lesions. The features of the ischemic cell change, pseudolaminar necrosis, and predilection for cerebral cortex and hippocampus are essentially those seen with anoxia. This close neuropathologic similarity between hypoglycemic and hypoxic-ischemic encephalopathy may reflect a final common pathway of neuronal death.

Endogenous neurotoxins

Uremic Encephalopathy. Renal failure from any cause can be associated with a number of specific neurologic syndromes (e.g., hypertensive encephalopathy, peripheral neuropathy) that are directly related to one of the protean metabolic, endocrine, circulatory, and nutritional disturbances that accompany acute and chronic kidney disease. In addition, uremia alone produces a rather characteristic encephalopathy that is attributed to the underlying failure of the kidneys to excrete the end products of metabolism.

Often heralded by a fluctuating and episodic confusional state, uremic encephalopathy usually becomes clinically manifest when the glomerular filtration rate falls below 20%–25% of normal. More extreme alterations in consciousness may appear with the rapid onset or progression of uremia and include an agitated delirium, stupor, and coma. Motor abnormalities are usually prominent and materialize in a well-defined pattern as tremor, asterixis, myoclonus, or generalized seizures. Often several types are combined in the same patient and are called the uremic twitch-convulsive syndrome. Nonfixed focal neurologic abnormalities (e.g., hemiparesis, aphasia) may occur in uremia. Cheyne-Stokes respirations appear early, but Kussmaul breathing develops concurrent with severe metabolic acidosis. Pupillary and oculomotor responses remain preserved. While reminiscent clinically of other metabolic cerebral depressions, uremic encephalopathy may be distinguished by the presence of the twitch-convulsive syndrome, the invariably co-existing azotemia (although the degree of neurologic dysfunction does not always correlate well with the blood urea nitrogen), and the reversal of symptoms with dialysis treatment.

The nature of the metabolic derangements in uremia remains obscure, but it is generally accepted that a combination of factors is involved as the identification of a single "uremic toxin" has been unsuccessful. The relative contribution of electrolyte disturbances, water transport abnormalities, glucose intolerance, hypertensive vascular changes, and malnutrition, all of which attend renal failure, is unresolved. However, as the brain has protective mechanisms that defend against a fall in cerebral pH, systemic metabolic acidosis does not appear to play a role in this regard. Since nitrogenous by-products of protein and amino acid metabolism are pathologically retained in uremia, it is these substances that have been examined for encephalopathic properties. It has been found that urea is capable of producing myoclonus by an unexplained action on the brainstem reticular formation. There is a lack of precise correlation of the blood urea nitrogen to other neurologic symptoms, however. The retention of phenolic acids may play a role as these compounds have been found to inhibit cerebral enzymes, including several involved in neurotransmitter synthesis. Increased cerebral membrane permeability in uremic conditions permits the accumulation of these neurotoxic acids in brain tissue.

Other metabolic alterations have been identified in uremic encephalopathy. Uremic brain shows an impairment in $Na^+–K^+$ ATPase activity with a subsequent reduction in ATP turnover. This probably results in deleterious effects on ion transport across the cell membrane that may contribute to the overall depression of neuronal activity. Other studies indicate that the elevation of parathyroid hormone levels in uremia produces a significant increase in total brain Ca^{2+} content. Several critical biochemical functions, including neurotransmitter release, are substantially dependent on Ca^{2+}-related processes, and the abnormal Ca^{2+} concentrations in uremic brain may consequently interfere with these activities.

The end result of metabolic derangements in uremic encephalopathy is a generalized neuronal depression characterized, much like hypoglycemic encephalopathy, by a decrease in overall cerebral metabolic activity and oxygen consumption with the preservation of high-energy compounds. A scanty hyperplasia of astrocytes in the cerebral cortex may sometimes be identified on neuropathological examination in uremic encephalopathy, but in contrast to severe hypoglycemic conditions, permanent parenchymal changes (exclusive of concurrent hypertensive cerebrovascular damage) are not manifested in uremia. This corresponds with the clinical experience that the neurologic syndrome is entirely reversible by restoration of kidney function.

Two complications of dialysis therapy of renal failure deserve brief mention. The dialysis dysequilibrium syndrome consists chiefly of headache and, less often, delirium, obtundation, and seizures. It occurs either during or just after hemodialysis, particularly if performed rapidly. Uremic solutes can be removed relatively quickly from blood but not from brain. As a result, brain becomes hyperosmotic during dialysis, causing water to move into brain. This increases intracranial pressure, leading in turn to headache. Progressive dialysis encephalopathy ("dialysis dementia") is a subacute dementia that transpires after several years of hemodialysis. It usually begins with a stuttering dysarthria, followed by dysphasic abnormalities, mental deterioration, and myoclonus. These neurological findings are accompanied by periodic polyspike activity super-imposed on normal or slowed background rhythms on the EEG. Often the disease is fatal within months. Studies have found an excessive concentration of aluminum in brain in this condition, and as dialysis centers have restricted aluminum content of dialysate this syndrome is largely disappearing.

Hepatic Encephalopathy. Normal metabolic degradation of protein and amino acids in the body creates potentially harmful nitrogenous substances (principally ammonia, or NH_3) that are detoxified by the hepatic urea cycle enzymatic system. The liver converts to urea both the NH_3 generated by ordinary catabolic activities and transported in the systemic circulation and that produced by the deamination of dietary protein by intestinal bacteria and carried in the portal circulation. The urea is then excreted through the kidney. Compromise of NH_3 metabolism either by intrinsic hepatocellular disease (reduced enzymatic capacity) or by portal-systemic shunts (nitrogenous products in the portal vein bypass the liver) results in hyperammonemia and an associated hepatic encephalopathy. The degree of serum NH_3 elevation usually correlates with the severity of cerebral dysfunction. Patients with hepatic encephalopathy may demonstrate an erratic and unpredictable course, however, since episodic gastrointestinal hemorrhage variably precipitates an increase in bacterial NH_3 production.

The initial neurologic finding in hepatic encephalopathy, like the other metabolic disorders, is a clouding of consciousness alternating with more severe cognitive disturbances. When the mental abnormalities are well established, the distinctive signs of asterixis and primary hyperventilation (respiratory alkalosis) are exhibited. In the presence of overt stigmata of liver disease, there is little doubt as to the diagnosis. The EEG typically reveals irregular slow activity, periodically organized into bilateral paroxysmal, high-

CEREBRAL AMMONIA DETOXIFICATION

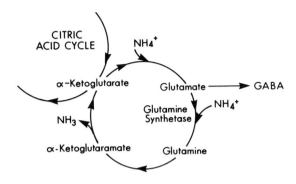

Key: NH₄⁺: ammonium ion
NH₃ : ammonia
GABA: ɣ-aminobutyric acid

Fig. 16–3. Cerebral ammonia detoxification. Blood ammonia (NH₃) readily crosses the blood-brain barrier, where the ammonium ion (NH⁺₄) is trapped by glutamate metabolism. Cerebral glutamine synthetase is a glial enzyme that is primarily involved in this process.

voltage slow waves. With severe or continued hepatic insufficiency, stupor or coma may supervene and be accompanied by extensor posturings and focal neurologic deficits. Pupillary and oculomotor responses are usually retained. Because of the severe nature of the nonneurologic complications of liver failure, hepatic coma not infrequently is a terminal event. If the fundamental hyperammoneic disorder can be corrected reasonably early, full neurologic recovery is expected. However, should hepatic encephalopathy persist for weeks or months, irreversible cerebral changes take place, culminating in a condition called chronic hepatocerebral degeneration. This is recognized clinically by dementia, dysarthria, cerebellar ataxia, and choreoathetosis. These signs remain prominent even if the patient recovers from liver failure. The manifestations of reversible hepatic encephalopathy may blend imperceptibly into those of the fixed disorder, implying that the basic metabolic derangement is responsible for both.

Similar to other metabolic encephalopathies, neuronal activity in hepatic failure is characterized initially by a diminished cerebral metabolic rate with preserved energy stores. As the disorder persists or becomes severe, cerebral ATP falls below vital levels. The precise manner in which these biochemical changes occur in hepatic encephalopathy its unresolved, but the neurotoxic effects of both NH₃ itself and its altered metabolism are thought to play a major role.

Because the brain lacks urea cycle enzymes, the NH₃ generated by cerebral amino acid catabolism is biotransformed by a portion of the glutamine metabolic pathway that is located principally within neuroglia (Fig. 16–3). Since NH₃ readily crosses the blood-brain barrier, hyperammonemia considerably increases total brain NH₃ content. The glutamine synthetase-dependent ammonium ion detoxification pathway is stimulated, thereby markedly depleting the substrate glutamate and increasing the concentrations of the metabolites, glutamine and alpha-ketoglutaramate; indeed, elevated levels of these metabolites are found in the CSF of patients with hepatic encephalopathy. As glutamate is a putative excitatory neurotransmitter, and since alpha-ketoglutaramate may act as a competitive inhibitor for its receptor site, the net effect of the heightened N_3 metabolic mechanisms may be to depress neuronal activity by prohibiting excitatory neurotransmission. Ammonia also retards the conversion of pyruvate into citrate and thus reduces the cerebral concentration of asparate, another excitatory neurotransmitter (see Fig. 16-1). Furthermore, hyperammonemia is associated with increased levels of octopamine, an amine produced by bacterial decarboxylase action on dietary protein. In hepatic failure increased circulating levels of octopamine and similar compounds may displace the customary neuroactive biogenic amines from nerve terminals and thus act as "false" neurotransmitters. These and other observations, taken together, suggest that the reversible neurological impairment seem in hepatic encephalopathy may be based, at least in part, on abnormalities in neurotransmitter function.

Prolonged or severe NH_3 intoxication appears to result in decreased mitochondrial levels of the hydrogen acceptor nicotinamide adenine dinucleotide (NAD), perhaps due to interference with the transport of reduced equivalents across the mitochondrial membrane. Therefore, the delayed fall in brain ATP production in hepatic encephalopathy may stem from insufficient mitochondrial oxidative phosphorylation due to disruption of the NADH-dependent electron transport system (see Fig. 16-1) and eventuate in "power failure" with cellular disintegration. This would explain the permanent neurologic changes evident in chronic hepatocerebral degeneration.

The histopathologic findings in acute or subacute hepatic encephalopathy are confined to a prominent increase in the size and number of astrocytes seen diffusely throughout the cerebral gray matter. This astrocytosis may represent a compensatory alteration of the cells to the stimu-

lated glutamine-linked NH_3 metabolic pathway that is contained in glia. In hepatocerebral degeneration, conspicuous astrocytic proliferation is also evident and typically includes giant protoplasmic astrocytes with pale, lobulated nuclei (Alzheimer type II astrocyte) (Fig. 16-4). At times, periodic acid-Schiff (PAS)-positive glycogen granules of unknown significance are identified within the astrocytic nuclei. Neuronal degeneration and loss are manifested primarily in the deeper layers of cerebral cortex, where it may assume a pseudolaminar appearance, as well as in the cerebellar cortex and basal ganglia, thus providing the neuroanatomic basis for the cardinal clinical elements (dementia, dysarthria, ataxia, and choreoathetosis) of this condition. The neuropathological features of cortical neuronal loss, diffuse astroyctosis with Alzhemier type II cells, and PAS-positive intranuclear inclusions are specific for chronic hepatocerebral degeneration.

Acid–base, water, and ionic disturbances

Acid–Base Imbalances. The kinetics of intracellular enzymatic reactions are pH-dependent, so that acid–base imbalances may have marked effects on the rate of neuronal metabolic processes. The degree of neurologic impairment in these conditions is proportionate to the extent of the cerebral pH shift from normal. However, there are three protective mechanisms by which the brain maintains pH homeostasis even in the presence of pronounced systemic acid-base disturbances: Unwanted charged particles, such as hydrogen and bicarbonate (HCO_3^-) ions, are excluded by the permeability characteristics of the blood-brain barrier; neurons contain buffering systems; and changes in the pH of the CSF that bathes the medullary respiratory centers rapidly promote compensatory adjustments in breathing patterns. In fact, in metabolic acidosis and

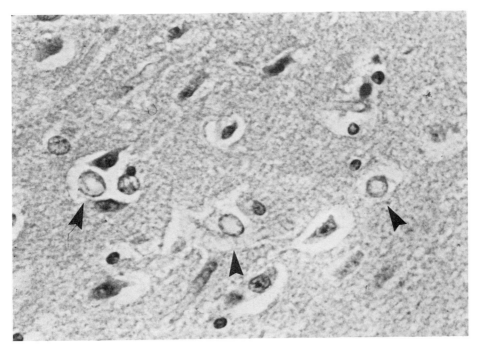

Fig. 16–4. Protoplasmic astrocytes undergo marked swelling as a result of chronic ammonia intoxication from liver failure. Arrows indicate characteristic Alzheimer type II astrocytes with large pale nuclei. Glycogen is increased within these nuclei. (Courtesy of K. Fulling, M.D.)

respiratory and metabolic alkalosis the cerebral tissue is safeguarded from all but the most extreme or prolonged shifts in pH. Encephalopathy in these conditions is generally attributable to the primary disorder (e.g., uremia) rather than the associated acid–base abnormalities. However, because of the diffusion properties of CO_2, respiratory acidosis does produce primary neurologic manifestations and merits special consideration.

Pulmonary failure produces an elevation of serum CO_2. Since this molecule readily crosses the blood-brain barrier and other cell membranes, the resultant acidosis is in equilibrium in blood, brain, and CSF. This causes a general cerebral depression, often termed CO_2 narcosis. Metabolic dysfunction may be related to decreased concentrations of glutamate and aspartate and other substrates as acidosis is known to inhibit enzymatic steps of the glycolytic pathway. Additional factors contributing to the brain dysfunction in pulmonary insufficiency may be the cerebral effects of hypoxia, as well as an increase in intracranial pressure that arises when CO_2 stimulates cerebral vasodilation. Neurologic manifestations are most prominent when the pulmonary deterioration is rapid, partly because the synthesis of brain HCO_3^- and other intracellular buffers lags behind the accumulation of carbonic acid.

The neurologic signs in this syndrome include a depressed level of consciousness (ranging from an irrritable confusional state to stupor or coma), headache (occasionally accompanied by papilledema), and various motor disturbances. Asterixis is particularly characteristic, and tremor and myoclonus are frequent. Once the cerebral pH returns to normal, there are no neurologic sequelae; CO_2 narcosis alone is not associated with irreversible damage.

Therapy of either chronic respiratory or metabolic acidosis may be complicated by "paradoxical" worsening of cerebral function. Chronic hypercapnea, for example, results in a decreased sensitivity of the medullary centers of CO_2 and leaves the ventilatory rate dependent on the hypoxic drive. Treatment of chronic lung disease with oxygen supplementation can remove this hypoxic stimulus and may produce profound hypoventilation, further rise in PCO_2, and advanced stupor or coma. Controlled mechanical ventilation may be required for this complication. At the other extreme, if elevations in $PaCO_2$ are corrected too rapidly patients can deteriorate neurologically. Chronic elevations in CO_2 result in a compensatory increase in brain HCO_3^-. When $PaCO_2$ is rapidly reduced, brain HCO_3^- becomes disproportionately elevated since it cannot diffuse from CSF to blood. Cerebral alkalosis occurs, encephalopathy worsens and seizures may appear. The use of exogenous bicarbonate in the treatment of metabolic acidosis may also lead to CNS depression in a directly opposite manner. Following HCO_3^- administration, there is an increase in serum CO_2, which rapidly diffuses into brain tissue. Cerebral bicarbonate ion accumulation occurs only slowly, however, and pH homeostatic mechanisms that had successfully operated against the metabolic acidosis are compromised. A neurologic syndrome similar to CO_2 narcosis results.

Disorders of Osmolality. The osmolality of body fluids is determined by the concentrations of osmotically active solutes (e.g., Na^+ and glucose) within a solvent (e.g., serum). The normal osmolality of serum is 290 mOsm per liter. Significant deviations from this norm produce corresponding shifts in the water content of body tissues in relation to the extracellular space. The subsequent volume changes in individual cells translate into either swelling or shrinkage of the entire organ. Because the brain is encased within the fixed compartment of the skull, these volume alterations can cause cerebral injury, and indeed the clinical expression of disorders of water balance is primarily neurological. Homeostatic mechanisms act to preserve cell volume by adjusting the intracellular osmotic environment (see Chap. 17). Neurological abnormalities occur in relation to either hypo-osmolar (essentially limited to hyponatremia) or hyperosmolar (due either to hypernatremia or hyperglycemia) disorders. If structural cerebral lesions can be avoided, the metabolic encephalopathies associated with these conditions are reversible.

Hypo-osmolality (hyponatremia) The normal serum concentration of Na^+ is 140 mEq per liter. Dilution of this concentration results either from the excessive retention of water (seen with the syndrome of inappropriate antidiuretic hormone; or with sudden inordinate water loads) or from the preferential depletion of Na^+ (seen with diuretic therapy and with salt-losing nephropathies). In either situation, the extracellular fluid becomes hypo-osomar relative to the intracellular environment, and the osmotic difference drives water into the cells with a subsequent increase in cell volume. In the brain, this water intoxication leads to a rise in intracranial pressure that is opposed only by the unyielding bony vault. Neurologic manifestations of hyponatremia may begin at concentrations of < 125 mEq per liter (serum osmolality < 260 mOsm). These include confusion, asterixis, myoclonus, generalized seizures, and coma. If hyponatremia is severe (serum Na^+ < 100 mEq per liter), brain edema and swelling can lead to herniation and permanent damage.

The appearance of hypo-osmolar encephalopathy is most likely when hyponatremia develops acutely. In chronic conditions, brain cells preserve cell volume by active depletion of intracellular osmoles, principally K^+, thereby equalizing the intracellular and extracellular osmotic pressures. Without an osmotic gradient, there is no net shift of water and normal volume is maintained. Regardless of the altered ionic composition, neuronal activity apparently remains stable and ATP levels are normal. There may be no clinical abnormalities with this cerebral compensation despite serum Na^+ concentrations of < 115 mEq per liter.

Hyperosmolality. (i) Hypernatremia: Illnesses associated with an abnormal loss of water (e.g., diabetes insipidus, profuse diarrhea) or excessive infusions of hypertonic solutions may produce hypernatremia, with serum sodium concentrations > 160 mEq per liter and serum osmolality > 330 mOsm. The neurologic manifestations are superimposed on the systemic signs of dehydration and include progressive obtundation, myoclonus, seizures, focal deficits, and coma. Permanent sequelae following recovery are not uncommon.

The pathophysiology of hypernatremic encephalopathy rests on the transudation of water from the intracellular milieu to the hyperosmolar extracellular compartments. Cell shrinkage and loss of brain volume result, and small bridging vessels that are anchored to the dura on the inner table of the skull may stretch and eventually tear. Hence, intracranial hemorrhage may be an important complication and perhaps is responsible for the permanent sequelae of hypernatremic encephalopathy. As with hypo-osmolar conditions, the neurologic manifestations are most probable when the hyperosmolality is sudden in onset and outpaces cerebral defense mechanisms.

With slower increases in extracellular osmolality, brain cells adjust to their altered environment by expanding concentrations of intracellular, osmotically active particles called idiogenic osmoles. These are principally amino acids (glutamate, glutamine, and aspartate) that increase in concentration during chronic hy-

pernatremia. These serve to keep water from leaving the intracellular space. Their increased concentrations may also contribute to the overall neurologic dysfunction, perhaps by affecting membrane excitability. Cerebral ATP levels remain normal in hypernatremic encephalopathy.

The presence of intracellular idiogenic osmoles in chronic hyperosmolality may perversely lead to acute water intoxication when the extracellular space suddenly is made normo-osmolar by precipitous rehydration with hypotonic fluids. This situation is closely related to that of the dialysis dysequilibrium syndrome.

(ii) Hyperglycemia: Diabetes mellitus is associated with a number of potentially neurotoxic systemic derangements, including metabolic acidosis. However, exclusive of hypoglycemia, the manifestations of diabetic metabolic encephalopathy are most directly related to hyperosmolar complications. Two distinct hyperglycemic abnormalities are associated with neurologic dysfunction and are distinguished by the presence or absence of serum ketone bodies. In diabetic ketoacidosis, a decrease in peripheral glucose utilization from insulin deficiency leads not only to hyperglycemia (often > 400 mg/dl), but also to increased hepatic conversion of free fatty acids into acetyl-CoA. Metabolic acidosis develops secondary to the accelerated production of the ketone acetoacetate and its metabolites, acetone and beta-hydroxybutyric acid. The syndrome of nonketotic, hyperglycemic, hyperosmolar coma, on the other hand, is seen in patients with mild, often non-insulin-requiring diabetes. In these cases insulin activity is adequate to prevent the hepatic ketogenic mechanisms but cannot effect sufficient glucose utilization to avoid hyperglycemia (800–1,200 mg/dl). In either condition, hyperosmolality is produced by the increase in serum glucose concentration accentuated by water loss that results from an osmotic diuresis. The neurologic manifestations are essentially those of hypernatremic encephalopathy. The concomitant metabolic acidosis in diabetic ketoacidosis produces the additional sign of Kussmaul breathing.

Ionic Disorders. Disturbances in magnesium and phosphate concentrations, while capable of producing neurologic abnormalities, are rarely encountered as primary disorders and thus will not be considered further. The role of Ca^{2+} as an essential factor in neurotransmission has already been discussed. In addition, altered extracellular Ca^{2+} concentrations may have significant effects on the neuronal membrane. As a divalent cation, Ca^{2+} is bound to negatively charged membrane phospholipids and thus creates a small stabilizing electric field that is independent of the transmembrane potential. Furthermore, membrane-bound Ca^{2+} has been demonstrated to influence the permeability characteristics of membrane ionic channels, particularly those for sodium. These passive electrochemical properties of membrane-bound Ca^{2+} are disrupted by abnormal extracellular Ca^{2+} concentrations and, combined with disordered Ca^{2+}-dependent neurotransmitter release, contribute to modifications of neuronal excitability in these conditions.

Hypocalcemia is characterized by tetany, where peripheral nerve fibers in a state of unstable depolarization produce the clinical features of paresthesias and muscular cramps. CNS correlates of irritable neuronal membranes include seizures, which are a frequent manifestation of hypocalcemia in children. Cognitive disturbances (e.g., delirium, lethargy) occasionally are evident, even in the absence of tetany. The usual cause of hypocalcemia is hypoparathyroidism.

Hypercalcemia is usually a complication of either neoplasia or hyperparathyroidism and becomes manifest primarily as a metabolic encephalopathy. Symptoms of confusion, hallucinations, and increasing obtundation in a setting of sys-temic cancer should direct attention to the serum Ca^{2+} concentration.

Exogenous neurotoxins

The list of exogenous chemical agents that may produce neurologic dysfunction is great, and poisonings from accidental and intentional drug intoxications form a substantial group of metabolic encephalopathies. Most of the drugs that affect the CNS do so by their actions at synaptic sites, although the exact toxic mechanisms are often incompletely understood. Of particular importance in these conditions is that if vital functions are maintained while the offending drug is being biotransformed and eliminated, complete recovery is the rule. It must also be emphasized that many drugs have a direct depressant effect on brainstem respiratory functions and can cause severe hypoxemia soon after ingestion. Barbiturates, opioids, and alcohol are potent in this regard. Other drugs, such as the antidepressants, can cause cardiac arrhythmias and also lead to secondary cerebral metabolic insults causing encephalopathy.

Sedative-Depressants

Alcohol. While alcohol disturbs practically every organ system in the body, it most affects the brain. The clinical features of acute alcohol intoxication reflect a widespread, general cerebral depression, and initially include disinhibited behavior, impaired coordination and motor performance, and dulled cognitive abilities; eventually, stupor or coma occurs. These manifestations occur with other CNS depressants, and not infrequently alcohol is ingested in combination with one or more sedative drugs with a subsequent potentiation of toxic effects.

With chronic abuse, the brain becomes habituated to ethanol so that the abrupt cessation of its intake leads to a predictable neurologic disorder: the alcohol withdrawal syndrome. This is characterized by signs of cerebral overactivity, appearing first as generalized tremulousness 12 to 24 hours following cessation of drinking. Alcohol withdrawal seizures ("rum fits") occur between 24 and 72 hours, usually as two to three generalized convulsions. Delirium tremens usually begins after three days and is characterized by vivid hallucinations and autonomic overactivity—tachycardia, fever, and sweating. This can last three to seven days with complete recovery. The cause of these syndromes is unknown, but one hypothesis suggests that metabolites of alcohol may form condensation products with catecholamines and disrupt catecholamine neurotransmission.

Chronic alcoholics are often malnourished, and the Wernicke-Korsakoff syndrome commonly occurs in this population. This disorder results from a specific deficiency of vitamin B_1, or thiamine, which is an essential cofactor for the enzymatic decarboxylation of pyruvate and alphaketoglutarate as well as necessaary for reactions in the pentose pathway. The disease presents acutely as a quiet confusional state that is almost always accompanied by conjugate gaze abnormalities, ataxia and peripheral neuropathy. Immediate replacement of thiamine induces resolution of encephalopathy and opthalmoplegia within days, but delay in therapy leads to permanent neurologic deficits. These include a profound inability to make new memories (Korsakoff psychosis) and a severe disorder of stance and gait. The patho-anatomic substrate of the Wernicke-Korsakoff syndrome involves lesions restricted to gray matter in the walls of the third ventricle (e.g., dorsomedial nucleus of the thalamus; mammillary bodies), periaqueductal region, vestibular nuclei, and superior vermis of the cerebellum (Fig. 16–5).

Barbiturates. Drugs in this class (e.g., pentobarbital, phenobarbital) also act as powerful general depressants of cerebral activity. Abuse of these compounds is re-

sponsible for one-fifth of all drug poisonings. The clinical features of barbiturate intoxication are primarily depression of consciousness and decreased respiratory drive. The ventilatory reduction occurs at drug levels that are only three times greater than those usually employed for hypnotic effects and is the major cause of death from barbiturate poisoning. The mechanisms of action of these drugs are not entirely known, but they may facilitate GABA-ergic inhibition of neuronal pathways throughout the brain. The widespread neuronal inhibition produced by barbiturates underlies their effective anticonvulsant properties and in severe intoxications may give rise to an isoelectric EEG that nevertheless returns to normal with clinical recovery.

Benzodiazepines. The benzodiazepines (e.g., diazepam) are the most frequently prescribed compounds in the world. Fortunately, their toxic potential is *relatively* low due to their comparatively mild respiratory depressive effects and their minimal addictive possibilities. They may be abused, however, in conjuction with other CNS depressants (e.g., ethanol) and therefore contribute to neurologic symptoms and signs. Benzodiazepines do not seem to be depressants of general neuronal systems, but rather exert their effects via an indirect enhancement of GABA-mediated presynaptic inhibition in discrete polysynaptic pathways. The reticular activating system appears particularly sensitive to this inhibition and may explain the hypnotic properties of these drugs.

Opioids. The discovery that natural and synthetic opioid substances (e.g., morphine, meperidine) bind to specific CNS receptors that also have endogenous ligands (the enkephalins) has suggested that the neurotoxocity of opioids is in some way related to an overactivity of normal cerebral functions subserved by these endogenous peptides. However, although enkephalins probably act to regulate neuronal activity through presynaptic mechanisms,

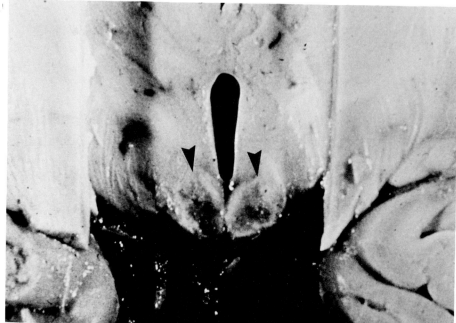

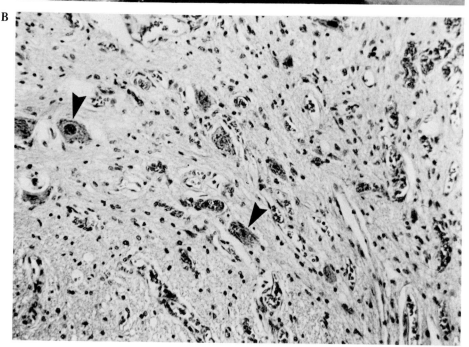

Fig. 16–5. **A.** Neuropathological charges in the Wernicke-Korsakoff syndrome (thiamine deficiency) are seen as increased vascularity and microhemorrhages in both mammillary bodies (arrows) surrounding the base of the third ventricle. Similar lesions occur in dorsal thalamus, periaqueductal gray, matter and brainstem. **B.** Histopathology shows marked increase in vascularity and gliosis. Note preservation of neurons (arrows). (Courtesy of K. Fulling, M.D.)

their precise role in the modulation of neurotransmission is unsettled. Based on their functional and anatomic distribution within the CNS, they do appear capable of influencing a wide variety of neurologic functions, including pain perception.

Opioid intoxication produces analgesia, mood changes (commonly euphoria), and eventually stupor and coma. The brainstem is quite sensitive to opioid actions, and nausea and vomiting (from stimulation of the medullary emesis center) are frequently early signs of intoxication. Even when consciousness is intact, the brainstem respiratory control centers may become depressed and apnea is the primary cause of death from these drugs. The hallmark of opioid poisoning is marked miosis ("pinpoint pupils"), which results from stimulation of the parasympathetic portion of the third nerve nucleus.

Psychoactive Drugs. The sympathomimetic compounds (e.g., amphetamine, cocaine) produce their clinical manifestations (e.g., mood elevation, appetite suppression, heightened energy) apparently by potentiating the activity of biogenic amines by blocking reuptake following their release as neurotransmitters. Multiple sites of action that are generally linked to neurotransmission have been postulated for the hallucinogenic agents (e.g., lysergic acid diethylamide, phencyclidine); their exact effects are unknown.

Other Drugs. Anticholinergic compounds (e.g., atropine) may cause a toxic cerebral disorder that is manifested by delirium and pronounced mydriasis (secondary to cholinergic blockade of the sphincter of the iris). Taken in excessive amounts, salicylates can produce an encephalopathy characterized by seizures, delirium, and eventual coma. Concurrent acid–base disturbances arise from a direct stimulation of respiratory centers (primary respiratory alkalosis) and also from an accumulation of organic and salicylic acids (metabolic acidosis).

SUMMARY

The metabolic encephalopathies comprise a vast, heterogeneous group of CNS disorders in which the neurologic manifestations reflect a diffuse disturbance in cerebral metabolic processes that results from an underlying systemic illness or intoxication. Typically, they are clinically expressed by abnormalities of consciousness, motor responses, and ventilatory control, but not by interruption of the pupillary light reflex arc. The degree of neurologic impairment generally parallels the rapidity of onset, severity, and duration of the fundamental disease.

The basic cerebral biochemical lesions in most of these disorders are not fully elucidated, but many appear related to disruption of normal neurotransmitter mechanisms. If cerebral energy production is not compromised, full metabolic and neurologic recovery is the rule. Thus, accurate diagnosis and prompt corrective measures are imperative, for the metabolic encephalopathies remain a significant class of treatable neurologic disease.

GENERAL REFERENCES

Cooper, J. D., V. C. Lazarowitz, and A. I. Arieff. Neurodiagnostic abnormalities in patients with acute renal failure. *J. Clin. Invest.* 61:1448–55, 1978.

Fahn, S., J. N. Davis, and L. P. Rowland (eds.). Cerebral hypoxia and its consequences. *Advances in Neurology,* Vol. 26. New York, Raven Press, 1979.

Fishman, R. A. and P. H. Chan. Metabolic basis of brain edema. Cervos-Navarro, J. In Ferszt, R. (eds.) Brain edema. *Advances in Neurology,* Vol. 28. New York, Raven Press, 1980.

Hoyumpa, A. M., P. V. Desmond, G. R. Avant, R. K. Roberts, and S. Schenker. Hepatic encephalopathy *Gastroenterology* 76:184–195, 1979.

Llinas, R. R. Calcium in synaptic transmission. *Sci. Am.* 247:56–65, 1982.

Passonneau, J. V., R. A. Hawkins, W. D. Lust, and F. A. Welsh (eds.). Cerebral metabolism and neural function. Baltimore, Williams and Wilkins, 1980.

Plum, F. (ed.) *Brain Dysfunction in Metabolic Disorders*. Research Publications Association for Research in Nervous and Mental Disease, Vol. 53. New York, Raven Press, 1974.

Plum, F. and J. B. Posner. *The Diagnosis of Stupor and Coma,* 3rd ed. Philadelphia, Davis, 1980.

Siesjo, B. K. Brain energy metabolism. Chichester, Wiley, 1978.

Victor, M., R. D. Adams, and G. H. Collins. *The Wernicke-Korsakoff Syndrome.* Philadelphia, Davis, 1971.

17.

Cerebrospinal Fluid, Blood-Brain Barrier, and Brain Edema

JAMES W. SCHMIDLEY

Brain edema contributes to the disability or death of patients suffering from a variety of diseases. Because brain edema is not an isolated phenomenon, a full understanding of its causes and consequences requires knowledge of the brain's barrier systems and the cerebrospinal fluid (CSF), as well as an appreciation of the dynamic relationships among the three main intracranial components—brain, CSF, and blood.

A detailed knowledge of CSF physiology is important to the understanding of brain edema for three reasons. First, CSF pressure, when measured at lumbar puncture or by intraventricular catheter, is a direct measure of intracranial pressure. Continuous recording of intracranial pressure enables clinicians to monitor the response to various therapies for brain edema. Second, a knowledge of CSF formation, circulation, and absorption is important for understanding and treating some types of brain edema. Finally, the CSF is in continuity with the brain extracellular fluid. Analysis of its constituents gives

us valuable data about both normal and pathologic CNS function.

Familiarity with the structure and function of the blood-brain barrier is important because (i) the most common form of brain edema, vasogenic edema, results from blood-brain barrier dysfunction, and (ii) the proper treatment of elevated intracranial pressure requires an understanding of both normal and abnormal blood-brain barrier function.

The cranial contents (brain parenchyma, blood, and CSF) are encased in nondistensible bone after the cranial sutures close in childhood. The contents of the spinal canal are similarly enclosed, although the spinal subarachnoid space is slightly distensible, especially in the lumbosacral region. The total volume of the three intracranial components must remain constant; an increase in any of them must be compensated for by reciprocal decreases in volume of one or both of the remaining components. This concept, first proposed in its complete form in 1846, remains important to understanding the

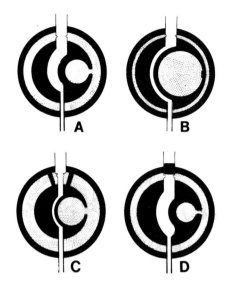

Fig. 17–1. Schematic representation of relationships among brain (shaded), CSF (stippled), and vascular (open at each end) compartments within the rigid cranium (heavy black sphere). **A.** The normal situation. **B.** The result of ventricular obstruction with noncommunicating hydrocephalus. **C.** The result of obstruction of the extraventricular CSF pathways, with communicating hydrocephalus. **D.** The vascular engorgement resulting from venous sinus obstruction. (From J. Foley, Benign forms of intracranial hypertension— "toxic" and "otitic" hydrocephalus. *Brain* 78:1–41, 1955, with permission of the author and Oxford University Press.)

extracellular fluid of the brain. Ependymal cells, which line the ventricular cavities, and pial cells, which invest the external surfaces of the brain, are joined by discontinuous intercellular junctions (maculae adherens and gap junctions), which allow molecules as large as ferritin (diameter 100 Å, mol wt 900,000) to diffuse between them. There are important exceptions to this generalization concerning ependymal cells. These will be discussed in the section on brain-barrier systems. The CSF and the extracellular fluid are therefore in continuity and can be thought of as one fluid compartment (Fig. 17–2).

Composition

The CSF resembles blood plasma, but the two fluids differ in a few important ways (Table 17–1). These differences reflect the distinctive anatomical features of the choroid plexus and the active transport mechanisms of its epithelial cells. Since the CSF is continuous with the brain extracellular fluid, mechanisms regulating the composition of extracellular fluid (e.g., astrocytes and the cerebral capillaries) will also affect CSF composition. Major differences between CSF and plasma are (i) lower

pathophysiology and treatment of elevated intracranial pressure (Fig. 17–1A).

THE CEREBROSPINAL FLUID

CSF occupies the cerebral ventricles, the central canal of the spinal cord, and the subarachnoid spaces around the spinal cord and brain. In adult humans, the total volume of CSF is 140–150 ml, and its composition closely resembles a plasma ultrafiltrate. (The differences are the result of specific properties of the choroid plexus and the blood-brain barrier, which will be discussed later.) There are no anatomical barriers between the CSF spaces and the

Table 17–1. Typical plasma and CSF levels of various substances[1]

Substance	Plasma	CSF
Na^+	145.0	150.0
K^+	4.8	2.9
Ca^{2+}	5.2	2.3
Mg^{2+}	1.7	2.3
Cl^-	108.0	130.0
$HCO_3{}^-$	27.4	21.0
Lactate	7.9	2.6
$PO_4{}^{3-}$	1.8	0.5
Protein	7000.0	20.0
Glucose	95.0	60.0

[1] Protein and glucose concentrations are in mg/100 ml; all others are in mEq/liter.

From R. Katzman, Blood-Brain-CSF barriers. In *Basic Neurochemistry*, 3d ed., G. J. Siegel et al. (eds.). Boston, Little, Brown, 1981, with permission of the author and Little Brown and Co.

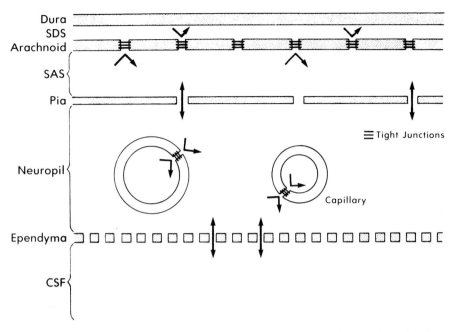

Fig. 17–2. Schematic representation of brain fluid spaces and CSF. The cells of the arachnoid and the endothelial cells of brain capillaries and of larger blood vessels are sealed by tight junctions, which restrict intercellular diffusion (deflected arrows). Water-soluble molecules are thus unable to enter the brain from the blood or from outside the arachnoid, which completely surrounds the CNS. These barriers do not impede transcellular diffusion of lipid-soluble molecules. The pia and ependyma present no barrier to diffusion (straight arrows); thus ventricular and subarachnoid CSF is in free communication with the extracellular space of the neuropil and brain extracellular fluid. SAS, subarachnoid space; SDS, subdural space (in vivo, a *potential* space).

concentrations of amino acids, Ca^{2+}, K^+, and glucose in CSF; (ii) markedly lower concentrations of protein in CSF (less than 0.5% of serum protein concentrations); and (iii) higher concentrations of Mg^{2+} and Cl^- in CSF. An example of CSF homeostasis is the control of CSF K^+ in the face of wide variations in serum K^+. When plasma K^+ is varied between 4 and 8 mEq per liter, CSF K^+ is kept below 4 mEq per liter by choroid plexus. By a similar process, astrocytes and capillary endothelial cells maintain the K^+ concentration of brain extracellular fluid at a relatively constant level. The CSF content of virtually every biologically important molecule has been analyzed in detail. The in-

terested reader should consult the works listed in this chapter's bibliography for specifics.

Functions

CSF literally keeps the brain afloat, providing protection and physical support. The 1.5-kg brain weighs only 50 g when suspended in CSF. CSF also serves as a metabolic "sink": Molecules can be removed from the CNS by bulk flow of brain interstitial fluid into CSF and subsequently across the arachnoid villi into the blood. Specific systems in the choroid plexus and capillary endothelial cells also transport substances out of the CSF (e.g., iodide,

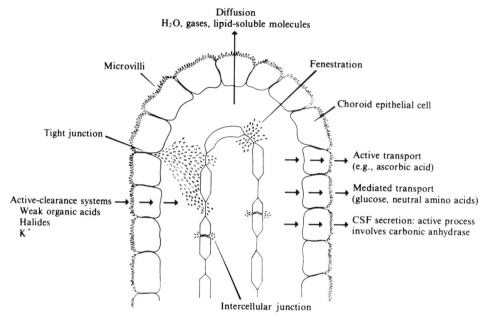

Fig. 17–3. Schematic representation of the anatomic and physiologic features of the choroid plexus. Protein molecules are shown crossing endothelial fenestrations and entering the choroid plexus stroma. Tight intercellular junctions prevent further diffusion into the CSF. (From R. Katzman, Blood-brain-CSF barriers. In G. J. Siegel et al. (eds.), *Basic Neurochemistry*, 3d ed. Boston, Little, Brown, 1981, with permission of the author and Little, Brown and Co.)

thiocyanate, and the weak organic acids such as penicillin, homovanillic acid, and 5-HIAA). The importance of this sink function for the resolution of some types of brain edema will be discussed later.

CSF may also serve a transport function. Hypothalamic releasing factors (e.g., TRH and LHRH) may be secreted into the third ventricular CSF and then be endocytosed by specialized ependymal cells called tanycytes. These cells have long processes contracting hyopthalamic-pituitary portal capillaries. The releasing factors may be transferred to the portal blood by the tanycytes, and then to the pituitary. The importance of this pathway in normal neuroendocrine regulation is uncertain.

Secretion

CSF is secreted by the choroid plexus epithelial cells of the lateral, third, and fourth ventricles. Substantial experimental evidence suggests that CSF is also formed extrachoroidally (i.e., within the brain parenchyma), presumably by cerebral capillaries; the relative importance of these two sources remains undefined.

The choroid plexus is composed of cuboidal epithelium, which overlies a vascular stroma (Fig. 17–3). The secretory cells of the choroid plexus have features typical of other secretory epithelia, i.e., apical tight junctions, apical microvilli, and basolateral infoldings. Unlike those of other brain capillaries, the endothelial cells of capillaries in the choroid plexus are fenestrated and do not act as a barrier (Fig. 17–3). Even large protein molecules (e.g., the electron-dense tracer horseradish peroxidase (HRP), Mol wt 40,000, molecular diameter, 50–60 Å), pass freely into the stroma of the choroid plexus when administered intravenously, but are prevented from reaching the CSF by the circumferential tight junctions between the epithelial cells. Although the processes of choroidal CSF secretion are still being studied, we know there is net transport of Na^+, with H_2O following passively, across the epithelial cell. Na^+–K^+ATPase, located on the apical membrane, is involved in this process because intraventricular ouabain can almost completely inhibit CSF secretion. Carbonic anhydrase, the enzyme that catalyzes the formation of H^+ and HCO_3^- from CO_2 and H_2O, is also important in CSF secretion. Acetazolamide, a carbonic anhydrase inhibitor, decreases CSF production by approximately 50% in animals.

Choroidal CSF secretion is subject to both neural and chemical control. The plexus is innervated by the sympathetic nervous system. Stimulation of the superior cervical ganglion in experimental animals causes a decrease in CSF formation. However, this decrease cannot be readily explained by changes in vasomotor tone of the vessels that supply the plexus. We do not know whether this pathway is important in the regulation of choroidal secretion *in vivo*. Cholera toxin, an activator of adenylate cyclase, results in elevated choroid plexus levels of cAMP and an increase in CSF production when infused intraventricularly. Biogenic amines stimulate the choroidal adenylate cyclase *in vitro*, but whether these agents and others that influence cAMP levels have an effect on CSF production is yet to be established. In normal humans, increasing CSF pressure does not inhibit CSF production, but in patients with communicating hydrocephalus, the rate of formation declines slightly with increasing CSF pressure.

Circulation and absorption

CSF produced in the lateral ventricles travels through the foramina of Monro to the third ventricle, then through the aqueduct of Sylvius into the fourth ventricle, from which it enters the subarachnoid space through the foramina of Luschka and Magendie (Fig. 17–4). It bathes the external surfaces of the spinal cord and brain and is then absorbed into the circulation by the arachnoid villi, which are invaginations of the arachnoid membrane into cranial venous sinuses and the epidural veins along spinal nerve roots. CSF must pass through the tentorial incisura to gain access to the cranial arachnoid villi, the major site of its absorption. CSF flow is often obstructed at the incisura by inflammatory exudate or fibrotic scarring in the subarachnoid space. This obstruction produces enlargement of the entire ventricular system, or communicating hydrocephalus, so named because the ventricles remain in free communication with one another and with the subarachnoid space (Fig. 17–1C). In noncommunicating hydrocephalus, CSF flow through the third ventricle, aqueduct, or fourth ventricle is obstructed, causing the ventricle(s) proximal to the obstruction to enlarge (Fig. 17–1B). Forces that aid in CSF circulation are the arterial pulsations of the choroid plexus and large vessels of the brain, movement of ependymal cilia, changes in posture, and fluctuations in cerebral venous volume with respiration. Functionally, the arachnoid villi act as "one-way valves," opening at a pressure of approximately 70 mm H_2O and venting increasing amounts of CSF as CSF pressure increases (Fig. 17–5). Although the cellular mechanisms that accomplish this are not fully understood, one theory suggests that giant vacuoles transport the CSF across the cells of the arachnoid villus into the vascular lumen.

BRAIN BARRIER SYSTEMS

To understand the concepts related to the cause and treatment of brain edema, it is essential to be familiar with the properties of the blood-brain barrier and with the anatomy of the CNS fluid compartments. There are obvious advantages of a constant extracellular milieu for neuronal function. The concept of a mechanism that

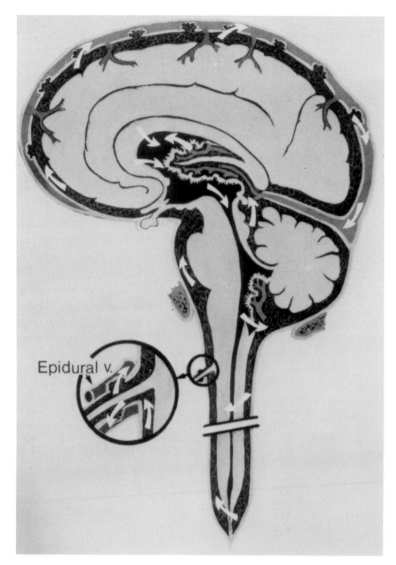

Epidural v.

Fig. 17–4. CSF circulation. In this depiction of a midsagittal section of the CNS, the third and fourth ventricles, with their choroid plexuses, are seen. CSF is shown leaving the ventricular system from the midline foramen of Magendie, at the caudal end of the fourth ventricle. The laterally placed ventricular foramina (of Luschka) are not illustrated, nor are the lateral ventricles. After leaving the ventricles and circulating in the subarachnoid space, CSF is absorbed into the bloodstream by arachnoid granulations along the superior sagittal sinus and on epidural veins along spinal roots. (From R. A. Fishman, *Cerebrospinal Fluid in Diseases of the Nervous System*. Philadelphia, Saunders, 1980, with permission of the author and W. B. Saunders Co.)

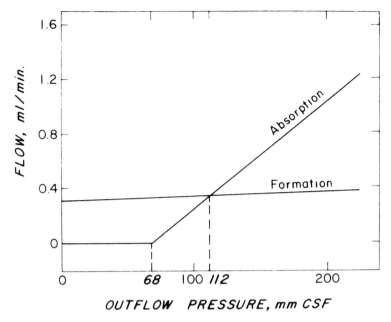

Fig. 17–5. Relationships among CSF formation, absorption, and pressure in humans. The rate of CSF formation is nearly constant, whereas that of absorption increases with CSF pressure once the "one-way valve" of the arachnoid villus opens, here shown at a pressure of 68 mm CSF. (From R. W. P. Cutler et al., Formation and absorption of cerebrospinal fluid in man. *Brain* 91:707–20, 1968, with permission of the author and Oxford University Press.)

selectively admits only certain bloodborne substances to the CNS (a blood-brain barrier) has had a long and embattled history, beginning with the discovery that intravenously administered dyes, such as trypan blue, stain all of the tissues in an animal *except* the CNS. After many years of debate and experimentation, it is now generally accepted that the blood-brain barrier is a reflection of the unique properties of the endothelial cells of CNS capillaries.

Tight junctions (fig. 17–2)

The CNS is surrounded by layers of cells with tight junctions that serve as a barrier between non-CNS tissues, such as the blood and pachymeninges, and the CNS. The arachnoid cells are united by circumferential tight junctions at the meningeal surface, preventing the intercellular diffusion of

water-soluble molecules such as the tracers horseradish peroxidase and microperoxidase (Mol wt, 1,900, molecular diameter, 20 Å). The endothelial cells of CNS capillaries are also joined at the interface between the brain and blood by tight junctions with similar properties (Fig. 17–6). In some tissues where cells are joined by tight junctions it is possible to study the permeability of the junctions to ions by using electrophysiological techniques. This approach has not yet been used to study the ion permeability of mammalian CNS capillaries, but work on frog CNS capillaries and arachnoid suggests that their tight junctions are capable of restricting the diffusion of ions. CNS endothelial cells lack fenestrations and have very few plasmalemmal vesicles. These structures are thought to play a role in transendothelial transport in non-CNS capillaries; the number of vesicles in CNS capillaries in-

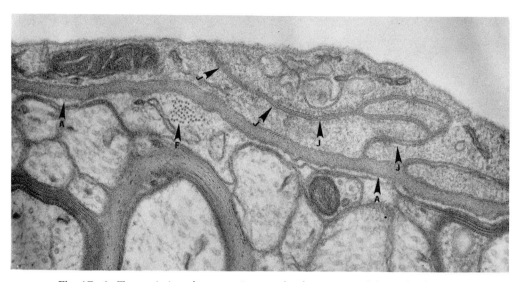

Fig. 17–6. Transmission electron micrograph of a portion of the wall of a capillary in rat cerebral cortex. In this specimen, fixed by vascular perfusion with aldehydes, the lumen (the clear area at the top of the micrograph) has been washed free of blood. A tight junction (J) seals the space between two endothelial cells. Astrocytes containing glial filaments (F) ensheath the vessel. At places (A) this sheath is quite thin, but it is always continuous. The homogeneous region between endothelium and astrocyte is the basal lamina, an extracellular matrix of glycosaminoglycans, collagen, and other molecules. The electron micrograph was prepared with the assistance of D. Crumrine in the laboratory of Dr. S. L. Wissig at the University of Calfornia, San Francisco.

creases in pathological states, such as acute hypertension, ischemia, and radiation injury.

No exception to the rule of arachnoidal cells being joined together by tight junctions is known. However, there are a few exceptions to the generalizations about the CNS capillaries (Fig. 17–7). Capillaries of the median eminence, the pineal, the area postrema in the floor of the fourth ventricle, and several other small regions of the CNS adjacent to the ventricles (the circumventricular organs) have fenestrated endothelial cells serving no barrier function. Only these regions become colored when dyes such as Evans blue and trypan blue (which are bound *in vivo* to serum proteins) are administered intravenously. Wherever fenestrated capillaries are found in the neuropil the junctions between the ependymal cells directly above

these regions are tight, which is not usually the case. These junctions prevent molecules that have escaped from the circulation from reaching the CSF. There is probably a small "leak" of such molecules into the CSF caused by diffusion out of the region below the ependyma having tight junctions into adjacent regions where the ependyma presents no barrier. This leak is minimal because the circumventricular organs make up only a tiny fraction of the CNS. We do not understand the function of most of the circumventricular organs and therefore can only speculate about why they lack a blood-brain barrier. The median eminence plays an important role in neuroendocrine regulation; perhaps the reason this area lacks a blood-brain barrier is to allow neurons within to "sample" the peripheral blood. The choroid plexus is another region in which a fenes-

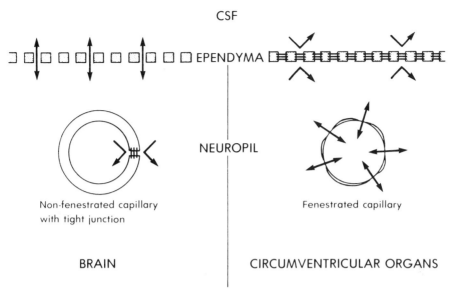

Fig. 17–7. Schematic representation of the distinctive features of ependymal and capillary endothelial cells in the circumventricular organs, such as the pineal, median eminence, and area postrema, contrasted with those in the remainder of the brain.

trated capillary bed lies beneath a layer of cells joined by tight junctions.

Properties of the blood-brain barrier

Strictly speaking there is no such thing as a single blood-brain barrier; the term is meaningless unless considered in the context of a particular molecule or class of molecules. Several factors determine whether a particular molecule can cross the barrier posed by the brain capillary endothelial cell and gain access to the extracellular fluid of the CNS. The biochemical characteristics of the molecule, its size, ionization at physiological pH, lipid solubility, and extent of binding to plasma proteins are all important. In some cases, the presence (or absence) of a specific transport system for a given molecule will be the determining factor.

We know from electron microscopic studies that CNS endothelial cells differ significantly from capillary endothelial cells outside the CNS (Fig. 17–8). Some of the differences responsible for the restrictive properties of the blood-brain barrier have already been mentioned: the absence of fenestrations, the sparse numbers of vesicles, and the tight intercellular junctions. Electron microscopic studies have also shown that CNS capillary endothelial cells contain more mitochondria per unit of cytoplasmic volume than do endothelial cells of capillaries in other organs. Therefore, the CNS endothelium probably requires more energy than other endothelia to support synthesis of proteins and other molecules associated with its various transport systems, or perhaps for the extrachoroidal formation of CSF. The microvasculature of the CNS is almost completely surrounded by a sheath of astrocytic processes (Fig. 17–6). These "foot processes" are not sealed by intercellular tight junctions and serve no structural barrier function. Whether they play a more subtle role in regulating passage of certain molecules into and out of the extracellular fluid is not known.

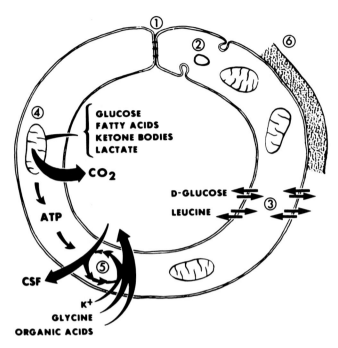

Fig. 17–8. Properties of the brain capillary endothelial cell. (1) Tight intercellular junctions, (2) few vesicles compared with continuous endothelia in other organs, (3) specific carrier-mediated transport of glucose and amino acids, (4) ability to use molecules other than glucose as sources of energy, (5) possible role in secretion of CSF and absorption of K^+ and other molecules from brain extracellular fluid, (6) basement membrane. (From G. W. Goldstein, Pathogenesis of brain edema and hemorrhage, role of the brain capillary. *Pediatrics* 64:357–60, 1979, with permission of the author and the American Academy of Pediatrics.)

Lipid-soluble nonpolar substances, such as alcohols and anesthetic gases, diffuse unimpeded across the blood-brain barrier. Some lipid-soluble molecules, such as the anticonvulsant phenytoin, are bound to a large extent to plasma proteins, which cannot cross the blood-brain barrier because of their size and charge. Only the free (non-protein-bound) fraction can diffuse into the brain. Water-soluble substances, except those for which a specific transport system exists, are generally excluded by the blood-brain barrier. Molecules with such a transport system are monocarboxylic acids (e.g., lactate), some amino acids, choline, and sugars. The best described among these is the monosaccharide transport system. This is a stereospecific system (D isomers only) mediated by a carrier molecule that facilitates diffusion of the hexose molecules across cell membranes. The carrier has a high affinity for glucose and a lower affinity for other sugars. The process is usually "downhill" from serum, where glucose concentration is 5–6 mM, to brain extracellular fluid where it is approximately 2 mM, and requires no energy. Because a finite number of carrier molecules is involved, the process is saturable and subject to competitive inhibition. In the therapy of brain edema advantage is taken of the minimal permeability of the blood-brain barrier to certain low molecular weight substances such as mannitol and glycerol. When these agents are administered to patients in concentrations sufficient to raise the plasma osmolality, an osmotic gradient between brain and plasma is established, causing H_2O to diffuse out of brain parenchyma, temporarily decreasing brain volume and lowering the intracranial pressure. Some amino acids, such as the essential amino acids and those that are neurotransmitter precursors, are transported into brain by well-defined endothelial carrier systems. Amino acids that can be synthesized readily from glucose metabolites (among them the putative neurotransmitters glycine, glutamate, aspartate, and gamma-aminobutyric acid) are not transported by the blood-brain barrier.

The CNS endothelial cells also provide an enzymatic barrier to neurotransmitters and their precursors. Monoamine oxidase and L-aromatic amino acid (dopa) decarboxylase are both present in CNS endothelial cells. When L-dopa is administered to a patient with parkinsonism, it is decarboxylated by aromatic amino acid decarboxylase in several sites outside the CNS (e.g., liver). It is also decarboxylated in the CNS microvessel wall, forming dopamine, which is then metabolized by monoamine oxidase while still in the endothelial cell. This efficient mechanism illustrates why very large doses of L-dopa, or the concomitant administration of a decarboxylase inhibitor, are required in the treatment of parkinsonism (see Chap. 19).

From this brief outline of a few aspects of the brain barrier systems it is clear that a knowledge of these systems is not only central to understanding the pathogenesis of brain edema, but is also important to physicians faced with the challenge of delivering drugs or enzymes into the sanctuary of the CNS.

BRAIN EDEMA

Brain edema occurs in patients with a variety of infectious, vascular, metabolic, neoplastic, toxic, and traumatic brain disorders. Brain edema can also occur in patients with no intrinsic brain pathology. For example, it may complicate the otherwise successful insulin treatment of diabetic ketoacidosis (see Chap. 16). Brain edema has been subdivided in many ways. The current concept includes three types of edema: vasogenic, cellular, and hydrocephalic. This classification is useful because it provides a framework for thinking about pathophysiology, yet also corresponds closely to the clinical realities. However, not all types of edema encountered in patients fit easily into one of these categories. For example, all three types probably coexist in purulent meningitis. The clinical features and pathophysiology of the various types of edema are summarized in Table 17–2. The clinical effects of brain edema can be catastrophic. Many patients still die of brain herniation—the result of uncontrolled edema—despite the best medical or surgical treatment for the underlying nervous system disease.

Brain edema is defined as an increase in brain volume caused by an increase in brain H_2O content. Seemingly small changes in brain H_2O content can produce large increases in volume; for example, a 2% increase in white matter H_2O from 70% to 72% represents a 6.7% increase in volume. Brain edema should be distinguished from brain *engorgement*, which is an increase in brain volume resulting from an increase in blood volume.

Cellular brain edema

The term *cellular brain edema* replaces the older term *cytotoxic*. While it is true that metabolic poisons cause brain cells to swell, other states, such as water intoxication, also bring about cell swelling. The newer term encompasses the essential features of this type of brain edema: The edema is intracellular, brain extracellular fluid volume is diminished, and the blood-brain

Table 17–2. Classification of brain edema

	Vasogenic	Cellular (cytotoxic)	Interstitial (hydrocephalic)
Pathogenesis	Increased capillary permeability	Cellular swelling—glial, neuronal, endothelial	Increased brain fluid due to block of CSF absorption
Location of edema	Chiefly white matter	Gray and white matter	Chiefly periventricular white matter in hydrocephalus
Edema fluid composition	Plasma filtrate including plasma proteins	Increased intracellular water and sodium	Cerebrospinal fluid
Extracellular fluid volume	Increased	Decreased	Increased
Capillary permeability to large molecules (RISA, inulin)	Increased	Normal	Normal
Clinical disorders	Brain tumors, abscess, infarction, trauma, hemorrhage, lead encephalopathy Ischemia Purulent meningitis (granulocytic edema)	Hypoxia, hypo-osmolality due to water intoxication, etc. Disequilibrium syndromes Ischemia Purulent meningitis (granulocytic edema) Reye's syndrome	Obstructive hydrocephalus Pseudotumor (?) Purulent meningitis (granulocytic edema)
EEG changes	Focal slowing common	Generalized slowing	EEG often normal
Therapeutic effects			
Steroids	Beneficial in brain tumor, abscess	Not effective (?Reye's syndrome)	Uncertain effectiveness (?pseudotumor, ?meningitis)
Osmotherapy	Reduces volume of normal brain tissue only, acutely	Reduces brain volume acutely in hype-osmolality	Rarely useful
Acetazolamide	?Effect	No direct effect	Minor usefulness
Furosemide	?Effect	No direct effect	Minor usefulness

From Fishman, *Cerebrospinal Fluid in Diseases of the Nervous System.* Philadelphia, Saunders, 1980, with permission of the author and W. B. Saunders Co.

barrier is intact. Cellular edema can be subdivided further into osmotic edema, caused by changes in plasma or brain osmolality, and metabolic edema, caused by toxins or substrate deprivation.

Osmotic edema is produced in experimental animals by administering antidiuretic hormone and free water, thereby causing an abrupt decrease in plasma osmolality. If the blood-brain barrier is intact, the resulting osmotic gradient will favor the movement of water into the brain. Acutely, brain water increases, but the brain content of solutes expressed as milliequivalent per kilogram *dry* weight remains unchanged. In the presence of con-

tinued plasma hypo-osmolality the brain adapts by losing intracellular solute, especially K^+, thus reducing intracellular osmolality and diminishing the osmotic gradient driving water into brain cells. The changes in brain water and electrolytes in acute hypo-osmolality have been studied extensively in animals. Clinically, acute hypo-osmolality is usually secondary to hyponatremia. Decreases in plasma sodium large enough and rapid enough to cause clinically apparent brain edema are rare in humans, but the few cases studied pathologically have had brain edema.

The brain adapts to chronic plasma *hyper*osmolality by accumulating intracellular osmotically active molecules, which diminish the osmotic gradient favoring water movement out of the brain. In some instances the identity of these molecules is known. For example, in hypernatremia, amino acids account for *some* of the increase in intracellular osmoles. In other hyperosmolal states, such as hyperglycemia, the molecules have not been identified. In both instances, those intracellular, osmotically active molecules that cannot be accounted for by measurable increases in amino acids, electrolytes, or other small molecules are termed *idiogenic osmoles*. The nature of these *idiogenic osmoles* is a fundamental question in the field of brain osmoregulation. They may represent changes in activity, rather than concentration, of intracellular cations brought about by changes in binding to intracellular macromolecules. When plasma hyperosmolality (due to hypernatremia) is corrected rapidly, idiogenic osmoles persist in the brain, creating an osmotic gradient favoring the movement of H_2O into brain and the development of edema. Brain edema occasionally complicates the insulin treatment of diabetic ketoacidosis. The mechanism is uncertain, but may involve the persistence of idiogenic osmoles in the brain or a direct effect of insulin on brain electrolyte concentrations.

Metabolic edema occurs when cellular energy production is compromised and the cell's ion pumps are deprived of ATP. Intracellular Na^+ accumulates in excess of the K^+, which passively leaks out of the cell. The intracellular osmolality increases: In response to this osmotic gradient the cell imbibes H_2O and its volume increases. Cellular energy production can be impaired by exogenous metabolic inhibitors, such as cyanide, 2,4,-dinitrophenol, and 6-aminonicotinamide or by substrate deprivation. Substances like ouabain that interfere with key membrane enzymes such as the $(Na^+ - K^+)$-ATPase, can also cause edema. The edema is characterized by in-

creased intracellular concentrations of Na^+, decreased intracellular K^+, and evidence of cellular swelling on light microscopy. Of particular clinical note is that when the brain is deprived of glucose and O_2 by circulatory arrest, its cells swell as their ion pumps fail and the volume of the extracellular space decreases. Strictly speaking this state is not brain edema since there is no net increase in the volume of the brain. Because circulation has ceased, any increase in the volume of cells must come at the expense of either the extracellular fluid volume or the intravascular volume, which is not being replenished.

In certain clinical conditions the major part of cellular edema is thought to occur in astrocytes. When cerebral infarction or severe head trauma results in an increase in extracellular K^+, protoplasmic astrocytes respond by taking this up with subsequent swelling. A situation that is thought to be analogous occurs when the cerebral cortex of an animal is superfused with high concentrations of KCl (>10 mM). Cellular edema develops that is confined almost exclusively to astrocytes. This selective swelling seems to be triggered by the elevated extracellular K^+, rather than indirectly via an effect on neurons (such as neurotransmitter release). Part of the astrocytic swelling develops as a passive response to the higher concentration of K^+ and the lower concentration of Na^+ in the extracellular fluid. The remainder of the swelling is accounted for by a K^+-dependent, HCO_3-stimulated, carrier-mediated transport of Cl^- ion, coupled with cation, into astrocytes.

Reye's syndrome is an acute disorder characterized by an encephalopathy with severe brain edema and elevated intracranial pressure, along with fatty degeneration on the liver. The brain edema of Reye's syndrome is most likely metabolic, but the exact biochemical pathology is not understood. There is some disagreement as to whether the liver disease is primary (with the encephalopathy secondary to the elevated levels of NH_3 resulting from liver dysfunction), or whether the disease is caused by a generalized, temporary mitochondrial dysfunction, perhaps triggered by short-chain fatty acids affecting liver and brain mitochondria simultaneously. Exogenous substances, including aspirin, have also been implicated in Reye's syndrome. Although the disease usually follows a viral infection, there is no evidence of direct viral hepatitis or encephalitis. The most consistent neuropathological finding is cerebral edema. Ultrastructural studies show swelling of astrocytes, abnormal mitochondria, and focal expansions of the myelin sheath. There is no sign of inflammation or viral inclusions. Despite our lack of knowledge about the cause of Reye's syndrome, the elevated intracranial pressure can often be lowered (see later discussion).

Recent work suggests that free radicals (chemical species with a lone electron in the outermost orbital), polyunsaturated fatty acids, and excitatory neurotransmitter amino acids may be important inducers of the brain edema associated with ischemia, hyperosmolal states, trauma, tumors, and infections. These compounds induce cellular edema in brain slices in *in vitro*, but their role *in vivo* has yet to be established. Free radicals such as superoxide ion, hydroxyl radical, and singlet oxygen cause degradation of membrane phospholipids and may perturb key membrane-associated enzymes by peroxidation of membrane lipids. Recent studies show that arachidonic acid, a major membrane phospholipid component, inhibits $(Na^+ + K^+)$-ATPase activity in synaptic membranes and cortical slices. The *in vivo* action of polyunsaturated fatty acids, free radicals, and excitatory amino acids is currently under investigation.

Vasogenic brain edema

The most common type of brain edema encountered in clinical practice is vasogenic brain edema. This type of brain edema is a frequent and severe complication of primary and metastatic tumors, focal and diffuse CNS infections, all types of CNS trauma, and the encephalopathy of lead poisoning in children. You will recall that, unlike other vascular beds, the endothelial cells of the brain microvasculature have tight junctions and sparse plasmalemmal vesicles and thus allow very little protein to enter the brain extracellular fluid. Vasogenic brain edema differs from cellular brain edema in that the fluid that accumulates is *extra*cellular and high in plasma protein. The proteinaceous nature of vasogenic edema has been confirmed by two morphological techniques. Protein tracers such as Evans blue-albumin (which fluoresces under ultraviolet light) and HRP (which can be cytochemically converted into an electron-dense reaction product) have been shown to accumulate in the extracellular space of regions rendered edematous by cerebral injury or inflammation. These large molecules are ordinarily confined to the plasma and do not cross the normal blood-brain barrier. More recently, direct biochemical analysis of minute amounts of edema fluid has confirmed its high protein content.

Endothelial ultrastructure has been studied extensively in animal models of vasogenic edema. The observed changes, thought to allow the leakage of protein, Na^+, and water across the microvessel wall, range from subtle changes in endothelial cell structure to total necrosis of the vessels. These changes include increases in the numbers of vesicles in the endothelial cytoplasm and the appearance of fenestrae or transendothelial channels, structures not seen in normal brain endothelial cells.

Vasogenic brain edema shows a predilection for white matter and tends to extend from gray matter into, and along, adjacent white matter tracks. The extension along white matter is probably a reflection of the organization of this tissue. It is believed that the parallel bundles of myelinated axons making up white matter offer less resistance to the flow of extracellular fluid than the dense network of neuronal and glial processes composing gray matter. Vasogenic edema fluid spreads by bulk flow rather than by diffusion, i.e., solutes of different molecular weights move at the same rate as each other and as the solvent (in this case, H_2O). Thus, in the edema spreading from a necrotic lesion, molecules such as sucrose (mol wt 342) and albumin (mol wt, 70,000) move at the same rate. The rate of this spread is proportional to the systemic arterial blood pressure. One of several factors affecting the resolution of vasogenic edema is the bulk flow of H_2O and solutes into the CSF. This will occur as long as there is a pressure gradient between brain and CSF. Other factors such as the "back transport" of H_2O and proteins across the blood-brain barrier into the circulation and the uptake of extravastated serum proteins by astrocytes have also been proposed as mechanisms of resolution. The quantitative significance of each of these processes in a given clinical situation is unknown, although all have been demonstrated in experimental animals.

Vasogenic edema is most often associated with focal, rapidly expanding lesions of the brain (e.g., metastatic tumors and pyogenic abscesses). In these situations the edema component may contribute as much (or more) to the "mass" effect exerted by the lesion. Edematous mass lesions can exert pressure on the microvasculature of surrounding normal brain, thereby producing an ever-expanding zone of ischemia and further edema in a self-perpetuating cycle. Effective therapy for edema will stop or delay these changes and allow time for definitive therapy of the underlying pathology. The pathogenesis and clinical manifestations of brain herniation are discussed more completely in Chapter 10.

Table 17–3. Causes of hydrocephalus

Obstruction of CSF pathways: intraventricular (noncommunicating) or extraventricular (communicating or noncommunicating)
  Postinflammatory or posthemorrhagic obstruction
  Congenital malformations:
    Arnold-Chiari malformations, meningomyelocele
    Occlusion of outlets of fourth ventricle (Dandy-Walker syndrome)
  Neoplasms obstructing the ventricular system

Overproduction of CSF:
  Choroid plexus papilloma (may also cause ventricular obstruction)

Defective absorption of CSF:
  Impaired venous drainage
  Defective arachnoid villi (congenital or acquired)

From R. A. Fishman, *Cerebrospinal Fluid in Diseases of the Nervous System*. Philadelphia, W. B. Saunders, 1980, with permission of the author and W. B. Saunders Co.

Hydrocephalus and hydrocephalic brain edema

Hydrocephalus is the dilation of one or more of the cerebral ventricles, with an increase in CSF volume. The distinction between communicating and noncommunicating hydrocephalus, explained earlier (Fig. 17–1), is clinically useful because it serves as a guide for placement of shunts designed to bypass the obstruction to CSF flow. The causes of hydrocephalus are summarized in Table 17–3. Clinically, the most important cause is obstruction of the CSF pathways either within or beyond the ventricular system. A rare intraventricular tumor, the choroid plexus papilloma, has been shown to secrete CSF at a rate about four times normal and may cause hydrocephalus.

The ventricular enlargement in hydrocephalus occurs at the expense of the periventricular white matter. The first event that follows acute obstruction of CSF flow is the transependymal movement of CSF into the periventricular white matter. This extracellular accumulation of CSF is termed hydrocephalic brain edema. As intraventricular pressure increases, the periventricular white matter begins to lose myelin lipids. These changes are reversible if the obstruction is relieved and CSF pressure is reduced to normal within several weeks (the exact time limit is unknown).

The treatment of hydrocephalic edema is actually the treatment of the underlying hydrocephalus. It is possible to relieve elevated intraventricular pressure by diverting (or "shunting") CSF into the circulation or the peritoneal cavity.

INTRACRANIAL PRESSURE

Normal intracranial pressure is 65–195 mm H_2O, or 5–15 mm Hg. Clinically, CSF pressure is usually measured during lumbar puncture with the patient lying on his side so that the cranial compartment and lumbar sac are at the same level. The pressure in the lumbar subarachnoid sac is equal to the intracranial pressure if the patient is horizontal and there is no obstruction to free flow of CSF between the two compartments such as a spinal tumor that has obliterated the subarchnoid space around the cord. In recent years, direct recording of subarchnoid or intraventricular pressure has been possible by using surgically implanted devices. Direct isovolumetric recordings from these devices provide immediate information about intracranial pressure in disease and the effects of measures directed at controlling its increase.

CSF pressure varies from moment to moment, with the variation best appreciated in recordings made from the ventricles. It can be seen in a manometer attached to a needle in the lumbar subarachnoid space, but the excursions are highly damped. CSF pressure varies with the cardiac cycle; the pressure during systole is 20–30 mm H_2O higher than during diastole. It is believed that these pulsations reflect the pulsations of the major intracranial conducting arteries. Respiration also influences CSF pressure. During quiet breathing CSF pressure fluctuates by

10–20 mm H_2O. This respiratory variation illustrates that CSF pressure depends on cerebral blood volume as well as on the volume of brain tissue and CSF (Fig. 17–1D), an important and clinically useful point. Central venous pressure falls on inspiration. Since the jugular venous system is in direct communication with the right atrium, pressure in the intracranial venous sinuses also falls. Thus, with inspiration, CSF pressure falls with the decrease in intracranial venous pressure. The reverse happens with expiration. The changes during expiration are accentuated during forced expiration against a closed glottis (Valsalva maneuver). The increased intrathoracic pressure decreases venous return, including that from the cerebral venous sinuses. Cerebral blood volume increases and is reflected in an elevation of CSF pressure.

CSF pressure also varies with changes in the arterial blood gases. Hypoxemia and hypercarbia both cause cerebral vasodilatation, an increase in cerebral blood volume, and increased CSF pressure (Fig. 17–1D). Hypocarbia produces cerebral vasoconstriction and thus decreased blood volume and CSF pressure. This decrease in CSF pressure evoked by a decrease in arterial PCO_2 is clinically useful. Mechanical hyperventilation lowering PCO_2 to 25 mm Hg is the fastest way to lower raised intracranial pressure. The maneuver can be used to control potentially life-threatening intracranial pressure elevations in patients with intracranial masses until more definitive therapy is started.

Each of the preceding examples demonstrates the exquisite dependence of intracranial pressure on cerebral blood volume and serves to emphasize that elevated intracranial pressure (intracranial hypertension) is not synonymous with brain edema. Even in the absence of brain edema, intracranial pressure can be elevated by an increase in the blood volume of the intracranial compartment (brain engorgement). Furthermore, the presence of brain edema does not necessarily imply an elevated intracranial pressure. For example, a tumor may induce edema in the surrounding brain, but if it develops slowly and is not extensive, overall intracranial pressure may not be increased.

Increased intracranial pressure

Increased intracranial pressure may result from increases in the volume of any of the normal constituents of the intracranial compartment (brain, blood, or CSF) or the addition of new tissue (e.g., hematoma or tumor) to the intracranial compartment. Intracranial pressure is a function not only of the *volume* of these components, but also of the *rates* of CSF formation and outflow, the pressure in the venous sinuses, and the compliance of brain tissue. For example, consider a patient with an expanding intracranial mass such as a tumor. As the tumor grows, two compensatory mechanisms come into play. CSF outflow through the "one-way," low-resistance valves of the arachnoid villi increases and its volume diminishes. The lumbar meninges (which are slightly distensible) and large veins (which have low intraluminal pressures and are easily compressed) also enable the system to adjust to the expanding mass without an initial increase in intracranial pressure. The tumor's growth, however, will reach a point at which these processes can no longer compensate. If the tumor grows slowly, pressure atrophy of the brain will result. If the tumor grows rapidly, elevated intracranial pressure will eventually supervene. The relationship between changes in the volume of the intracranial contents and intracranial pressure is shown in Figure 17–9. If one starts with normal intracranial pressure (left side of Fig. 17–9), large increments in the volume of intracranial constituents result in little or no change in intracranial pressure because of the pre-

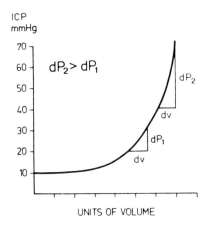

Fig. 17–9. Theoretical intracranial volume-pressure curve. (From J. D. Miller, Volume and pressure in the craniospinal axis. *Clin. Neurosurg.* 22:76–105, 1975, with permission of the author and the Congress of Neurological Surgeons.)

viously mentioned compensatory mechanisms. With continuing increases in volume, progressively larger increases in intracranial pressure result from smaller increments in volume (the steep, right-hand portion of the curve in Fig. 17-9). These pressure–volume relationships can be expressed numerically as *compliance* (dV/dP). With expanding intracranial masses, compliance decreases.

Compliance can be determined in the clinical setting by injecting a known volume of artificial CSF into a ventricular catheter and observing the resulting change in intracranial pressure. This information complements data on intracranial pressure because it tells the neurosurgeon the patient's status on the pressure-volume curve. Some neurosurgeons have used this intracranial compliance monitoring as an indicator of response to medical therapy for elevated intracranial pressure and as an aid in determining when surgical intervention is needed.

Continuous recording of CSF pressure in patients with high intracranial pressure has shown marked fluctuations. Several

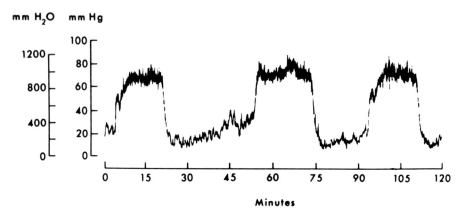

Fig. 17–10. Recording of intracranial pressure from a patient with a brain tumor shows three prominent plateau, or "A," waves. From N. Lundberg, Continuous recording and control of ventricular fluid pressure in neurosurgical practice. (*Acta Psych. Neurol. Scand.* Supp. 149, vol. 36, 1960, with permission of the author and Minksgaard International Publishers, Ltd.)

types of fluctuations have been described, the best known being "A" waves, or plateau waves (Fig. 17–10). These usually last many minutes. Patients may be symptomatic with vomiting, headache, depression of consciousness, or rigidity during these acute severe elevations in intracranial pressure. Blood pressure is sometimes concomitantly elevated. Plateau waves can be induced in patients with increased intracranial pressure by the inhalation of 5% CO_2 or by the injection of small amounts of saline into the ventricles. However, they may occur spontaneously in patients who are mechanically ventilated with constant arterial PCO_2 and intrathoracic pressure values. Cerebral arteriograms performed during plateau waves show arterial dilatation. Although cerebral blood *flow* is diminished during these episodes, cerebral blood *volume* is increased. Plateau waves occur when a patient with elevated intracranial pressure is on the steep portion of the pressure–volume curve, i.e., when minimal increases in cerebral blood volume (brought about by disordered autoregulation of cerebral blood flow, CO_2 retention, or other factors we do not

understand) evoke sharp increases in intracranial pressure.

THERAPY OF BRAIN EDEMA AND ELEVATED INTRACRANIAL PRESSURE

The treatment of brain edema and elevated intracranial pressure is far from ideal and is likely to remain so until their pathogenesis is better understood. In considering the treatment of these conditions it is important to remember the distinction between brain edema and its consequence, elevated intracranial pressure. Much of the current therapy for patients with brain edema is actually directed at lowering the intracranial pressure and exerts its effect on normal brain tissue.

While specific therapies such as adrenal corticosteroids and osmotic agents can be very effective in some patients with elevated intracranial pressure secondary to brain edema, general measures that are often overlooked can be equally important. In caring for patients with elevated intracranial pressure, knowledge of pathophysiology dictates that CO_2 retention, hypoxia, serum hyposomalality, and the use of drugs that cause cerebral vaso-dilatation (e.g., halothane) should be scrupulously avoided. As mentioned ear-lier, the cerebral vasoconstriction induced by a low arterial PCO_2 is the quickest way to lower intracranial pressure. However, the cerebral vasculature of patients with severe elevations in intracranial pressure does not always respond as expected. These patients, especially those with severe head injuries, often suffer cerebral vasomotor paralysis, rendering hyperventilation ther-apy ineffective.

Adrenal corticosteroids

Adrenal corticosteroids have proven to be effective therapy for the vasogenic edema associated with primary and metastatic CNS tumors, but have been much less ef-fective when used to treat patients with other types of edema. Although used al-most universally in patients with severe head trauma, their effectiveness and the dosage required are still debated. Steroids have never been shown to be useful in ce-rebral infarction or the cellular edemas (with the exception of alkyl tin edema, a laboratory model with little applicability to the clinical problem of brain edema). Steroids have been widely used in patients with Reye's syndrome but have not been studied in a controlled fashion in this con-dition. The action of these powerful drugs is not understood and it is even uncertain whether the observed effects are the result of a decrease in edema per se or of a sep-arate action on damaged neural tissue. Since steroids are most useful in the vaso-genic edemas, it seems reasonable that they work by stabilizing the microvascular en-dothelium in some undetermined way. Al-though there is evidence for this concept, other mechanisms have been proposed, such as effects on lysosomes, electrolyte transport, or phospholipase A_2 (the en-zyme responsible for the release of polyunsaturated fatty acids from neural membranes). In addition, the effectiveness of steroids in patients with brain tumors may be due to their ability to reduce the size of the tumors themselves.

Osmotherapy

The treatment of elevated intracranial pressure with osmotic agents is based on the tendency of the blood-brain barrier to exclude lipid-insoluble substances for which no specific transport system exists. These agents increase the plasma osmolal-ity; because they cross the blood-brain barrier to a minimal extent, they create an osmotic gradient favoring the movement of H_2O out of brain and into plasma. Brain volume will fall only if this gradient exists. The areas of brain that lose water are those with a normal blood-brain barrier. Re-gions of brain with a damaged blood-brain barrier do not lose water because no gra-dient favoring water movement out of brain is ever established. Thus osmotherapy lowers intracranial pressure in patients with brain edema, but does nothing to dehy-drate regions of the brain with an abnor-mally permeable blood-brain barrier.

In patients with intracranial mass le-sions osmotherapy is most useful when it can be used to temporarily lower in-creased intracranial pressure until defini-tive surgical therapy can be performed. Chronic osmotherapy is less effective for several reasons. First, the osmotic gra-dients between blood and brain are tran-sient due to two factors: (1) None of the solutes employed is completely excluded by the blood-brain barrier and eventually there is equilibration between plasma and brain; and (2) the solutes are also cleared by the kidneys. Second, as we have seen in the section on cellular edema, normal brain adjusts to chronic plasma hyperosmolality by increasing its intracellular osmolality, which tends to minimize the magnitude of any osmotic gradient between plasma and brain. Finally, pathological regions of brain that lack a normally functioning blood-brain barrier will not exclude the osmotic agent in the first place. When plasma osmolality declines as a dose of osmotic agent is excreted, a reverse gradient is established with the osmolality of the edematous region exceeding that of plasma. This is responsible for the rebound increases in intracranial pressure that sometimes follow single doses of osmotic agents.

Patients being treated with osmotherapy should be clearly monitored. Ideally, intracranial pressure, plasma osmolality and electrolytes, central venous and arterial blood pressures, and urine output and electrolytes should be followed in an intensive care unit. Severe plasma hyperosmolality must be carefully avoided because it is not beneficial to brain function. Gradients of as little as 10 mOsm per liter are effective.

The agents used for osmotherapy include urea, mannitol, and glycerol; currently the latter two are most widely used. Mannitol is more effectively excluded by the blood-brain barrier than glycerol, but, unlike glycerol, it cannot be given orally. Mannitol is not metabolized, whereas glycerol is converted to CO_2 and H_2O with the production of 4.3 calories per gram. Although these drugs exert their primary effects on brain water content, chronic plasma hyperosmolality also reduces CSF secretion, which would be beneficial in patients with elevated intracranial pressure.

Diuretics

Acetazolamide and furosemide inhibit CSF secretion by different mechanisms. These drugs have been used to reduce interstitial brain edema in hydrocephalic patients and to enhance the clearance of vasogenic edema fluid from brain into the CSF "sink." Ethacrynic acid, which inhibits Cl^- transport in astrocytes, may prove to be useful in some patients with head injuries, but its place in the treatment of edema is yet to be defined.

GENERAL REFERENCES

Bradbury, M. W. B. *The Concept of a Blood-Brain Barrier.* John Wiley and Sons, Chichester, 1979.

Cervos-Navarro, J., and R. Ferszt (eds.). *Brain Edema, Advances in Neurology,* vol. 28. New York, Raven Press, 1980.

Fishman, R. A. *The Cerebrospinal Fluid in Diseases of the Nervous System.* Philadelphia, Saunders, 1980.

Katzman, R., and H. M. Pappius. *Brain Electrolytes and Fluid Metabolism.* Baltimore, Williams and Wilkins, 1973.

Klatzo, I. Neuropathological aspects of brain edema. *J. Neuropath. Exper. Neurol.* 26:1–14, 1967.

Pappius, H. M., and W. Feidel (eds.). *Dynamics of Brain Edema.* New York, Springer-Verlag, 1976.

Rapoport, S. I. *Blood-Brain Barrier in Physiology and Medicine.* New York, Raven Press, 1976.

Siegel, G. J., R. W. Albers, B. W. Agranoff, and R. Katzman (eds.). *Basic Neurochemistry,* 3d ed. Boston, Little, Brown, 1981.

Wood, J. H. (ed.). *Neurobiology of Cerebrospinal Fluid.* New York, Plenum Press, 1980. (vol. 1; vol. 2 in press).

Wright, E. M. Transport processes in the formation of the cerebrospinal fluid. *Rev. Physiol. Biochem. Pharmacol.* 83:1–34, 1978.

18.

Infections

LAWRENCE D. GELB

In this chapter the pathophysiology of central nervous system infections is reviewed: how they arise, how they produce neurologic damage, and how the clinical presentation and sequelae derive from this damage. The major classes of CNS infection under consideration are meningitis, encephalitis, brain abscess, and parameningeal infections.

The manifestations of CNS infections can be very subtle, especially early in the course of disease. Patients can present with symptoms ranging from a slight lack of well-being to a bewildering array of clinical abnormalities. The most frequent presentation is the sudden onset of fever (sometimes slight), headache, and lethargy. Nausea, vomiting, and other symptoms related to elevation in CSF pressure may also be prominent. Another important clue to CNS infection is the presence of infection elsewhere. CNS infection does not usually arise de novo; it is often accompanied by adjacent infection involving the ears, mastoid, or paranasal sinuses, or by distant infections, such as those of the pulmonary parenchyma or endocardium.

Meningitis, the most common CNS infection, is characterized by inflammation of the pia-arachnoid membranes, with symptoms of headache, confusion, and resistance of the neck to passive flexion. Encephalitis, on the other hand, involves the brain parenchyma itself and is characterized by disorders of mentation and focal abnormalities related to the area of damage. It is frequently accompanied by some degree of meningeal inflammation (meningoencephalitis or encephalomyelitis). A brain abscess is a localized suppurative process within the brain substance. It presents primarily as an expanding mass lesion with focal neurologic abnormalities that often overshadow the signs of infection. The parameningeal infections are those infections that are adjacent to, but do not involve, the meninges. These include epidural abscess, subdural empyema, and dural sinus thrombosis. Symptoms include headache and fever, confusion, and focal abnormalities related to the location of disease.

PATHOPHYSIOLOGY

The presentation and course of CNS infections are closely related to the anatomy of the skull and spinal canal. The physical relationships determine the route of infection, the organisms involved, the location of the infectious process, and the ultimate containment or spread. The nature of the infecting organism and the physical constraints of the calvarium and spinal canal largely determine the extent of damage.

The anatomy of the CNS and its coverings both protect it from infection and promote extensive damage once infection occurs. The calvarium and bony spinal canal protect the brain and cord from trauma and, along with the dura mater and leptomeninges, protect the CNS from direct invasion by pathogenic organisms. The blood-brain barrier protects the CNS from hematogenous infection. Infection of brain parenchyma rarely follows bacteremia alone, since healthy cerebral tissue is quite resistant to infection; direct intracerebral inoculation of bacteria in animals does not result in abscess formation unless large volumes are used or necrosis is induced first.

These same protective mechanisms contribute to spread and increased damage once infection occurs. The calvarium and spinal canal are rigid and do not allow significant expansion of the infected tissue. This adds pressure necrosis to the damage produced by the invading organism itself. The meninges generally contain the infection and prevent spread across them, but they also allow free spread in the spaces they enclose. All structures within these spaces, such as the choroid plexus and the cranial and spinal nerve roots, are trapped with the infectious agent, inflammatory cells, and various toxins for extended periods of time. Similarly, adjacent structures such as pial blood vessels and underlying cerebral and cerebellar cortices may be involved. The blood-brain barrier, while generally protective, also inhibits the ingress of phagocytes, antibodies, and antibiotics. In addition, cerebral tissue lacks effective phagocytes and lymphatic drainage to combat infection

when it does occur. Thus once infection is established in the CNS, it tends to be virulent and destructive. Central nervous system infections are consequently a true medical emergency. The prognosis is strongly correlated with the time elapsed between onset and the start of effective therapy.

Routes of infection

The most common route of CNS infection is via the bloodstream. Bacteremia, viremia, rickettsemia, or fungemia usually precede or occur simultaneously with CNS invasion. Pneumococci, *H. influenzae,* and meningococci, the three most common pathogens in bacterial meningitis, have an apparent predilection for the meninges, but it is unclear how and in what circumstances these organisms are able to cross the blood-CSF barrier. It seems that some preceding disruptive event may be required. Infection in this instance is usually caused by a single virulent organism. Blood-borne infection of the CNS can also result from septic emboli, particularly from the lung and the endocardium. The range of organisms tends to be wide and, with pulmonary foci, mixed.

The most common route of parameningeal infection is from a contiguous focus of disease such as otitis, mastoiditis, paranasal sinusitis, or cranial osteomyelitis. In these cases, infection can erode through the inner table of the skull, across the dura, and into the subdural space, the subarachnoid space, or the brain itself. Contiguous infection also results in CNS invasion by involvement of the diploic veins and retrograde extension to the dural sinuses and brain. These infections reflect the flora of the parameningeal focus and therefore tend to be mixed.

The third major route of CNS infection is via direct invasion. Direct invasion may accompany or follow trauma, or it may occur as a consequence of an acquired or congenital defect such as an old

Table 18–1. Organisms commonly responsible for bacterial meningitis

Neonatal Meningitis	Childhood and Adult Meningitis

1. Organisms acquired at birth
  a. Gram positive:
     Streptococci especially groups A, B, & D
     Listeria monocytogenes
	1. Respiratory commensals
	  a. Limited pathogenic subtypes
	     H. influenzae, type B
	     N. meningitidis groups A, B, & C
	     Resistance develops with
	     exposure to nonpathogens;
	     incidence maximal at 1 year

b. Gram negative:
     Enterobacteriaceae (e.g., *E. coli*)
	b. Multiple pathogenic subtypes
	     S. pneumoniae (pneumococcus),
	     80 + capsular types
	     No definite cross-protection
	     Most common adult pathogen

2. Organisms acquired in the nursery
  a. Gram positive:
     S. aureus
	2. Disseminated pathogens
	  a. Gram positive:
	     Streptococci, groups A & D
	     S. aureus

b. Gram negative:
     Environmental commensals
     (e.g., pseudomonas)
     Respiratory pathogens are not
     seen because of passively
     acquired immunity
	b. Gram negative:
	     salmonella
	
	  c. Acid fast:
	     M. tuberculosis

fracture of the cribiform plate or a dermoid sinus tract.

Organisms encountered

A wide variety of pathogens has been associated with CNS infection, including bacteria, protozoa, viruses, fungi, mycobacteria, rickettsia, and even metazoan parasites. Although almost any organism can produce neural inflammation, the organisms involved can often be predicted on the basis of the area of the CNS involved and the route of infection. In bacterial meningitis, the vast majority of infections is presumed to be hematogenous; 85% of the adult cases are due to pneumococci, *H. influenzae,* and meningococci. *H. influenzae* is the most common organism overall and is especially likely in children under six years of age. The organisms that frequently cause bacterial meningitis are listed in Table 18–1.

Special circumstances increase the probability of other organisms causing CNS infection. Concomitant pulmonary infection is often associated with mixed bacterial CNS infections. Similarly, endocarditis increases the likelihood of *Staphylococcus aureus* infection. Transplacental infection producing CNS disease has been reported with such viruses as rubella and cytomegalovirus, protozoans such as *Toxoplasma gondii,* and bacteria such as syphilis and *Listeria monocytogenes.* Neonatal CNS infections with group B, beta-hemolytic streptococci and herpes simplex virus are apparently acquired during passage through the birth canal and strongly correlate with vaginal carriage of the organism by the mother.

The infections of the CNS that are associated with contiguous foci generally contain the flora and pathogens of the primary site. CNS infections originating in paranasal sinusitis are usually mixed infections due to mouth flora such as anaerobic streptococci and *Bacteroides* species. Infections associated with trauma are often staphylococcal, while those resulting from CSF leaks are frequently pneumococcal. Despite these predilections, however, the etiologic agent of CNS infection cannot be reliably predicted solely on clinical grounds. Laboratory confirmation is essential.

Factors predisposing to CNS infection

Many of the factors that lead to infection of the central nervous system are identical to those that predispose to infections elsewhere. Most of these are related to the host—both to the "normal host" and to the "abnormal host." Factors relating to the invading organism and the environment are also important. An environmentally fostered organism exploits some defect or deficiency in the host to establish infection in the central nervous system.

Host factors

It is useful to discuss the defenses of the central nervous system first and then to consider how they are breached. The major defenses of the CNS against infection include general good health, an intact anatomic barrier between the outside and the CNS, adequate blood flow, and a functioning immune system, both humoral and cellular. But deficiencies in these defenses occur, even in the host that is otherwise normal. The most clearly defined "normal" deficiency is that related to immunologic immaturity and lack of exposure. Newborns are always deficient in specific IgM antibody since it does not cross the placenta. Consequently, they are uniquely susceptible to infection with enteric Gram-negative rods, and these organisms account for a significant percentage of neonatal bacterial meningitis (and sepsis). Other factors must also be involved, however, since enteric meningitis is quite uncommon even though the neonatal deficiency of serum IgM is universal.

Older infants begin to lose their placentally acquired IgG, and because of lack of exposure, become increasingly susceptible to CNS infection by meningococci and *H. influenzae*—both neurotropic organisms with limited pathogenic serotypes. These "deficiencies" largely disappear by the age of 6 as adult patterns emerge. The adult is still compromised by lack of exposure, however, and meningitis due to organisms with multiple pathogenic serotypes like the pneumococcus becomes more prevalent. Finally, as individuals age, immunity wanes and the incidence of CNS infection again increases.

As with most infections, males are significantly more at risk for CNS infection than females. Premature infants account for 48% of infected neonates although they represent only 8% of live births. Prematurity and even the normal immaturity of the newborn contribute to an increased susceptibility to CNS infections and tend to make those infections that do occur more severe. The trauma of even a normal vaginal delivery seems to increase the risk of infection, although the incidence is still higher with premature rupture of the membranes, prolonged or difficult labor, and infection in the mother in the week prior to delivery.

Frequently, CNS infection occurs in a host that has either a congenital or acquired defect in its immunologic or anatomic defenses. Both congenital immune defects and those produced by diseases or medications that suppress the immune system increase the likelihood of CNS infections. Absent or decreased IgG increases the incidence of CNS invasion by pneumococci and *H. influenzae*; suppression or absence of thymus-derived (T) lymphocytes increases the incidence and severity of viral and fungal infections of the CNS. Absence of T-cell function occurs in Di George's syndrome (absent thymus and parathyroids), Nezelof's syndrome (absent thymus), ataxia telangiectasia (dysplastic thymus, neurologic abnormalities, and reduced serum IgA), Wiskott-Aldrich syndrome (eczema, thrombocytopenia, and recurrent infections), and combined immunodeficiency disease (deficits in both humoral and cellular function). Even such normally non-virulent agents as live, attenuated vaccines can cause CNS involvement in these patients and should therefore not be administered.

Other immune defects are also possible etiologic factors in CNS infection. Abnormalities in polymorphonuclear leukocyte function have been noted in the newborn, but the importance of this observation with regard to neonatal meningitis is unclear. Congenital defects in phagocytic cell function or a decrease in the number of neutrophils during the treatment of neoplastic disease lead to an increased incidence and severity of many infections, but a similar increase in CNS infections has not been documented. Congenital or acquired asplenia is associated with an increased incidence of sepsis and CNS invasion, particularly with the pneumococcus. The risk is extremely variable and depends on the age of the host, the interval since spleen removal, and the indication for the procedure (trauma, staging for Hodgkin's disease, autosplenectomy of sickle cell disease, etc.). The risk of sepsis is quite high in patients who have had a splenectomy as a result of a hematologic disorder (up to 33% in thalassemia major), but virtually zero with splenectomy necessitated by trauma.

Malignancies, particularly of the reticuloendothelial system, also predispose the patient to infections of the central nervous system. Hodgkin's disease, leukemia, multiple myeloma, and lymphoma are all associated with decreased levels of circulating immunoglobulins, delayed antibody response, and depression of the functions of the fixed macrophages. These disorders, as well as the immunosuppressive agents, irradiation, and cytotoxic drugs that are used to treat them (and other malignancies or diseases), produce global deficits in the immune system and lead to an increased incidence of CNS infection.

Some deficits in the host's defenses are difficult to quantitate. For example, malnutrition and debilitation appear to be of significance in the etiology of CNS infections, but this association arises primarily from the clinical impression that all infections are more common and severe in the diseased and infirm. Defects in the immune response and in the anatomic barriers have been noted, but they have been variable and of questioned significance. Such chronic conditions as renal failure, alcoholism, and diabetes mellitus all predispose to infections in general and to CNS infections in particular. Again, the mechanisms are unclear and undoubtedly multiple.

Congenital or acquired anatomic defects are also important risk factors in the development of CNS infection. Meningomyeloceles are usually quite obvious, but smaller defects such as a neurodermal sinus can be difficult to detect. Acquired defects usually entail some form of CSF leak that is produced by accidental or surgical trauma, or by a tumor such as a craniopharyngioma. Foreign bodies, including the various shunts, wires, and patches introduced in neurosurgical procedures, should be included in the category of anatomic defects that predispose to CNS infection. The infections tend to be indolent and caused by relatively nonpathogenic organisms that normally constitute part of the flora of the skin. *Staphylococcus epidermidis* has been particularly common in shunt infections.

The presence of an infection in another site is a major factor predisposing to CNS infection. The importance of distant sites of infection such as pneumonia or bacterial endocarditis has already been discussed. Infections in contiguous sites are especially important in the pathogenesis of parameningeal infections. Epidural abscess, subdural empyema, and dural sinus thrombosis as well as brain abscess are frequently associated with infection in adjacent structures. Infection from subacute or chronic otitis media and mastoiditis spreads to the temporal lobe, cerebellum (usually in children with mastoiditis), epidural space, subdural space, lateral dural sinus, and to the meninges. Infections from the nasal area and the sinuses spread to the frontal lobes and cavernous sinus and occasionally to the temporal lobe. All localized CNS infections can extend. Brain abscess can produce ventriculitis and meningitis; epidural abscess can rupture across the dura and produce a subdural empyema. Thus, the presence of an infection that is localized either within or adjacent to the central nervous system is often the first stage in the production of more extensive disease.

Factors related to the infecting organism

Certain organisms with neurotropic predilection, such as those responsible for acute bacterial meningitis, possess virulence factors that are independent of deficiencies in the host's defenses. These factors influence both the likelihood and the severity of CNS infection. Other organisms that only occasionally infect the CNS lack special virulence. These organisms produce disease only when the host is compromised in some way. As discussed earlier, *S. epidermidis,* although usually nonpathogenic and part of the skin flora, is especially prone to infect ventriculoatrial shunts placed for the treatment of hydrocephalus. Low-virulence organisms such as corynebacteria, *Serratia marcescens,* nocardia, and cytomegalovirus only infect the CNS when there are abnormalities of the lymphoid or reticuloendothelial system.

Defects in the host's defenses are not necessary for the virulent organisms to produce infection of the CNS. The disease picture that a given virulent organism produces and the sequelae are closely related to the pathogenic qualities of the particular infecting organism. Pyogenic bacteria, such as *H. influenzae* and the

pneumococcus, produce meningitis that is characterized by a tremendous outpouring of inflammatory cells in the subarachnoid space. This in turn leads to fibrin deposition, venous thrombosis, and arteritis with subsequent cerebral infarction and edema. Vasculitic organisms like the meningococcus rarely produce significant purulence and therefore meningococcal meningitis is largely reversible. Meningoencephalitic organisms, such as staphylococci and amoebae, cause CNS infection only rarely, but are especially virulent when they do. In particular, they tend to produce intracerebral involvement, rather than just meningeal inflammation, and are often fatal.

There are some clues as to how each of these organisms expresses its particular pathogenic qualities, but the mechanisms are not fully understood. The pneumococcus is essentially a nontoxic organism that produces disease solely by local invasion. Its capsule makes it resistant to phagocytosis, which may lead to the development of an exuberant inflammatory response. The meningococcus, on the other hand, produces a particularly active endotoxin that rapidly induces disseminated intravascular coagulation and vascular changes that lead to an early clinical presentation. There may not be time for a purulent response to develop. Staphylococci are more invasive than the pneumococcus but less resistant to phagocytosis. These features might result in less inflammation in the CSF but in greater penetration into the brain parenchyma.

Indolent organisms like *M. tuberculosis* and fungi also have neurotropic propensities. They tend to produce a chronic granulomatous meningitis with complications secondary to fibrin deposition and organization, resulting in obstruction to CSF circulation, cranial nerve damage, and cerebral infarction. Thus, the intrinsic properties of the various micro-organisms determine not only the likelihood of CNS invasion, but also the type of disease produced once they get there.

Environmental influences

Environmental factors are closely related to the transmission of CNS pathogens. Both meningococcal and *H. influenzae* disease are strongly correlated with close contact between individuals. For example, nasopharyngeal colonization by *N. meningitidis* greatly increases when military recruits are put together in a barracks situation. An increased incidence of meningococcal sepsis and meningitis soon follows. A similar situation has been seen with *H. influenzae* in daycare centers, where bacteria of a particular strain apparently spread from child to child. These colonized children are much more likely to develop *H. influenzae* meningitis than those cared for individually in the home. Antibiotic prophylaxis is indicated for all close contacts when either meningococcal or *H. influenzae* meningitis is identified.

Other environmental factors increase the possibility of CNS infection. For example, amoebic meningoencephalitis has been associated with swimming in freshwater ponds filled with free-living amoebae. Arbovirus encephalitis occurs when there is contact with an infected arthropod vector. Consequently, this encephalitis only occurs when the arthropod vector and the reservoir host coexist. Household pets are often infected with leptospires and *Toxoplasma gondii;* CNS infections with these organisms are more common in people who have close contact with infected animals. Several other CNS infections that are not usually encountered in the United States are acquired as a consequence of exposure during travel. A history that includes questions about environmental contacts and travel is therefore essential for evaluating a patient with a CNS infection.

Factors influencing morbidity and mortality

The morbidity and mortality rates associated with CNS infections are influenced primarily by anatomic considerations and by the time elapsed before effective therapy is begun. The CNS is unique in that once infection occurs, there are few mechanisms available to contain it. The actual and potential spaces defined by the meninges allow relatively free spread throughout the system. All structures that penetrate these spaces both incoming and outgoing, are at risk for damage. These include the cranial nerves, particularly III, IV, VI, VII, and VIII, and the penetrating blood vessels. Vessel involvement may then produce ischemic or hemorrhagic injury to the brain or cord, with or without subsequent suppuration.

The brain parenchyma is also unique in its inability to handle infection. It is sequestered from the circulation and from circulating antibodies by the blood-brain barrier, although this is disrupted somewhat in infection. There are "watershed areas" of borderline blood supply that are especially vulnerable to ischemic injury. There are no lymphatics within the brain and little effective phagocytosis. The inflammation that does occur is largely due to infiltration of microglial cells and proliferation of astrocytes. Even this is reduced by ischemia. Abscess encapsulation does occur but is slower and less complete than elsewhere in the body, since it occurs not by fibrosis but by gliosis. All of this combines to make CNS infections especially virulent and difficult to treat.

In light of these considerations, the single most important determinant of morbidity and mortality is the speed with which appropriate therapy is instituted; the more prolonged the interval between onset and effective therapy, the greater the likelihood for death or permanent residua. The range of pathogenic organisms and the specificity of most of the available therapeutic regimens emphasize the importance of a rapid etiologic diagnosis and serve to underscore the critical role of the physician in diagnosing and treating CNS infections.

CLINICAL SYNDROMES

Meningitis

Acute meningitis is a medical emergency. As many as one-third of the patients with bacterial meningitis die. Clearly, if these statistics are to change, the syndrome must be recognized and treated more rapidly.

Inflammation of the subarachnoid space produces symptoms that include headache, backache, and stiff neck (the resistance of the neck to passive anterior flexion). Passive flexion of the neck will often result in flexion of the legs at the knees (Brudzinski's sign) and resistance to complete extension of the knees when the hips are flexed to 90° (Kernig's sign). These are presumably protective reactions to minimize stretching of the inflamed meninges.

Symptoms of meningitis may be quite subtle, especially in infants and the elderly. There may be little more than fever, a mild headache, and irritability or lethargy. The earlier the presentation, the less specific the symptomatology but the better the chance of complete recovery with appropriate treatment. It is also worth noting that noninfectious forms of meningitis, such as carcinomatous involvement, chemical irritation, or hypersensitivity reaction, can produce an identical clinical picture.

Photophobia, nausea, and vomiting (related to the elevation of CSF pressure), and mental dysfunction ranging from lethargy through confusion to coma, are other signs and symptoms of meningitis. CSF pressure is almost always elevated (300–600 mm H_2O). In infants the elevation of CSF pressure is indicated by

bulging fontanels that have lost their normal pulsations. However, papilledema is rare in meningitis; when present it suggests other conditions, such as brain abscess or subdural empyema, associated with a more prolonged elevation of CSF pressure.

The severity of the clinical syndrome depends on both the type of organism infecting the meninges and the duration of the infection prior to treatment. The pyogenic organisms, such as H. influenzae, pneumococcus, and L. monocytogenes, produce an intense purulent exudate in the meninges. Obtundation or stupor is a relatively early manifestation, and focal neurologic signs are common. The mortality rate associated with these infections is high. CSF pressure is quite elevated due to communicating or, less frequently, noncommunicating hydrocephalus and also because of inappropriate release of antidiuretic hormone with subsequent brain swelling. Purulent complications including subdural empyema and dural venous sinus thrombosis are common. Permanent sequelae are also more common in the pyogenic meningitides. Significant deficits in mental function (estimated to occur in 30%–50% of H. influenzae meningitis), including retardation, have been observed in patients who had purulent meningitis in childhood. Seizures are common in the acute stages, particularly in infants, but do not generally persist. Epilepsy develops in 2%–3% of pediatric cases and less often in adults.

Vasculitic organisms (e.g., meningococcus) produce somewhat different syndromes. Brain swelling with associated headache, nausea, and vomiting may be severe; it is more a manifestation of an altered blood-brain barrier than extensive subarachnoid inflammation. The associated vasculitis affects the cranial nerves, particularly VIII. Purulent complications are unusual, but permanent cerebral dysfunction can follow the vasculitis. Meningococcemia is also associated with shock,

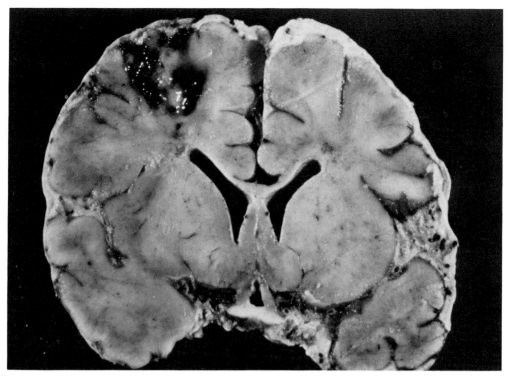

Fig. 18–1. *E. coli* meningitis in a newborn child. The subarachnoid space is filled with purulent material, and there is a large area of venous infarction on the left superiorly.

consumption coagulopathy, and infection at distant sites.

The meningoencephalitic organisms (staphylococci, streptococci, enteric Gram-negative bacilli, and amoebae) produce similar, but more severe, symptoms. The patient is often left with significant permanent residua since the brain substance as well as the meninges are involved (Fig. 18–1). Disseminated infection is also common.

The indolent organisms, *M. tuberculosis* and the fungi (especially coccidioides and cryptococci), usually produce a subacute or even a chronic picture, with prognosis inversely related to the time (after presentation) required to make a diagnosis. The signs and symptoms are the results of a chronic, organizing, inflammatory process at the base of the brain, leading to hydrocephalus, cerebral infarction, and cranial nerve defects, particularly III, IV, and VI. Permanent disturbance of ADH secretion and endocrine function may also occur.

Viral or "aseptic" meningitis generally presents with a mild meningitic picture characterized by headache, fever, and photophobia. Although varying degrees of encephalitis may also be present and lead to transient alterations in consciousness or nerve paralysis, these results are infrequent. Signs and symptoms of generalized viral disease such as chest or abdominal pain and rash are often associated. Enteroviruses cause the majority of the proven cases of viral meningitis; they occur in a distinct late summer–early fall pattern. With the possible exception of herpes simplex meningitis, no therapy is available.

However, most cases of viral meningitis run a short, benign course with no permanent sequelae.

Encephalitis

Encephalitis is a nonsuppurative inflammation of the brain parenchyma. Since meningeal inflammation usually accompanies encephalitis, the terms *meningoencephalitis* or *encephalomyelitis* are often used. The infectious agents involved reach the CNS primarily by the bloodstream, but migration may occur along peripheral and cranial nerves (e.g., with rabies and herpes simplex virus). The clinical picture reflects the area of the CNS involved. Most encephalitides tend to be diffuse, but asymmetrical involvement and preference for certain locations are not unusual (e.g., herpes simplex encephalitis and temporal lobe involvement).

Disturbances in mentation including abnormal behavior and alterations in consciousness are the dominant symptoms of encephalitis. Motor and sensory deficits and seizures are also commonly observed, along with symptoms of meningitis. Depending on the site of disease, abnormalities of temperature regulation and endocrine function may also occur. Involvement of the spinal cord produces flaccid paralysis, depressed deep tendon reflexes, bowel and bladder paresis, and sensory changes.

A wide variety of pathogenic agents have been associated with encephalitis. Some, like the herpes simplex virus, produce severe tissue destruction and necrosis. Others, like the so-called slow virus diseases, e.g., Creutzfeldt-Jakob and kuru, produce minimal, if any, inflammation. Still others, like the postinfectious encephalitides that follow measles, varicella, rubella, and vaccinations, are associated predominately with tissue reactivity, including perivascular infiltration of mononuclear cells and perivenous demyelination.

The time course of encephalitis depends on the infectious agent involved. Bacterial encephalitis and rickettsial disease are usually acute in onset, whereas infections like neurosyphilis can be quite insidious. Viral infections likewise may be either acute or chronic. Typical viral encephalitides such as those arising from herpes simplex or the arboviruses often present abruptly, but postinfectious encephalitis follows the primary infection in 2–12 days. The slow virus infections (subacute sclerosing panencephalitis, rubella panencephalitis, progressive multifocal leukoencephalopathy, kuru, and Cruetzfeldt-Jakob disease) appear years after the presumed exposure as an insidiously progressive and invariably fatal disease. The first three are apparently related to conventional viruses, but the precise nature of the infectious agent responsible for the latter two is unknown.

Determining the etiologic agent in encephalitis is of clinical importance since effective therapy is available at present for herpes simplex infection and may soon be available for others. The precise definition of the organism involved requires laboratory confirmation, but will be suggested by the epidemiology, temporal sequence of the signs and symptoms, and localization as deduced by diagnostic studies and the physical examination.

Brain abscess and parameningeal infections

Brain abscesses and parameningeal infections, including subdural empyema, epidural abscess, and suppurative intracranial phlebitis, may occur alone or in conjunction with other CNS infections. Brain abscesses and parameningeal infections are largely bacterial processes. Most follow contiguous infection. The clinical picture depends on the site of the lesion(s); the location is largely determined by the route of infection.

Blood-borne infection rarely seeds the epidural or subdural spaces (except the spinal epidural space). The brain parenchyma also resists infection unless it is produced by septic emboli rather than bacteria per se, presumably reflecting a requirement for some degree of ischemic damage before infection can become established. Brain abscesses produced in this manner are distributed according to blood flow, primarily in the branches of the middle cerebral artery. Emboli that are secondary to pulmonary infectious foci or associated with congenital right-to-left shunts are relatively large; they tend to produce abscesses that are centrally located at the junction of the white and gray matter. Emboli that are secondary to bacterial endocarditis are smaller and less commonly produce a brain abscess. When they do, however, the abscesses tend to be multiple and located peripherally in the distribution of medium-sized vessels.

Brain Abscess. Brain abscess is approximately one-tenth as common as acute bacterial meningitis. Otogenic abscesses are the majority (up to half) with about 10% rhinogenic, 10% from direct inoculation, 10% without identifiable cause, and the remainder hematogenous. The microbiology is distinctly different from that of acute meningitis. Pneumococci, meningococci, and *H. influenzae* account for 60% of the cases of meningitis but only 8% of brain abscesses. Streptococci are involved in 40%, *S. aureus* in 20%, enteric Gram-negative bacilli in 15%–20%, and bacteroides species in 10%. The infections are often mixed; at least 25% have an anaerobic component.

The clinical picture of brain abscess is usually insidious, developing over days or even months. It is rarely fulminant. Signs and symptoms include low-grade fever and evidence of elevated CNS pressure: headache, nausea, vomiting, drowsiness, confusion, papilledema, and VI nerve palsy. Seizures and focal neurologic signs may occur late in the syndrome. Specific neurologic signs and symptoms depend on the location of the abscess. In addition to actual destruction of nervous tissue, brain abscesses may rupture into a ventricle or the subarachnoid space, extend, or lead to uncal herniation. The prognosis is related to size and location, but the mortality rate approaches 40%.

Epidural Abscess. The cranial epidural space is actually just a potential space, since the dura is closely adherent to the inner table of the skull. Infection here is extremely limited and often produces no specific neurologic symptoms unless it is associated with CNS infection elsewhere. One exception is Gradenigo's syndrome, in which mastoid infection invades the petrous ridge of the temporal bone and produces ipsilateral involvement of cranial nerves V and VI. Since cranial epidural abscesses arise from contiguous infection, the bacteriology and treatment are those of the primary infection.

The spinal epidural space is quite different. It is a real space filled with loose, vascular, fatty tissue that runs the length of the spine. The majority of spinal epidural abscesses are hematogenous, either from a genitourinary source via the vertebral venous plexus or from a generalized bacteremia, perhaps due to a furuncle or dental infection. Spinal epidural infection is especially common in children; 75% of childhood cases are due to *S. aureus*. Minor back trauma often precedes the infection, suggesting that tissue damage that is peculiarly susceptible to secondary infection may have occurred. Epidural abscesses in adults can also result from contiguous osteomyelitis (pyogenic and tuberculous).

The danger of spinal epidural abscess arises from the anatomy of the epidural space. There is little to limit the spread of infection once it is established so that it is able to spread up and down the spine quickly. Local extension results in nerve root and cord compression and eventual vascular compromise. If the pressure is not quickly relieved by laminectomy, permanent damage, including paraplegia, can occur. A spinal epidural abscess is a true surgical emergency, since irreversible damage can occur within hours.

There are four phases in the clinical progression of spinal epidural abscess that may overlap. Symptoms begin with local pain; root pain and paresthesias develop next, followed by weakness, sensory loss, and reflex changes. There is often local evidence of infection at this point. If symptoms progress to the fourth or paralytic stage, the damage is often permanent. Antibiotics are helpful but are clearly secondary to operative drainage.

Subdural Empyema. Subdural empyema is also a serious infection. As the term *empyema* implies, it is an infection of a true space, and like spinal epidural infection, once established, can spread freely. In this case the infection spreads over the entire cerebral hemisphere, limited only by the falx. The usual origin is from chronic sinusitis, especially of the frontal sinus, which spreads via the penetrating veins. Subdural empyema also results from direct inoculation, hematogenous spread, or secondary infection of the sterile subdural effusions that often occur in bacterial meningitis. The organisms involved in subdural empyema resemble those of brain abscess more closely than those of meningitis. Streptococci and staphylococci account for the majority of cases.

The clinical presentation is characterized by the rapid development of symptoms including severe headache, nausea, vomiting, and meningismus progressing over hours or a few days to obtundation and coma. Focal neurologic deficits and seizures are common. Spread of infection produces a mass effect, with marked elevation of CSF pressure. Uncal herniation is a distinct possibility and, as with brain abscess, may be precipitated by a lumbar puncture. Like spinal epidural abscess, the

primary treatment is surgical drainage; antibiotics are clearly secondary.

Major Dural Sinus Thrombosis. Infection and thrombosis of the venous sinuses may follow meningitis, subdural or epidural abscesses, and contiguous infection spreading along the extracerebral emissary veins. Thrombosis may occur in the cavernous, lateral, and superior sagittal sinuses. The likelihood of thrombosis is increased by conditions that alter blood viscosity or coagulability. *S. aureus* is the most frequent bacterial isolate.

The clinical findings of dural sinus thrombosis vary with the sinus involved, the extent of propagation, and the associated CNS conditions. Cavernous sinus thrombosis follows oculonasal infection. It is characterized by abrupt onset, diplopia, orbital edema, exophthalmos, and palsies of cranial nerves III, IV, V, and VI. Obstruction of venous return leads to papilledema, retinal hemorrhages, and visual loss. Infection may also spread to the contralateral cavernous sinus. Superior sagittal sinus thrombosis is less common. It produces hemiplegia, convulsions, and (occasionally) communicating hydrocephalus. Lateral sinus thrombosis is associated primarily with chronic mastoid infection. The initial signs and symptoms are those of increased intracranial pressure, including headache and papilledema, but often little else.

DIFFERENTIAL DIAGNOSIS

Although the diagnostic considerations presented by a patient with possible CNS infection are quite extensive, treatment, not precise diagnosis, should be the first concern. Mortality in CNS infections often exceeds 50% and is clearly related to the time elapsed before effective therapy is begun. In the case of acute fulminant meningitis, a lumbar puncture should be performed and effective antimicrobial therapy instituted within 30 minutes of the time the patient enters the emergency room. With a less fulminant presentation or after empiric therapy has begun, a more precise evaluation can be performed. A detailed history and physical examination along with a careful neurologic evaluation are, of course, essential, but the most helpful procedure in the differential diagnosis of CNS infections is a lumbar puncture and analysis of the CSF.

A lumbar puncture carries some risk, however, particularly if the intracranial pressure is markedly elevated, as with a space-occupying lesion like a tumor or brain abscess. Sudden reduction of the lumbar intrathecal pressure could lead to herniation of the cerebellar tonsils or the uncus of the temporal lobe with fatal results. A lumbar puncture is usually not indicated in the presence of papilledema, at least until a space-occupying lesion can be ruled out by computerized axial tomography (CT). Nevertheless, it is worth emphasizing that meningitis is much more common than parameningeal infections or mass lesions, and the diagnostic value of a lumbar puncture far outweighs the relatively small risk of harm. If there is reason to suspect increased intracranial pressure, an intravenous needle should be placed before beginning the procedure, and mannitol or urea should be readily available for infusion. If, in a patient with the clinical picture of meningitis, it seems prudent to rule out a mass lesion prior to lumbar puncture, empiric antibiotics should be started first.

Cerebrospinal fluid examination

Meticulous study of the cerebrospinal fluid is mandatory in the diagnosis of CNS infection. The examination must include measurement of the pressure, determinations of the protein and glucose, counts of the cells, and a careful search for organisms. The resulting patterns of findings often suggest the diagnosis and permit the design of antibiotic therapy. Therapy determined by these laboratory findings can be different from the initial empiric therapy and should be further modified when culture results are known.

The CSF pressure is measured before any fluid is removed; normal pressure is less than 200 mm H_2O. Normal spinal fluid is clear and colorless. Only a few hundred cells per cubic centimeters will produce an opalescent turbidity if the cells are neutrophils. CSF that appears frankly purulent will contain several thousand neutrophils per cubic centimeter. Lymphocytes rarely produce a change in the appearance of the fluid, even in large numbers.

Cytologic examination is a critical step in the evaluation of CSF. Cell numbers are determined in a counting chamber before and after the addition of a dilute solution of acetic acid to lyse the red cells. Cerebrospinal fluid pleocytosis can be detected even after a traumatic lumbar puncture if the ratio of white cells to red cells exceeds that of the patients blood. A differential cell count should not be attempted in the counting chamber since it is easy to confuse the cell types, even with the addition of a stain such as methyl green. Rather, a separate Wright-stained smear of the spun sediment should be performed. This is also necessary in examining the CSF for the presence of malignant abnormal cells. A smear performed with a cytocentrifuge is an acceptable alternative. Recently, immunologic techniques have been employed to identify specific antigens on fresh or cultured cells obtained from the CSF. This technique will perhaps permit the rapid etiologic diagnosis of many CNS infections including viral encephalitis, but it is not yet ready for general use.

Increased CSF protein content is one of the most common abnormalities in neurologic disease and consequently one of the most difficult to interpret. An elevation of several hundred milligrams per deciliter is the norm in inflammatory meningitis and tends to persist for some weeks. The rise in more subacute or chronic processes such as tuberculous meningitis may persist for years. Modest elevations of protein, less than 100 mg per deciliter, may be found in a variety of infectious and noninfectious conditions such as encephalitis, cerebral infarction, parameningeal infection, demyelinating disease, and neurosyphilis. Particularly high levels of CSF protein are found with obstruction of CSF flow in the spinal subarachnoid space.

Most CSF protein appears to be albumin, which crosses the blood-brain barrier. Gamma globulins, often in excess of the 1:8 globulin to albumin ratio of serum, are probably produced within the central nervous system and are especially elevated in certain diseases such as multiple sclerosis. The amount and composition of the CSF protein are strongly correlated with the magnitude and type of CSF pleocytosis. Organism-specific antibodies, antigens, and enzymes have all been detected and have proven useful for diagnosis. Latex agglutination, countercurrent immunoelectrophoresis, immunofluorescence, radioimmunoassay, and ELISA (enzyme-linked immunosorbent assay) are all techniques that are employed.

Abnormally low CSF glucose is a common finding in bacterial, tuberculous, fungal, carcinomatous, and occasionally early viral meningitis. The exact mechanisms that produce low CSF glucose are not fully understood, but the major factor is thought to be an alteration of glucose transport across the blood-brain barrier. Bacterial metabolism, leukocyte metabolism, and even CNS metabolism are thought to contribute to the low glucose levels, but their role is probably minimal. Optimally, CSF glucose levels are determined in the fasting state. Since this option is usually not available in a rapidly evolving clinical situation, a simultaneous blood sugar should be drawn for comparison. As it takes approximately 2 hours for equilibration between the serum and CSF, even this value must be interpreted cautiously. An extremely low CSF glucose is usually a very poor prognostic sign.

Definitive microbiologic diagnosis is made by culture, which should be done whenever a CNS infection is even remotely suspected, since the absence of cells in the CSF in no way precludes an infectious etiology. Cerebrospinal fluid should be inoculated onto a variety of media capable of growing all of the pathogens known to be associated with meningitic infection: blood agar, chocolate agar, special H. influenzae plates, and thioglycolate broth, with special incubation conditions when indicated. If tuberculous or fungal meningitis is a possibility, specific media such as Dubos' (TB) or Saboraud's (fungi) can be employed. The isolation of viruses requires inoculation of cells in tissue culture or injection into mice or embryonated eggs. Cultures should also be taken from the blood and any other site of possible involvement. However, since rapid treatment is so critical in CNS infections, special importance is attached to smears and immunologic techniques that will provide at least a tentative etiologic diagnosis within minutes or hours.

A Gram-stained smear of the spun sediment is especially valuable in acute bacterial meningitis since at least 60% of such disease is caused by the pneumococcus, the meningococcus, and H. influenzae. In most cases (80%–90% of bacterial meningitides), bacteria are visible on the smear, which takes only a few minutes to prepare. Quellung and agglutination reactions were previously used for type-specific diagnosis but these have now been supplanted by countercurrent immunoelectrophoresis utilizing specific antibodies to most serotypes of pneumococcus, meningococcus, and H. influenzae type B. Bacterial antigen can often be detected in less than an hour even in patients who have been partially treated with antibiotics. Thus, the diagnosis can be made even when the CSF culture is negative. Occasional false positives, false negatives, and cross-reactions occur.

Ziehl-Neelsen or Kinyoun stains should be performed if tuberculous meningitis is a possibility. These smears may be positive in 10%–90% of cases. The yield is considerably increased if large fluid volumes are used and the smear made from the protein pellicle that often forms upon standing. Similarly, the CSF should be examined for *Cryptococcus neoformans* by the India ink method. Particular attention should be paid to the presence of budding forms since even experienced observers have difficulty in distinguishing yeast from lymphocytes.

Cerebrospinal fluid findings characteristic of various CNS inflammatory diseases are presented in Table 18–2. There are three major groups: the purulent profile, which is most representative of bacterial meningitis; the low-glucose, lymphocyte-predominant profile typical of indolent meningitis (TB and fungi); and the normal-glucose, lymphocyte-predominant profile characteristic of parameningeal disease, encephalitis, viral meningitis, and partially treated bacterial meningitis. A fourth group, that of eosinophil-predominant pleocytosis, is uncommon and is seen mainly in parasitic or hypersensitivity diseases. There is considerable overlap among the groups and several infections can produce several different CSF profiles, depending on the stage of the disease at the time of the examination. Nevertheless, the CSF profile can often provide the etiologic diagnosis or at least suggest appropriate ancillary tests.

Ancillary clinical and laboratory data

Serology. There are several situations in which it is not possible to establish a diagnosis of CNS infection by either culture or immunochemical identification of the pathogen. Some organisms, such as viruses, leptospires, or protozoans, cannot

be cultured with the facilities available in most institutions. Other organisms like syphilis cannot be cultured at all. With some organisms, like *M. tuberculosis* and some of the fungi, culture is possible but the yield may be low. And with still others, like arbovirus encephalitides, the etiologic agent is not usually accessible for culture. Consequently, diagnosis is often made retrospectively by serology. A single serologic titer is generally of no value for diagnostic purposes, but a fourfold rise in titer between the acute and convalescent serum samples provides strong evidence for etiology. It is therefore reasonable to draw and store an acute-phase serum in all suspected cases of CNS infection, particularly of possible viral origin. In the absence of an alternative diagnosis (or to provide confirmation), this can be analyzed along with a specimen drawn two or three weeks later.

Microbiology. Since it is sometimes not possible to establish a definitive diagnosis from the clinical evaluation nor from examination and culture of the CSF, every effort should be made to obtain additional data. This includes culturing every fluid or organ that might be helpful. Blood cultures are especially important, since they are positive in over half the cases of bacterial meningitis. Cultures of skin lesions may also suggest the pathogen in CNS infection. Smears or biopsies of these same lesions can reveal bacteria, fungi, or rickettsia, while respiratory secretions may reveal the source of hematogenous CNS infection. Throat washings or stool samples can suggest the etiology of aseptic meningitis or encephalitis. It may even be worthwhile on occasion to culture patient contacts since the results may suggest the pathogen.

X Ray. X Rays of the skull, sinuses, chest, and spine do not indicate CNS infection per se but may be useful insofar as they can define a relevant contiguous or distant

Table 18–2. Cerebrospinal fluid profiles in CNS inflammation

	Pressure (mm H₂O)	Cell count (WBC/mm³)	Differential	Stains		Culture	Glucose	Protein
				Gram	Other			
1. Purulent profile								
a. Bacterial	220–1,000	500–20,000+	PMNs>>mono	85%	—	85%+	Low, <40 (occ, <10)	100–1,000
b. Chemical	200–500	100–1,000	PMNs>>mono	—	Keratin?	—	20–40	50–100
c. Early phase viral	Normal	<1,000	PMNs>>mono	—	IF	Virus	Normal	Normal
d. Early phase TB	200–500	25–500	PMNs>>mono	—	10% + AFB	—	Normal	Normal
e. Amoebic	200–500	500–20,000+	PMNs>>mono	—	wet mount	Special culture	Low	50–100
2. Lymphocyte predominance, low glucose								
a. TB	200–500	25–500	90% monos	—	10–90% + AFB	40–90%+	20–40	25–500
b. Fungal	200–500	25–500	90% monos	—	Budding yeast + india ink	80%+	20–40	25–500
c. Leptospires, syphilis	200–500	100–500	90% monos	—	Dark field	—	Low–normal	50–400
d. Tumor	Normal–elevated	0–100+	90% monos	—	cytology	—	20–40	50–1,000
e. Sarcoid	Normal–elevated	0–100+	90% monos	—	—	—	Low–normal	25–500
f. Some viruses (e.g., mumps, LCM)	Normal	<1,000	90% monos	—	IF	Virus	20–40	50–1,000
3. Lymphocyte predominance, normal glucose								
a. Partially treated bacterial meningitis	Normal	0–100+	Usually monos	—	—	Rarely+	Normal	50–100
b. Parameningeal infection	Low—markedly elevated	0–100+	Usually monos	—	—	Neg	Normal	50–500
c. "Aseptic" encephalomyelitis	Normal	0–1,000	Usually monos	—	IF	Virus	Normal	100
d. Hemorrhagic encephalitis	Elevated	0–1,000+	Variable PMSs, monos, RBCs	—	—	—	Normal	Elevated

AFB, acid-fast bacillus (mycobacteria); IF, immunofluorescence; monos, mononuclear cells (lymphocytes, monocytes); PMNs, polymorphonuclear leukocytes; RBCs, red blood cells.

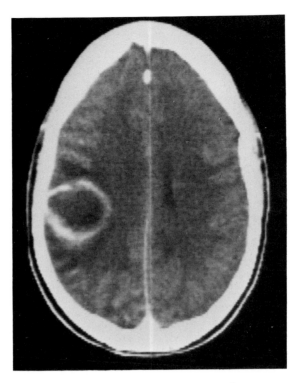

Fig. 18–2. CT scan after intravenous administration of contrast material, demonstrating a large brain abscess in the left temporal lobe. The contrast material accentuates the zone of increased vascularity in the capsule. Edema is evident around the abscess, and the left lateral ventricle is compressed.

infectious focus. CT scans can be extremely helpful for both the diagnosis and followup of CNS infection. It is especially useful in brain abscesses and parameningeal infections. Brain abscess characteristically produces a lucent area surrounded by a faint rim. After intravenous administration of contrast, the dense ring is enhanced and seen to be surrounded by a lucent area of cerebral edema. Various degrees of compression and shift of cerebral structures are indicative of the mass effect (Fig. 18–2).

CT scans are also useful in the diagnosis of subdural empyema, CSF leaks, cranial osteomyelitis, some forms of encephalitis, and the complications of meningitis, such as subdural effusion/empyema and hydrocephalus. The CT scan has largely replaced other radiologic procedures in CNS infections, but arteriograms or radionuclide studies may complement the CT scan or be used for primary diagnosis when a CT scanner is not available. While arteriography can be used to define a brain abscess or subdural empyema, it is not reliable in the early phases of the disease. Cerebral angiography is the most specific test for venous sinus thrombosis, although static and dynamic radionuclide scans can be helpful. Radionuclide brain scans and indium-111 leukocyte scans have been helpful in the early diagnosis of cerebral abscess and may show the location of lesions in encephalitis, even when the CT scan is normal. Localization is particularly helpful in herpes simplex encephalitis, since a biopsy may be necessary to confirm the diagnosis. Spinal myelography is the procedure of choice in the diagnosis of spinal epidural abscess.

Biopsy. Biopsy is seldom required for the diagnosis of CNS infection but there are circumstances in which it is helpful and even essential. Peripheral biopsy is useful in such disorders as sarcoidosis or toxoplasmosis, where specific microscopic findings can suggest the etiology of the CNS disease. Brain biopsy is not a trivial procedure, but it is necessary for the diagnosis of herpes simplex encephalitis and some of the slow virus diseases. Biopsies are indicated in suspected herpes simplex encephalitis, not only because effective therapy is available (adenosine arabinosine and probably acyclovir), but also because almost half the cases thought to be herpes encephalitis on clinical grounds prove to be due to something else and the alternative diagnosis is often treatable. Whenever tissue is obtained for histological study, it should also be cultured for infectious agents and examined, where facilities permit, by electron microscopy and fluorescent antibody techniques.

GENERAL REFERENCES

Baker, A. S., R. G. Ojemann, M. N. Swartz, and E. P. Richardson, Jr. Spinal epidural abscess. *New Eng. J. Med.* 293:463–8, 1975.

Berk, S. L., and W. R. McCabe. Meningitis caused by gram-negative bacilli. *Ann. Int. Med.* 93:253–60, 1980.

Brewer, N. D., C. S. MacCarty, and W. E. Wellman. Brain abscess: A review of recent experience. *Ann. Int. Med.* 82:571–6, 1975.

Colding, H., and I. Lind. Counterimmunoelectrophoresis in the diagnosis of bacterial meningitis. *J. Clin. Microbiol.* 5:405–9, 1977.

Dodge, P. R., and M. N. Swartz. Medical progress. Bacterial meningitis—a review of selected aspects. II. Special neurologic problems, postmeningitic complications and clinicopathologic correlations. *New Eng. J. Med.* 272:954–60, 1003–10, 1965.

Johnson, R. T. *Viral Infections of the Nervous System.* New York, Raven Press, 1981.

Kalbag, R. M., and A. L. Woolf. Cerebral Venous Thrombosis. London, Oxford University Press, 1967.

Kaufman, D. M., M. H. Miller, and N. H. Steigbigel. Subdural empyema: analysis of 17 recent cases and review of the literature. *Medicine* 54:485–98, 1975.

Meyer, H. M., Jr., R. T. Johnson, I. P. Crawford, H. E. Dascomb, and N. G. Rogers. Central nervous system syndromes of "viral" etiology. *Am. J. Med.* 29:334–47, 1960.

New, P. F. J., and K. R. Davis. The role of CT scanning in diagnosis of infections of the central nervous system. In *Current Clinical Topics in Infectious Diseases*, J. S. Remington and M. N. Swartz (eds.). New York, McGraw-Hill, 1980, pp. 1–33.

Swartz, M. N., and P. R. Dodge. Medical progress. Bacterial meningitis—a review of selected aspects. I. General clinical features, special problems and unusual meningeal reactions mimicking bacterial meningitis. *New Eng. J. Med.* 272:725–31, 779–87, 842–8, 898–902.

19.

Parkinsonism

G. FREDERICK WOOTEN

Parkinsonism, or Parkinson's disease, is a clinical syndrome consisting of tremor, rigidity, brady- and hypokinesia, and deficits in equilibrium and posture. The tremor is most prominent at rest and is usually interrupted by volitional movement. Parkinsonian rigidity is characterized by a uniform resistance to the passive stretch of muscle throughout the full range of motion of a joint. Often an examiner is able to feel a rhythmic interruption of the hypertonus when testing muscle tone. This is called the "cogwheel phenomenon." Both a slowing of volitional movements (bradykinesia) and an overall reduction of spontaneous movements (hypokinesia) are characteristic of parkinsonism. Disorders of equilibrium and posture are most apparent in the flexed truncal position and the shuffling gait, which is punctuated by unsteady *en block* turns. Along with these four cardinal signs and symptoms of parkinsonism are less common features including speech abnormalities, autonomic symptoms, abnormalities of ocular control, and a variable degree of reduction in intellect and alteration of mood.

Parkinsonism is but one of a group of symptom complexes that emerges as a consequence of dysfunction in the basal ganglia. The basal ganglia are a group of neuron-dense structures consisting of the caudate-putamen (corpus striatum), globus pallidus, subthalamic nucleus, and substantia nigra. These structures are highly interrelated anatomically and physiologically (see Chap. 9). The striatum receives afferents from the neocortex substantia nigra pars compacta and the centromedianum of the thalamus (Fig. 19–1). The striatum, in turn, projects to the globus pallidus externa and interna as well as to the substantia nigra pars reticulata. The subthalamic nucleus receives afferents from the external segment of the globus pallidus and, in turn, projects to both segments of the globus pallidus and the substantia nigra reticulata. The major extrinsic source of afferents to the basal ganglia is from neocortex. The major outputs from the basal ganglia are from globus pallidus interna and substantia nigra reticulata to the ventral anterior and ventral lateral thalamic nuclei, which in turn project back to the neocortex. A major portion of this thalamocortical projection is to cortical regions involved in motor control. Thus the basal ganglia may be viewed as a sub-

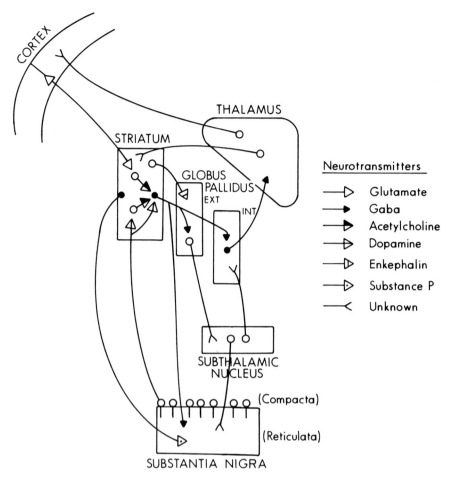

Fig. 19–1. Major connections and neurotransmitters in the basal ganglia. Cell bodies are indicated by circles, axon terminals by arrowheads. The output from the substantia nigra pars reticulata is thought to be GABAergic, with projections to thalamus, tectum, and brainstem reticular nuclei.

routine or loop for modifying motor output as the region receives its major input from cortical motor areas and its major output is directed back to cortical motor areas via the thalamus.

Much new information has accumulated in recent years about the identity of neurotransmitters in the basal ganglia. Corticostriate projections are thought to be primarily glutamergic. There are numerous cholinergic interneurons in the striatum. Striatal efferents to globus pallidus interna, externa, and substantia nigra reticulata are at least in part GA-BAergic. Projections from globus pallidus interna and substantia nigra reticulata to the thalamus are also primarily GA-BAergic. Dopamine is the principal neurotransmitter in the nigrostriatal pathway. More recent studies have identified a substance P projection from striatum to substantia nigra and an enkephalin projection from striatum to globus pallidus externa. Thus the identity of many of the projections within the basal ganglia circuit is known and provides the potential for selective modification of activity in basal ganglia circuits with drugs.

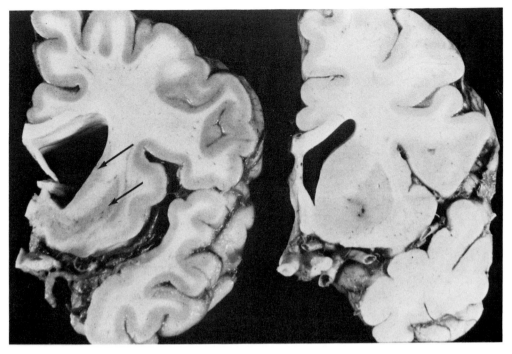

Fig. 19–2. Anterior unilateral coronal sections through the brain of a patient with Huntington's disease (left) compared to a normal brain (right). Note the marked atrophy of the caudate (upper arrow) and the putamen (lower arrow) and the secondary dilation of the lateral ventricle in Huntington's disease. (Fig. 19–2 and 19–3 reproduced by permission of Merck Sharp and Dohme Division of Merck and Company, Incorporated.)

CLINICAL-PATHOLOGICAL CORRELATIONS

In 1912 the English neurologist S. A. Kinnier Wilson reported the original clinical-pathological correlation between selective disease of the corpus striatum and the occurrence of a unique, basal ganglia motor syndrome: ". . . with pure bilateral lesions . . . of the corpus striatum, . . . the clinical symptoms are bilateral involuntary movements, practically always of the tremor variety; weakness . . . hypertonicity and dysarthria; but without any sensory disturbance, without any true paralysis, and without any alteration in the cutaneous reflexes. If the . . . plantars are of the extensor type, then the syndrome is no longer pure." This description of Wilson's disease paved the way for several subsequent clinical-pathological correlations. For example, it is now recognized that selective lesions of the subthalamic nucleus may result in hemiballismus, a striking movement disorder characterized by violent involuntary flinging movements of the contralateral limbs. Huntington's chorea, an inherited degenerative disease that initially and predominately affects the striatum (Fig. 19–2) produces quick, jerk-like, irregular involuntary movements called chorea. Pharmacological studies have led to the suggestion that the selective striatal pathology in Huntington's disease results in a relative excess of dopamine for the viable cells remaining in the striatum. It is of interest that patients with Parkinson's disease sometimes develop similar choreatic movements if they are treated with excessive amounts of dopaminergic drugs. Finally, choreatic movements also occur as a consequence of chronic treatment with antipsychotic drugs that block dopamine receptors. This movement disorder, called tardive dyskinesia, is thought to be caused by the development of supersensitivity at dopamine receptors secondary to chronic dopamine antagonist exposure. Because none of these syndromes share the signs and symptoms of pyramidal system disease (i.e., paresis, spasticity, and extensor plantar responses), they have been referred to collectively as extrapyramidal movement disorders.

Our understanding of the pathophysiology of signs and symptoms in these disorders depends on knowing how pathological lesions affect neurotransmitter metabolism and alter physiological activity within extrapyramidal circuits.

Pathophysiology of Parkinsonism

It was over 50 years ago that the first reports of reduced numbers of pigmented neurons in the substantia nigra of patients with idiopathic parkinsonism appeared. In the 1950s Swedish scientists identified the presence of large concentrations of dopamine in the striatum, noted that the treatment of laboratory animals with reserpine depleted brain stores of dopamine and produced symptoms similar to those of parkinsonism and discovered that treatment with dihydroxyphenlalanine (DOPA) reversed the clinical syndrome caused by reserpine. Intrigued by these experimental findings, Hornykiewicz and colleagues measured the concentrations of dopamine and its metabolites in post-mortem brain material from patients with idiopathic parkinsonism and discovered that there was a large reduction in the content of dopamine compared to age-matched controls. Furthermore, these workers demonstrated a strong positive correlation between the severity of parkinsonian features and the degree of dopamine depletion in the corpus striatum. Thus, the current working

hypothesis regarding the pathophysiology of parkinsonism evolved: The symptoms of parkinsonism are a consequence of the reduction in the dopamine content of the striatum. In addition, this same line of work has served to establish a general set of criteria to define the clinical-pathological entity, Parkinson's disease. In the most general terms, Parkinson's disease is characterized clinically by idiopathic parkinsonism and pathologically by selective degeneration of pigmented brainstem neurons (Fig. 19–3), resulting in reduction of the striatal concentration of dopamine.

Subsequent anatomical and biochemical studies have demonstrated that the pigmented neurons of the substantia nigra project widely and diffusely to the striatum and are specialized to synthesize and release dopamine. Selective death of the dopamine-synthesizing cells of the substantia nigra thus results in a reduction in striatal dopamine content. The dopamine-depletion hypothesis of the pathophysiology of Parkinson's disease was further supported by the observations that drugs that caused Parkinson-like symptoms in experimental animals interfered with dopamine synthesis (α-methyl-tyrosine), storage (reserpine), or receptor interaction (phenothiazine, butyrophenones); furthermore, selective destruction of the substantia nigra with a depletion of striatal dopamine content produced parkinsonism in laboratory animals (Table 19–1). The most recent major observations to support the dopamine hypothesis of Parkinson's disease have been those demonstrating that clinical symptoms could be attenuated by administration of the dopamine precursor L-dopa as well as a variety of direct-acting dopamine agonist drugs.

Recent physiological studies have focused on the synaptic effects of dopamine on striatal neurons. Based on intracellular recording of striatal neurons, it is now apparent that stimulating substantia nigra causes release of dopamine resulting in a short latency excitatory postsynaptic potential (EPSP) succeeded by inhibition (IPSP). Direct cellular recordings, however, from substantia nigra pars compacta neurons during a variety of voluntary movements in awake monkeys failed to identify any neurons that discharged with movement. These data strongly suggest that the nigrostriatal dopamine pathway functions primarily as a tonic modulator of striatal neurons and not as a phasic, binary signal. By contrast, recordings in the striatum, globus pallidus, and subthalamic nucleus show groups of neurons that fire in phase with movement. Of particular note for understanding parkinsonism is that physiologic studies have found that depletion of dopamine from the striatum results in a dramatic alteration in the firing rates of pallidal neurons. Instead of firing phasically with movement they now discharge tonically at high rates. In addition, metabolic studies have found an increase in the rate of glucose utilization in the external segment of the globus pallidus. These physiologic and metabolic changes are reversed by the systemic administration of L-dopa or dopamine agonist drugs. The increase in firing rates of pallidal neurons presumably disrupts the normal motor integration by the basal ganglia to produce the symptoms of Parkinson's disease. There obviously remains a huge gulf in the understanding of how dopamine depletion in the striatum results in the clinical syndrome of parkinsonism.

Pathogenesis and etiology

The cause of idiopathic parkinsonism is unknown. Since the first description of "shaking palsy" by James Parkinson in 1817, neurologists have recognized the illness to be fairly common. A prevalence rate of 1.7 per 1,000 was found in Rochester, Minnesota. Most studies indicate a slight preponderance of males. There is a striking positive correlation between age and the incidence of idiopathic parkinsonism; in the oldest group studied in Rochester, the prevalence of the disease approached 2%. About two-thirds of all patients with idiopathic parkinsonism experience the onset of symptoms between the ages of 50 and 69. Tremor is most frequently the presenting symptom, and patients who experience this tend to have a more benign course than those patients who present with bradykinesia or loss of postural reflexes. Prior to the introduction of L-dopa therapy in 1967, idiopathic parkinsonism substantially shortened life expectancy with a mortality rate approximately three times that of age-matched controls.

The signs and symptoms of parkinsonism begin to appear when striatal dopamine levels fall below 20% of control values. The central question regarding the pathogenesis of idiopathic parkinsonism is what causes the selective "premature" death of substantia nigra neurons resulting in striatal dopamine depletion. Three hypotheses have been suggested (Fig. 19–4). First, there could be a genetic deficiency in the number of substantia nigra neurons. Although experimental studies in mice have found that the number of tyrosine hydroxylase-containing neurons in different strains is genetically determined, there are only scattered reports of several members of the same family having parkinsonism. A recent national twin study found a very low concordance rate for parkinsonism, suggesting that there are no significant genetic factors in the majority of cases.

Second, several investigators have suggested that Parkinson's disease may represent an abnormal acceleration of the normal brain-aging process. Indeed, in the control population there exists a progressive, age-related decline in the number of substantia nigra neurons and in the concentration of dopamine in the striatum. A third hypothesis is that Parkinson's disease represents an acquired deficiency of substantia nigra neurons, such as occurs

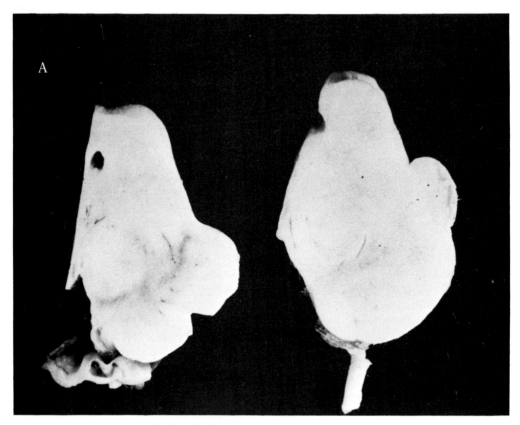

Fig. 19–3. A. Pathological changes in Parkinson's disease. Unilateral coronal sections through the midbrain of a normal brain (left) and a patient with Parkinson's disease (right). Note the absence of "black substance" (substantia nigra pigment) in the Parkinson's brain.

following encephalitis, vascular disease, or trauma. Surviving neurons would then be reduced by the normal aging process to a critical, or symptomatic, level sooner than normal.

In recent years much interest has been found focused on the role of viruses, particularly slow viruses or virus-like particles, in the pathogenesis of neurological disease. The prototype illness was the encephalitis lethargic epidemic in the early 1920s (von Economo's encephalitis), in which subsequent development of parkinsonism was common. Today sporadic cases

of parkinsonism still occur as a result of a variety of encephalitides. It is thought that an infectious agent with a predilection for pigmented neurons of the brainstem may cause Parkinson's disease, but convincing evidence is still lacking for the majority of cases.

Clinical features of parkinsonism may be a prominent aspect of other degenerative neurological illnesses that affect areas in addition to, or outside of, the substantia nigra. These include progressive supranuclear palsy, striatonigral degeneration, olivo-ponto-cerebellar atrophy and

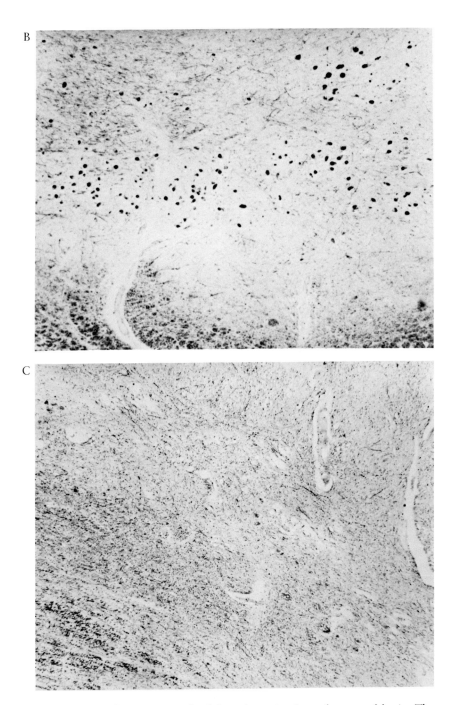

Fig. 19–3. B. Photomicrograph of the substantia nigra of a normal brain. The dark pigment is melanin within dopamine neurons of pars compacta. **C.** The substantia nigra of a brain with Parkinson's disease typically shows marked reduction of pigmented neurons in substantia nigra. Here the neurons of pars compacta have degenerated and been replaced by gliosis.

Table 19–1. Drugs that affect dopamine metabolism and neurotransmission

Mechanism of action	Drugs
1. Inhibit tyrosine hydroxylase	α-methyl-tyrosine
2. Dopamine precursors	L-Tyrosine, L-dopa
3. L-Aromatic amino acid decarboxylase inhibition	Carbidopa, alphamethyldopa
4. Block intraneuronal vesicular-concentrating mechanism	Reserpine, tetrabenazine
5. Facilitate synaptic release of dopamine	Tyramine, d-amphetamine
6. Antagonists that compete for dopamine receptor binding sites	Butyrophenone, phenothiazines, benzamides
7. Direct dopamine receptor agonists	Apomorphine, piribidel, 6,7–dihydroxy amino tetraline (ADTN), bromocriptine, pergolide, lisuride
8. Inhibitors of neuronal membrane reuptake process	Trihexyphenidyl, d-amphetamine
9. Monoamine oxidase inhibitors	Deprenyl, d-amphetamine
10. Catechol-O-methyltransferase inhibitors	Pyrogallol, tropolone

the Shy-Drager syndrome of idiopathic orthostatic hypotension. In contrast to patients with Parkinson's disease, patients with these other degenerative disorders show little or no response to replacement therapy with L-dopa.

Less common causes of parkinsonism are manganese toxicity and multiple small ischemic strokes. Rarely a mass lesion may produce clinical features of parkinsonism as part of its presentation. One of the most common causes of parkinsonism today is the use of major tranquilizers that block dopamine receptors (phenothiazines and butyrophenones) or deplete intraneuronal stores of catecholamine (reserpine).

Treatment strategies

The modern era of central nervous system pharmacology was greatly stimulated by the recognition of dopamine's role in the pathophysiology of parkinsonism and the successful amelioration of parkinsonian symptoms by treatment with L-dopa. Dopamine is ordinarily synthesized in the brain from the essential amino acid L-tyrosine (Fig. 19–5). Tyrosine hydroxylase, the enzyme that catalyzes the conversion of L-tyrosine to L-dopa, is the rate-limiting step in dopamine synthesis. In addition, this enzyme is highly localized to catecholamine-synthesizing neurons and is frequently used as a specific marker for these neurons by investigators. α-methyl-para-tyrosine is an inhibitor of tyrosine hydroxylase and is used both clinically and experimentally to inhibit the synthesis of dopamine, thereby reducing dopamine tissue levels. In contrast, L-aromatic amino acid decarboxylase (L-AAAD), the enzyme that catalyzes the conversion of L-dopa to dopamine, has relatively low substrate specificity and is present in many cells that are not specialized to synthesize catecholamines. Once synthesized, dopamine is concentrated in storage vesicles (Fig. 19–6). The membranes of these storage vesicles contain a high-affinity, energy-dependent, carrier-mediated transport system that sequesters dopamine within the vesicles against a concentration gradient. This transport mechanism at the vesicle membrane is blocked by drugs such as tetrabenazine and reserpine, the effect of which is to deplete tissue levels of dopamine. Under physiologic conditions dopamine is released by a calcium-dependent process from dopaminergic neurons. Dopamine thus released into the synaptic cleft is inactivated primarily by a high-affinity, carrier-mediated reuptake mechanism into

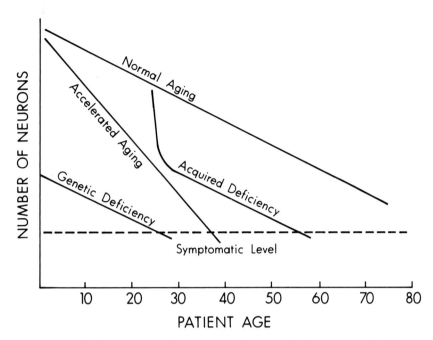

Fig. 19–4. Three hypotheses for understanding neurologic degenerative disease have been suggested: a genetic deficiency of neurons; accelerated aging; and acquired deficiency with normal aging. The appearance of signs and symptoms in each case would be variable and would occur when the number of neurons (or neurotransmitter products) reached a critical level.

dopamine terminals and may again be sequestered against a concentration gradient in storage vesicles for reuse. The neuronal membrane reuptake process may be blocked by a variety of drugs including D-amphetamine and trihexyphenidyl. The effect of these drugs is to prolong the period in which dopamine remains in the synaptic cleft, thereby prolonging the action of dopamine. Newly released dopamine in the synaptic cleft may bind to a cell surface receptor for dopamine on the same neuron from which it was released (autoreceptor) or on another neuron (postsynaptic receptor). Some dopamine surface receptors, particularly in the striatum, appear to be closely linked to a dopamine-sensitive adenylate cyclase enzyme. When dopamine occupies this receptor, the rate of synthesis of cyclic AMP is increased. Other cell-surface dopamine

receptors may not be associated with dopamine-sensitive adenylate cyclase. A variety of antagonist drugs compete with dopamine for the dopamine cell-surface receptor, including the phenothiazines (e.g., chlorpromazine, fluphenazine) and the butyrophenones (e.g., haloperidol). The effect of these drugs is to block the synaptic action of dopamine. Among their side effects is the production of drug-induced parkinsonism. Dopamine is enzymatically inactivated by the action of both monoamine oxidase (MAO), an enzyme highly localized to mitochondria, or catechol-O-methyltransferase (COMT), an enzyme localized primarily in glial cells in the brain. Numerous relatively specific inhibitors of MAO are in clinical use. Deprenyl is one that blocks the enzymatic inactivation of dopamine and prolongs its synaptic action. There is a variety of COMT inhibi-

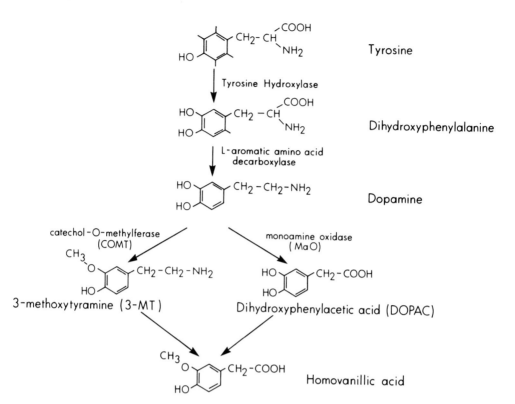

Fig. 19–5. Metabolic pathway of dopamine.

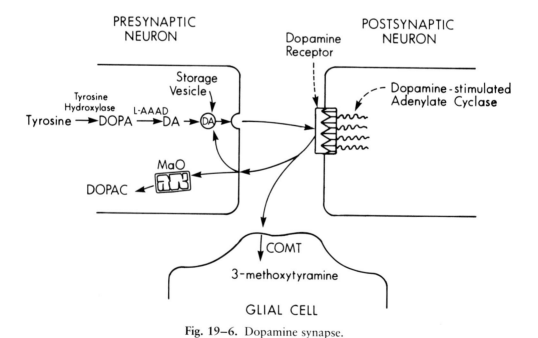

Fig. 19–6. Dopamine synapse.

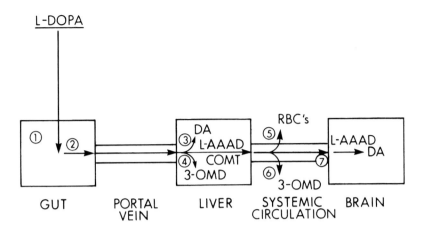

1. Subject to variations in gut motility, gastric emptying.
2. Saturable, carrier-mediated neutral amino acid transport system.
3. L-AAAD activity present in liver.
4. Catechol-O-methyl transferase activity present in liver.
5. Uptake of L-DOPA into red blood cells.
6. Catechol-O-methyl transferase activity present in red blood cells.
7. Blood-brain-barrier: carrier-mediated, saturable, stereospecific neutral amino acid transport system.

Fig. 19–7. Pathway of L-dopa passage from gut to brain.

tors available for experimental use but they are too toxic for administration to humans.

The direct administration of dopamine to patients with Parkinson's disease is ineffective because the passage of unaltered dopamine from blood to brain is prevented by a blood-brain barrier to dopamine. Because no such barrier exists for L-dopa, it may be administered systemically and is converted to dopamine by L-AAAD after entering the brain. The pharmacokinetics of L-dopa are complicated; serum levels reflect many independent metabolic steps (Fig. 19–7). The absorption of L-dopa from the gut into the portal circulation is carrier mediated and may be inhibited by the presence of other neutral amino acids or by decreased gut motility. In the liver L-dopa is subject to enzymatic conversion to dopamine by L-AAAD or

to 3-O-methyldopa by COMT. Today neurologists usually coadminister L-dopa with carbidopa, a peripheral L-AAAD inhibitor, to prevent the systemic conversion of L-dopa to dopamine. In the systemic circulation L-dopa may be taken up into and sequestered by red blood cells or converted into 3-O-methyldopa (OMD) by COMT in red blood cells. The passage of L-dopa through the blood-brain barrier is again carrier mediated, and high circulating blood levels of neutral amino acids will compete with L-dopa for this uptake site. Having entered the brain, L-dopa must then be converted to dopamine. Though ubiquitous, L-AAAD is present in particularly high concentrations in dopaminergic neurons, especially in the striatum. As dopaminergic neurons progressively die in parkinsonian patients, the number of potential sites for the conversion of L-dopa to dopamine may be reduced, thereby potentially reducing the efficacy of L-dopa in advanced Parkinson's disease.

Since the pathway for L-dopa passage from the gut to the dopamine synapse in the brain is complex and vulnerable, treatment with L-dopa is often inefficient, and the efficacy of L-dopa often declines as the disease progresses. In an effort to avoid some of the problems inherent in such precursor therapy, pharmacologists have been working to develop dopaminergic agonist drugs that stimulate dopamine receptors directly without requiring metabolic conversion. Such drugs include the substituted aporphines (e. g. apomorphine), piribedil, and ergot derivatives such as bromocryptine, pergolide, and lisuride. At the present time, however, L-dopa coadministered with a peripheral decarboxylase inhibitor represents the most potent, safe, and specific form of pharmacotherapy for Parkinson's disease.

CURRENT PROBLEMS IN THE MANAGEMENT OF PARKINSON'S DISEASE

With the advent of L-dopa therapy, the life expectancy of a patient with newly diagnosed Parkinson's disease is only a year or two less than that of a person in the general population. Furthermore, the quality of life of patients surviving with Parkinson's disease has been dramatically improved. These improvements for patients with Parkinson's disease are primarily due to the ability of L-dopa therapy to prevent morbidity and mortality from early complications. Despite this clear progress since the introduction of L-dopa, several major problems usually develop during the course of L-dopa treatment.

On the average, patients progressively lose their response to L-dopa after five years of continuous treatment with the drug. This may be due in large part to the progressive loss of the capacity to synthesize and store dopamine as a consequence of the progressive death of dopaminergic neurons.

This hypothesis of presynaptic failure for dopamine transmission may be only partly correct. Additional observations using direct-acting postsynaptic drugs have also found a progressive failure of response. A second hypothesis is a "desensitization" of dopamine receptors caused by chronic L-dopa treatments. In some patients, intermittent withdrawal of treatment appears to result in transient resensitization to L-dopa and to direct-acting agonists. The recent observation that dopamine receptors are reduced as a function of age provides a third, rather more pessimistic explanation for the phenomenon of decreasing drug efficacy with time.

Another major problem often encountered in the management of patients with Parkinson's disease is the emergence of marked fluctuations in symptomatology. After a period of relatively smooth responses to L-dopa, patients begin to develop fluctuations between "on" (i.e., response to L-dopa) and "off" (no response) periods during the day. The majority of these fluctuations are a result of the dosing interval and can be managed by reducing the interval between doses. The progressive shortening of the time-action response is probably a function of the reduced capacity to synthesize and store dopamine in the striatum. In perhaps 10%–15% of patients, however, rather sudden fluctuations occur that are difficult to attribute to pharmacokinetic causes. There is little understanding of the mechanism of these sudden, frightening fluctuations between "on" and "off" states. At least in part these changes may be a consequence of the continued progression of brain pathology that is little affected by treatment with dopaminergic drugs.

THE FUTURE

Recent progress in understanding the pathophysiology of parkinsonism and the strides made in patient management provide hope for future progress. The most important fundamental question facing researchers is why dopamine neurons die selectively and prematurely. Could this process be selectively altered by the discovery and therapeutic use of "trophic factors"? When does the process begin? Is the initial insult during the prenatal period or early life, or is the insult acquired during the adult years? What role may slow viruses or virus-like particles play in the selective vulnerability of dopaminergic neurons?

A secondary, but no less important issue revolves around the question of the physiologic consequences of dopamine depletion in the local neuronal circuits of the basal ganglia. Could a better understanding of the physiological basis for parkinsonian signs and symptoms lead to the development of pharmacologic probes aimed selectively at sites "downstream" from the neurons containing dopamine receptors? Could transplantation of cells capable of synthesizing and releasing dopamine result in physiologically effective dopaminergic reinnervation of the striatum?

Each of these questions can be answered. The recognition of this possibility adds to the challenge, excitement, and certainty of rich dividends that research in the pathophysiology of neurologic disease holds.

GENERAL REFERENCES

Carpenter, M. B. Anatomy of the striatum and brainstem integrating systems. In *Handbook of Physiology*. Section I *The Nervous System*, Vol. 11, *Motor Control*, Chap 19. Am. Physiol. Soc., Bethesda, Maryland, 1981.

Chase, T. N., N. S. Wexler, and A. Barbeau. Huntington's disease. *Adv. in Neurol.* 23, 1979.

Cotzias, G. C., M. H. van Woert, and L. M. Schiffer. Aromatic amino acids and modification of parkinsonism. *N. Eng. J. Med.* 276:374–9, 1967.

DeLong, M. R. and A. P. Georgopoulos. Motor functions of the basal ganglia. In *Handbook of Physiology*. Section I *The Nervous System* Vol. 11, *Motor Control*, Chap. 21. Am. Physiol. Soc., Bethesda Maryland, 1981.

Hoehn, M. M., and M. D. Yahr. Parkinsonism: onset, progression, and mortality. *Neurology* 17:427–42, 1967.

Hornykiewicz, O. Dopamine and brain function. *Pharmacol. Rev.* 18:925–64, 1966.

Marsden, C. D., and S. Fahn. *Movement Disorders*. Butterworth's International Medical Reviews. London, Butterfield Scientific, 1981.

Marsden, C. D., and P. Jenner. The pathophysiology of extrapyramidal side effects of neuroleptic drugs. *Psychol. Med.* 10:55–72, 1980.

Marsden, C. D., and J. D. Parkes. "On-off" effects in patients with Parkinson's disease on chronic levodopa therapy. *Lancet* 1:292–6, 1976.

Penney, J. B., Jr., and A. B. Young. Speculations on the functional anatomy of basal ganglia disorders. *Ann. Rev. Neurosci.* 7:73–94, 1983.

Tatton, W. G., and R. G. Lee. Evidence for abnormal long-loop reflexes in rigid parkinsonian patients. *Brain Res.* 100:671–6, 1975.

Index

Depression, 212
Dermatomyositis, 69–70
Densensitization, in treatment of Parkinson's disease, 376
Deuteranopia, 111
Diabetes insipidus, 321
Diabetes mellitus, hyperglycemia, 321
Dialysis encephalopathy, 316
Diencephalic syndrome, 188
DiGeorge's syndrome, 350
Diplopia
  evaluation of, 136–38
  lesions producing, 132–36, 149
  in myasthenia gravis, 137–38
  red glass test for, 136–37
Disconnection syndromes, 214
Diuretics, for brain edema, 346
Doll's head maneuver, 144–45
  in coma, 305
Dopamine
  action, 167
  in aging, 253
  in basal ganglia, 336
  in cortex, 224
  in Parkinson's disease, 368, 372–76
Drinking behavior, 183
Duchenne's dystrophy, 67–68
  creatine kinase in, 67–68
  electromyography of, 67
  muscle biopsy of, 67
Dural sinus thrombosis
  angiography in, 363
  clinical features, 347, 358
  in meningitis, 354, 358
Dyesthesias
  with demyelination of axons, 21
  with neuropathies, 34
Dysmetria, ocular, 141
Dystonia
  in lesions of basal ganglia, 166
Dystonia musculorum deformans, 163, 166

EMG (See electromyography)
Eating behavior, 183–85
Eaton-Lambert syndrome, 51–54
  acetylcholine release, 52
  with autoimmune disorders, 52
  clinical features, 51–52
  electromyogram, 52–53
  with malignancy, 52
  treatment, 53–54
Edinger-Westphal nucleus, 116, 134
Edrophonium hydrochloride, 44, 50
  in diagnosis of myasthenia gravis, 138
Electroencephalogram (EEG), 233
Electromyography, 59
  of cramps, 64
  of dermatomyositis, 69
  of Duchenne's dystrophy, 67
  of fasciculations, 64
  of fibrillations, 64
  of limb girdle dystrophy, 68
  of myotonia, 66
  in neuropathies, 38
  in phosphorylase deficiency, 70
  of polymyositis, 69
Emergency response, hypothalamic physiology, 191
Emmittance tests, 102
Encephalitis
  clinical features, 347, 356
  CSF profile, 361–62
  CT scan in, 363
  with herpes simplex, 356

  postinfectious, 356
  with slow viruses, 356
End-plate potential, 43
  in botulism, 43
  miniature, 42
  in myasthenia gravis, 45
Endoneurial pressure, 26–27
Endoneurium, 25
Endorphins, 79
Energy metabolism
  feeding behavior, 188
  in seizures, 245–49
Enkephalins, 79
  in basal ganglia, 366
Epidural abcess
  clinical features, 347, 357–58
  myelography in, 364
  spinal, 357–58
  tuberculous, 357
Epilepsy (See seizures)
Epileptic neuron, 235, Figs. 12–4 and 12–6
Epineurium, 25
Experimental allergic encephalomyelitis (EAE), 284
Extraocular muscles
  antagonistic pairs, 132
  actions, 132–33
  in diplopia, 136
  innervation, 134–36
  in myasthenia gravis, 137–38
  yoke muscles, 133
  in restrictive orbital diseases, 138
Extrapyramidal system, 165–66
Eye movements
  control centers
    cerebellar, 141–42
    cerebral, 147–48
    midbrain, 140–41
    pontine, 138–40
    superior colliculus, 141
    vestibular, 142–47
  conjugate, 133, 147
  convergence, 148
  disjunctive, 133, 148
  divergence, 148
  ductional, 132
  horizontal, 147–48
  saccadic, 138, 147–48
  smooth pursuit, 138, 147–48
  torsional, 149
  types, 138, 147–49
  vertical, 140, 148

Facilitation
  at neuromuscular junction, 43
    in Eaton-Lambert syndrome, 52
Fasciculations, 64
Fatty acid oxidation
  in exercise testing, 59, 63
  in phosphorylase deficiency, 70
Fever, mechanisms, 189
Fibrillations, 32, 64, 154
Flutter-like oscillations, 141
Fovea, 112
Friedreich's ataxia, 27–28, 36
Fusimotor system (See motoneurons, gamma)

GABA
  cortex, 206
  in epilepsy, 237–39
  terminations of, 116–18
Ganglion cells, retinal, 112
Gegenhalten, 164